AIDS, PHILOSOPHY AND BEYOND

FOR SHARYN

AIDS, Philosophy and Beyond

Philosophical dilemmas of a modern pandemic

JOSEPH WAYNE SMITH
Queen Elizabeth II Research Fellow, Bioethics
The Flinders University of South Australia

Avebury

Aldershot · Brookfield USA · Hong Kong · Singapore · Sydney

© Joseph Wayne Smith, 1991

All rights reserved. No part of this publication may be reproduced, stored in a retrieval system, or transmitted in any form or by any means, electronic, mechanical, photocopying, recording, or otherwise without the prior permission of Gower Publishing Company Limited.

Published by
Avebury
Gower Publishing Company Limited
Gower House
Croft Road
Aldershot
Hants GUII 3HR
England

Gower Publishing Company
Old Post Road
Brookfield
Vermont 05036
USA

Printed and Bound in Great Britain by
Athenaeum Press Ltd., Newcastle upon Tyne.

ISBN 1 85628 138 8

Contents

Preface		vi
1	Introduction - The AIDS Pandemic: Science and Controversy	1
2	AIDS, Ethics and the Limits of Philosophy	28
3	Public Policy and AIDS: Paradoxes of Social Choice	98
4	AIDS, Heroin and IV Drug Abuse: Philosophical Issues	160
5	Privacy, Medical Confidentiality and AIDS (with Rodney Allen)	195
6	AIDS, Egalitarian Justice and the Allocation of Scarce Medical Resources (with Rodney Allen)	237
7	AIDS, the Environmental Crisis and Beyond: A Study of Global Catastrophes	282
Index		340

Preface

The author is grateful for a National Health and Medical Research Council/Australian National Council on AIDS, Commonwealth AIDS Research Grant, through the Department of Community Services and Health, for 1988/89, and ARC for a Queen Elizabeth II Research Fellowship, 1990. The views expressed in this book are solely the author's (or where indicated, authors') and not necessarily, or by any way of endorsement, the views of the above social bodies, or constituent individuals of the mentioned bodies.

I am grateful to Rodney Allen, Dr. David Lamb and Dr. Richard Sylvan for their support and philosophical example, to Ina Cooper and Molly Scrymgour for word processing, and to Ingrid Birgden, Murray Bramwell, Theresa Francis, Elizabeth Jansson and Lindsay Webb for proof reading and comments.

1 Introduction – the AIDS pandemic: science and controversy

0   Introduction - The AIDS Pandemic

1   Statement of the Argument

2   Controversial Issues

      (1) Cameron's Statistical Argument for Casual Transmission of HIV in Zaire

      (2) The Masters, Johnson and Kolodny Report

      (3) Holistic Health Critique

      (4) Duesberg

3   Conclusion

0. INTRODUCTION - The AIDS Pandemic

"The social meaning affects the consequences of AIDS, especially for AIDS sufferers and their families and the gay community but also for medicine and the public as well.

The greatest consequences of AIDS are of course for AIDS sufferers. They must contend with a ravaging disease and the stigmatized social response that can only make coping with it more difficult. In a time when social support is most needed, it may become least available. And in the context of the paucity of available medical treatments, those with AIDS must face the prospect of early death with little hope of survival.

People with ARC or those who test antibody-positive must live with the uncertainty of not knowing what the progression of their disorder will be. And living with this uncertainty, they must also live with the fear and stigma produced by the social meanings of AIDS. This may mean subtle disenfranchisement, overt dis-crimination, outright exclusion, or even total shunning. The talk of quarantine raises the anxiety of "why me?" Those symptomless seropositive individuals, who experts suggest have a 5 to 20 percent chance of developing full-blown AIDS, must live with the inner conflict of who to tell or not to tell, of how to manage their sexual and work lives, and the question of whether and how they might infect others. The social meanings of AIDS make this burden more difficult". [1]

"Medicine has always had a distinct function in culture. Today, fears about iatrogenic disease and the failures of modern medicine need to be read in their historical context. The sick human body does not need some new spiritual magic, but it does, as always, need something made by human beings, namely a certain kind of practice which, in part, constitutes what we mean by healthy, normal or natural. This practice is not the trancendent power of nature or technology, it is an historical attitude which rests on both knowledge and its application, on both that which is moral in its activity and that which is fallible in its knowledge". [2]

"... the arguments over who got theirs first. The whiff of dishonest behaviour; the rush to announce results prematurely; the ugly nationalism of the Americans; the unwillingness and inability to conduct good controlled trials of possible treatment; the failure to research properly some of the less glamorous, but important, aspects of AIDS (such as the opportunistic infections); and the inability to explain to the public the difficulties inherent in much of the work. In the work on AIDS, science has finally lost its aura of innocence and unsullied objectivity." [3]

"AIDS presents, in short, a constellation of issues encompassing racism, poverty, homophobia, sexism, commodified health care (and its availability), censorship, sex, drugs, and death. It is clear that attacking AIDS cannot be left to the scientific and medical establishments, whose best effort to date, the drug AZT, can cost a thousand dollars a month for a life-sustaining dose. The efforts of a capitalist medical, insurance, and drug manufacturing conglomerate may prolong lives - some lives - but will never address the social issues which are the heavy baggage of AIDS. And AIDS activists have their work cut out for them just filling the holes in the public's knowledge, trying to dilute hysteria, and providing support services and advocacy to the sick and the dying.

An effective assault on AIDS needs to address the above-mentioned social issues as well as the relatively straightforward medical facts of the disease. AIDS as a social phenomenon in the United States cries out for broad-based analysis and activists capable of steering between the shoals of community denial and dread. The struggle against AIDS needs the voice and efforts of the Left; it needs the unified participation of progressives. [4]

"... the fears and vulnerabilities of people who are HIV-positive or have AIDS are being exploited by drug companies and opportunists. Drug companies have kept the results of drug trials confidential, have released information selectively, or have even delayed trials, in the interests of profitability. Some haven't bothered with trials at all before peddling cures or palliatives of no value". [5]

"The politics of AIDS is not primarily about either money or law. It is to do with morals, ethics, individual freedom, and communications - areas where governments tend to stumble". [6]

"The fear of AIDS - rather than AIDS itself - is part of the wave of reaction that is spreading across the Western democracies, a retreat from the freedom - or, depending on your point of view, the licence - that overwhelmed us in the 1960s and early 1970s. It is not just a medical but also a political phenomenon. How one reacts to AIDS is a measure of what one believes about sexual pluralism - and, even more importantly, what one believes about the individual's freedom in all ways, not just sexual, to be different. AIDS tests how a society balances the rights of a few with the good of the many". [7]

1. Statement of the Argument

There exists, at the time of writing, no <u>cure</u> for AIDS (in the sense of a process of effectively removing individually, HIV DNA from human chromosomes) [8], no overwhelmingly successful <u>non-toxic</u> antiviral drug [9] or effective immunization measure for HIV. [10] Consequently AIDS must be viewed, not only as a medical and public health problem, but as the introductory quotations indicate, as a socio-political moral problem as well. [11] Indeed AIDS is a problem of global proportions. [12] In June 1989, the World Health Organization said that by 1991, more than 1 million people world wide would be infected by AIDS, with 2-3 million cases by the late 1990s if no "cure" or vaccine was found. J.M. Mann, Director of the Global AIDS Programme of the World Health Organization, estimated that for early 1988, the number of actual AIDS cases worldwide was between 100,000 and 150,000 with an additional 50 to 100 HIV infected people for each actual case. [13] This gives an alarming statistic for the world as it approaches the year 2000. Africa had an estimated 200,000 cases in 1988, and by 1991 is expected to have 575,000 cases. In equatorial Africa 20% or more of the population in cities are now seropositive. To the end of April 1989 in Australia, more than 6,500 people have been officially notified as HIV antibody positive, although the actual number of untested people infected by HIV may total 50,000, approximately 8 times the number of known carriers. It is possible however to find in the writings of "futurists", even more alarming statistics and scenarios. The biophysicist John Platt gives one vision of the future:

> "The continued spread of AIDS into the 1990s would transform the whole state of the world. It could make overpopulation, famine, environmental destruction, or the extinction of species seem like minor complaints - especially in the developing nations likely to be hit hardest.
>
> AIDS may even transform the purposes of international politics. If the barriers do not become too high to communicate, the major powers will find a life-and-death interest in responding together to a mutual danger that laughs at the nation-state. Many of our nongovernmental organizations and networks, such as those

interested in environmental protection, women's rights, and nuclear disarmament, could also shift their focus toward concern with AIDS and providing help across national boundaries.

Eventually, if it continues, AIDS will change the balance of power. Some countries will be destroyed by it, some badly hurt, and some almost unharmed. Those that suffer least will tend to dominate afterwards as in previous epidemics". [14]

This situation will synergetically become worse with the influence of the other "horsemen" of the environmental crisis - the greenhouse effect, ozone depletion, forest destruction and the destruction of biological diversity (diversity that ironically may hold the key to the AIDS crisis), the increasing chemical toxicity of environments, and so on. (For a discussion cf. final chapter).

This "crisis of civilization" illustrates a fundamental truth that has been lost to the mind of modern Western techno-industrial society, but was well known and accepted by ancient civilzation - human beings, despite intelligence and culture are still biological organisms in an environment which by no means requires human beings to exist, and does not guarantee the eternal existence of the human race. From an evolutionary perspective, new species have emerged, and others have become extinct. Evolution has not stopped. Consequently we can predict with a degree of probability approaching 1, that the most successful survivors on earth - the viruses, bacteria and parasites will also continue to evolve, and new species shall continue to strike the human race. Pandemics, as Joshua Lederberg points out, are natural evolutionary phenomena:

> "Will AIDS mutate further? Already known, a vexing feature of AIDS is its antigenic variability, further complicating the task of developing a vaccine. So we know that HIV is still evolving. Its global spread has meant there is a far more HIV on earth today than ever before in history. What are the odds of its learning the tricks of airborne transmission? The short answer is, "No one can be sure". But we could make the same attribution about any virus; alternatively the next influenza or chicken pox may mutate to an unprecedented lethality. As time passes, and HIV seems settled in a certain groove, that is momentary reassurance in itself. However, given its other ugly attributes, it is hard to imagine a worse threat to humanity than an airborne variant of AIDS. No rule of nature contradicts such a possiblity; the proliferation of AIDS cases with secondary pneumonia multiples the odds of such a mutant, as an analogue to the emergence of pneumonic plague.

Such cases warrant and receive close-isolation precautions; but who will ensure that in Africa? We must particularly look more deeply into the biological mechanisms that govern how AIDS can or cannot be transmitted; our current assessments are crude empricisms. And with so much at stake we must multiply our vigilance for evidence of extraordinary channels of spread.

Our preoccupation with AIDS should not obscure the multiplicity of infectious diseases that threaten our future. It is none too soon to start a systematic watch for other new viruses before they become so irrevocably lodged. The fundamental bases of virus research can hardly be given too much encouragement - and they have made extraordinary leaps, particularly with the help of recombinant DNA technology. Such research should be done on a broad international scale, both to share the progress made in advanced countries and to amplify the opportunities for fieldwork in the most afflicted ones." [15]

From this perspective, the search for a "magic bullet" or effective treatment for AIDS will not necessarily mean that AIDS will cease to be a problem for all time - syphilis has persisted, despite the effectiveness of penicillin. [16] There will also be other pandemics ...

It is the aim of this book on the philosophy of AIDS, to cover more general and perhaps eschatological concerns, than the standard texts on AIDS, ethics and social policy. Although I shall address most of the standard questions, I view them within the framework sketched by Lederberg and in the context of the other crises threatening human civilization. Just as Camus in <u>The Plague</u> used the metaphor of the plague to comment on the ills of his society as he saw it, and the human condition as he saw it, so too, do I view the philosophy of AIDS. To seriously deal with this problem, in the wider context as a problem of the "crisis of civilization", will ultimately involve a radical change in the nature of the modern world. A world consisting of vast inequalities, of the sick and the poor living in filth and disease, and a world increasingly tending towards one globally connected city - is a world highly vulnerable to pandemics. I explore these wider ramifications of AIDS, and the environmental crisis in the last chapter of the book. It is not my claim that AIDS as such, necessitates the sorts of changes that are described in this book, rather it is the challenge posed by AIDS and the other pandemics that will almost certainly arise in the next century within the context of a highly polluted and toxic world (given present trends) that necessitates radical revisions in our ways of living and thinking. If this book is of any value, I believe it will be because of its no doubt stumbling, but sincere attempt to sketch a view of the wider scheme of things - the place of AIDS in the on going trauma of human life, that teaches us our limits.

2. Controversial Issues

It is not my intention in this book to give any summary of the bio-medical aspects of AIDS, as this material is available in accessible forms elsewhere. [17] A philosopher though is naturally drawn towards controversial issues, so I shall mention some before moving on to my principal argument.

Whilst in most of my philosophical framework I have tended to support controversial views, believing that science best develops by constant challenge and response, there is a limit to even this metascientific position. With respect to a highly political topic such as AIDS, researchers have a moral responsibility to be absolutely cautious in the expression of their positions. It is not immoral for example, to set out to challenge the Special Theory of Relativity on experimental and logical grounds, or to criticize the theory without producing an alternative or to argue for crazy things, just for the fun of it. In the case of AIDS though, this sort of sceptical free-wheeling scholarship, unless supported by the most overwhelming experimental evidence and logical argument, can function so as to cause the general public to become complacent about the AIDS issue, to adopt more readily a "it-won't-happen-to-me" attitude with respect to "unsafe" sexual practices. This is most clearly seen in the influential view advanced by some segments of the "new right" in Australia, that AIDS is merely a "gay disease" and that heterosexuals who engage in vaginal sex with multiple partners are at no risk of contracting the disease. This dangerous position is examined and refuted in chapter 3. For the moment I consider other controversial views, that I believe are equally lacking in argument and truth.

1 Cameron's Statistical Argument for Casual Transmission of HIV in Zaire

Cameron [18] is concerned with what he takes to be a statistical error in the 1986 paper by Mann (et al) published in the Journal of the American Medical Association. [19] Cameron says this about the 1986 study:

> "Specifically, 204 household members of 46 AIDS patients were compared with 155 household members of 43 patients without AIDS seropositivity. Spousal seropositivity was set aside as being almost certainly due to sexual commerce - no quarrel here. However, then the remaining group of 186 AIDS household members was statistically compared with the remaining control group of 128 non AIDS household members. The authors concluded

that "seroprevalence did not differ significantly between case and control-household contacts" and "these data ... do not support the hypothesis that nonsexual transmission occurs in households".

By incorrectly choosing <u>individuals</u> rather than <u>households</u> as the unit of analysis, the authors used a 9/186 (4.8%) vs 2/128 (1.6%)) 'no statistically significant difference' rather than a 15.2% vs 4.7% or 2.3% statistical judgement against stated conclusions. The appropriate comparison would have been between 'households exposed to AIDS in-home' vs 'households not exposed to AIDS in-home'. Ignoring the nonrandom nature of the samples, members of the comparison groups <u>were not drawn independently</u> but, rather in clusters, i.e. households. The t test and cannot be blindly applied here, since the correlation between members of the same household with regards to health status and seropositivity is unknown". [20]

The author concludes:

"Excluding spouses, there were 7 (15.2%) of 46 households exposed to AIDS in which one or more members were seropositive vs 2 (4.7%) of 43 households not exposed to AIDS in which one or more members were seropositive; Fisher's exact test is .095, implicating household transmission. If we exclude the domestic workers (who would seem considerably more likely to have picked up the virus from nonfamily encounters), we end up with 7 (15.2%) of 46 AIDS families vs 1 (2.3%) of 43 non-AIDS-families in which one or more members were seropositive; Fisher's exact test is .036, strongly implicating familial transmission. Taken at face value this study suggests horizontal (or casual) transmission of the AIDS virus within families". [21]

Cameron appears to be correct in his statistical fine point that the the comparison groups were not drawn independently. However, all that can be inferred from a use of Fisher's exact test, is some familial transmission. This need not be taken to be evidence for casual transmission of HIV within families, as it could be very well due to incest within the family, which is not rare in any part of the globe. If an error is found in such a report, then what is required is further research. A premature conclusion is unwarranted.

2 <u>The Masters, Johnson and Kolodny Report</u>[22]

This survey by the famous sex researchers involved 800 sexually active heterosexual adults 21-40 years of age who: (a) had no blood transfusions since 1977; (b) no use of illicit drugs by injection; (c) no homosexual or bisexual contact since 1977. The 800 adults consisted of 200 men and 200 women who had been in long-term monogamous relationships for at least five years; 200 men and 200 women who had a minimum of six sexual partners a year over the preceding five years. The prevalence of the AIDS virus among 400 strictly monogamous men and women was low - only one out of the 400 had evidence of AIDS contact (although precisely how is not specified by the authors). The prevalence of infection among the 400 sexually active group was high: 14 women (7 percent) and 10 men (5 percent). In a sub-group with more than 12 sexual partners annually, the prevalence of infection was higher at 14 percent for women and 12 percent for men. On this basis Masters, Johnson and Kolodny predicted a "trickle down" effect, so that infection will be common even in heterosexuals with relatively few sexual partners. They predicted that the number of AIDS cases in America will exceed 500,000 with more than 300,000 deaths, and worldwide with 2 million cases of AIDS with over 1 million deaths.

The problem with the Masters, Johnson and Kolodny Report is that it is so unrepresentative a sample as to be virtually useless for inferring anything about the wider heterosexual community. Tables 1 and 2 show that Australia's heterosexual HIV infection percentage is quite contrary to the predictions of Masters, Johnson and Kolodny. [23] The Report has been briefly, but widely criticized in the press by leading AIDS authorities. The book has now sunk without a trace into the stormy seas of AIDS controversies. It is mentioned here by way of completeness.

TABLE 1: CUMULATIVE NATIONAL CASES OF AIDS (AUSTRALIA) AND KNOWN DEATHS FROM AIDS BY AGE AND SEX (to 16th June, 1989)

	CASES				KNOWN DEATH			
AGE	M	F	TOTAL	(%)	M	F	TOTAL	(%)
0- 9	8	2	10	(0.7)	6	1	7	(70.0)
10-19	6	2	8	(0.6)	3	1	4	(50.0)
20-29	267	15	282	(20.8)	129	3	132	(46.8)
30-39	573	5	578	(42.7)	284	2	286	(49.4)
40-49	323	5	328	(24.2)	162	4	166	(50.6)
50-59	105	7	112	(8.3)	59	6	65	(58.0)
60+	26	11	37	(2.7)	22	10	32	(86.4)
	1308	47	1355	(100.0)	665	27	692	(51.1)

TABLE 2: CUMULATIVE NATIONAL CASES OF AIDS (AUSTRALIA) AND KNOWN DEATHS FROM AIDS BY TRANSMISSION CATEGORY (to 16th June, 1989)

TRANSMISSION CATEGORY	CASES				KNOWN DEATHS			
	M	F	Total	(%)	M	F	Total	(%)
1. Homo-/Bisexual	1198	0	1198	(88.4)	600	0	600	(50.1)
2. IV drug abusers	8	8	16	(1.2)	3	1	4	(25.0)
3. Homo-/Bi IVDU	36	0	36	(2.7)	17	0	17	(47.2)
4. Blood transfusion	32	23	55	(4.1)	25	22	47	(85.4)
5. Haemophiliac	15	0	15	(1.1)	8	0	8	(53.3)
6. Heterosexual trans	10	10	20	(1.5)	5	2	7	(35.0)
7. Under investig'n	4	2	6	(0.4)	3	0	3	(50.0)
8. None of the above	5	4	9	(0.7)	4	2	6	(54.5)
	1308	47	1355	(100.0)	665	27	692	(51.1)

3 Holistic Health Critique

The holistic health literature on AIDS has as its epistemological basis, a critique of physicalistic reductionism in medicine, as well as the "germ theory" of disease. [24] A typical such critique is summarized by McKee:

> "Germ theory provides a framework that promotes technology as the solution to disease, since technology is required to produce antibiotics, vaccines and other drugs to combat pathogens. With the cause of disease located in external pathogens, there is limitless demand for technology, since symptomatic treatment cannot cure the ailment that affects the whole body, and new imbalances result from the side effects of drugs designed to treat only the part rather than the whole. And as one pathogen is eradicated or becomes immune to a drug, a new more virulent pathogen often evolves, requiring an ever new wonder drug. Scientific medicine is more capital intensive than other forms of medicine, and is dependent on the clinical laboratory for diagnosis, and the industrial laboratory for its cures. To the extent that technology and drugs are promoted for the purpose of profit at the expense of health needs, health suffers.
>
> In the literature therefore, social researchers have demonstrated how the analytical reductionism of Western medicine - particularly germ theory -

serves the capitalist system, which is based on profit at the expense of health needs: (1) by obscuring the social determinants of illness, and (2) by promoting treatment that serves capital accumulation and the commodification of health needs." [25]

The Australian "alternative" health literature is largely concerned with treating AIDS by mega-doses of vitamic C (ascorbic acid), popularized by Linus Pauling's so called "orthomolecular medicine". [26] Herbert, writing in 1988 in the New Zealand Medical Journal has the following comments to make about this tradition:

"We have promoters of toxic megadoses of vitamins and minerals running rampant in the United States, and here in New Zealand as well. One of our leading promoters of nutrition nonsense, Linus Pauling, in his 1986 book, recommends that every American, for ordinary every day good health, should eat 25 000 international units of vitamin A a day. That is a toxic dose. He doesn't mention that. At that dose we are beginning to see infants born with nervous system damage and external ear deformities just like those we see when pregnant rats are given toxic doses of vitamin A. It is only five times the 1980 recommended dietary allowance in the United States of vitamin A, but it may be a teratogenic dose. Vitamin A is a known teratogen in large doses. We are trying to get warning labels put on all the pills in the United States that are sold in health food shops: If you are pregnant or contemplating pregnancy, 25000IU of vitamin A daily taken just before pregnancy and during the first month of pregnancy may give you a deformed baby. We need that labelling. The same dose taken daily by healthy adults, in 7-10 years can destroy their lives. We have seen patients in our VA hospitals, men who come in having taken this one health food capsule a day of 25000IU of vitamin A for 7-10 years. They come in with what looks like hepatitis, severe liver damage, and we do liver biopsies and, lo and behold, the liver has been replaced by deposits of vitamin A which have literally crushed the liver cells to death. The human body has no good modality for excretion of excesses of fat soluble vitamins, or excesses of minerals." [27]

In the Australian literature, [28] IV mega-doses of vitamin C ranging from 1 gram up to 60 grams is recommended. This is an absolutely incredible dosage which no doubt seeks to remove the blood and replace it by vitamin C solution! The reader should recall that the recommended daily dosage of vitamin C is about 30 milligrams, and scurvy arises with a prolonged dosage of less than 10 milligrams of vitamin C per day. Defenders of these insane doses of vitamin C argue that we should be seeing an epidemic of kidney stones in the West if mega-doses of such vitamins were harmful. According to Herbert, hospitals are seeing the results of vitamin abuse. There is no adequate evidence to support the claims of orthomolecular medicine, and such views may give AIDS sufferers false hopes if not make them sicker. [29] The orthomolecular nutritionists have not produced adequate experimental evidence, based upon rigorously checked, controlled tests to support their treatments. There is evidence that redox substances such as vitamin C, the vitamin K derivative menadione and ubiquinone may play a role in slowing down mitochondrial mutations in cells - but this is yet to be adequately tested, and if true does not involve insane mega-doses of vitamins. [30] The hopes lying behind the "new age" approach to AIDS, is that AIDS cannot be as deadly or as bad as the press would have us believe, and that if we get in balance with the cosmic force/nature/oureselves (take your pick), all will be well. The reality of the AIDS pandemic though shatters this cosy home-spun optimism - AIDS is a serious health and social problem. I agree that it can be controlled by "right living", that is by "safe" sexual practices and the avoidance of the use of "shared" IV needles, but the <u>seriousness</u> of the <u>threat</u> of AIDS cannot be diminished by such measures - that is a social problem.

4 <u>Duesberg</u>

<u>Peter Duesberg</u>: "If someone had a clean preparation of the virus [HIV] and could check its purity, I wouldn't mind injecting it. I wouldn't be afraid to be infected with HIV".

<u>Harry Rubin</u>: "There has been a bland and uncritical acceptance that HIV is the causative agent [for AIDS] looking for a simple, single causative agent for such an enormous complex of diseases is unrealistic".

<u>Robert Gallo</u>: "Peter can do a lot of disservice. He has now indicated to people that they can go out and fuck around and get infected by this virus and not worry. That's the part where I am mad at Peter". [31]

The views of Professor Peter Duesberg, that HIV is not the cause of AIDS, have generated extreme controversy. In a popular book, <u>AIDS: The HIV Myth</u> [32] Adams gives a summary of Duesberg's views and maintains that there is an "AIDS Establishment" whose scientific prestige and profit depends upon advancing what Adams describes as the "HIV myth". Duncan Campbell in his devastating review of this book published on 6th May 1989 in <u>New Scientist</u> says about Macmillan publishers, the publishers of Adams' book: "It is now many weeks since Macmillan became aware of the book's major errors. It is difficult to contemplate any motive, other than arrogance or greed, which can make a serious publisher so recklessly indifferent to accuracy in reporting". [33]

Duesberg summarizes his critique of the received position on AIDS as follows:

> "Lymphotropic retrovirus has been proposed to cause AIDS because 90% of the patients have antibodies to the virus. Therefore antibody to the virus is used to diagnose AIDS and those at risk for AIDS. The virus has also been suggested as a cause of diseases of the lung and the nervous system. Promiscuous male homosexuals and recipients of frequent transfusions are at a high risk for infection and also at a relatively high annual risk for AIDS, which averages 0.3% and may reach 5%. Others are at a low risk for infection and if infected are at no risk for AIDS. AIDS viruses are thought to kill T-cells although these viruses depend on mitosis for replication and do not lyse cells in asymptomatic infection. Indeed the virus is not sufficient to cause AIDS (a) because the percentage of symptomatic carriers is low and varies between 0 and 5% with the risk group of the carrier, suggesting a cofactor or another cause; (b) because the latent period for AIDS is 5 years compared to an eclipse of only days to weeks for replication and direct pathogenic and immunogenic effects; and (c) because there is no gene with a late AIDS function, since all viral genes are essential for replication. Moreoever the extremely low levels of virus expression and infiltration cast doubt on whether the virus is even necessary to cause AIDS or any of the other diseases with which it is associated. Typically, proviral DNA is detectable in only 15% of AIDS patients and then only in 1 of 10 to 10 lymphocytes and is expressed in only 1 of 10 to 10 lymphocytes. Thus the virus is inactive or latent in carriers with and without AIDS. It is for this reason that it is not transmitted as a cell-free agent. By contrast, all other viruses are expressed at high titers when they function as pathogens. Therefore AIDS virus could be just the most common occupational infection of those at risk for AIDS because retroviruses are not cytocidal and unlike most viruses persist as latent, nonpathogenic infections. As such the virus is an indicator of sera that may cause AIDS. Vaccination is not likely to benefit virus carriers, because nearly all have active antiviral immunity. [34]

The Duesberg critique can be summarized as follows:

13

1. Claims HIV cannot be isolated from 20 to 50% of AIDS cases.

2. "The virus would be a plausible cause of AIDS if it were reactivated after an asymptomatic latency, like herpes viruses. However, HIV remains inactive during AIDS. Thus the "AIDS test" identifies effective natural vaccination, the ultimate protection against viral disease". [35]

3. "The long and highly variable intervals between the onset of antiviral immunity and AIDS, averaging 8 years, are bizarre for a virus that replicates within 1 to 2 days in tissue culture and induces antiviral immunity within 1 to 2 months after an acute infection". [36]

4. "Retrovirus are typically not cytocidal. On the contrary, they often promote cell growth ... Yet HIV, a retrovirus, is said to behave like a cytocidal virus, causing degenerative disease by killing billions of T cells. This is said even though T cells grown in culture, which produce much more virus than has ever been observed in AIDS patients, continue to divide". [37]

Duesberg however has no specific causal mechanism for AIDS:

> "The 'A' in AIDS does not stand for <u>infectious</u>. It stands for acquired. You can acquire lung cancer by smoking. You can acquire death by living on this planet for eighty years. You can acquire a lot of trouble by having five hundred or a thousand sexual contacts. And you can acquire HIV by living however those at risk for AIDS live". [38]

The following points can be made in criticism of Duesberg:

1. The objection to the belief that HIV causes AIDS is based upon a reductionistic biological prejudice, namely that the inability to show an unequivocal molecular association between HIV and AIDS shows that nothing is known about AIDS' etiology. This objection though would mean that there is no noticeable scientific knowledge about any human viral disease for by the molecular reductionistic approach, no such etiology can be proved. As this is an absurd consequence, Duesberg's argument must be wrong. [39]

2. Finding antiviral antibodies in the blood does not <u>prove</u> effective antiviral immunity. The presence of antibodies no more indicates victory, than for example the presence of a country's army indicates a secure defense against an enemy force. The enemy force may be stronger, and sabotage the country's defenses.

3. Duesberg does not show that there is a single case of AIDS, where HIV is not present. If this could be done, the

received theory would be refuted. On the contrary, Duesberg is at a loss to explain AIDS infection arising from needle pricks and lab. accidents in otherwise low risk people. Acceptance of causality presupposes a <u>common cause</u>, and that common cause is HIV.

4. Duesberg ignores evidence that about 15% of the macrophage and monocyte cells are positive for HIV viral protein. A strategic attack on the very basis of the body's immune system would be sufficient to undermine the health of an organism.

5. Many viruses may hide in the body's cells for long periods in latent form e.g. herpes simplex viruses, visna virus. Even if there was no other examples of viruses which had such a long latency period, this would be a dangerous inductive inference to make about AIDS; if this disease is new, it may well challenge established principles, which after all were based on past experience. (The epistemological problem about induction is considered in the next chapter).

6. "The strongest evidence that HIV causes AIDS comes from prospective epidemiological studies that document the absolute requirement for HIV infection for the development of AIDS. It has been shown for every population group studied in the United States and elsewhere that, in the years following the introduction of HIV and subsequent seroconversion of members of the population, the features characteristic of progressive immunodeficiency emerge in a predictable sequence resulting in clinical AIDS. Furthermore, other epidemiological data show that AIDS and HIV infection are clustred in the same population groups and in specific geographic locations and in time. Numerous studies have shown that in countries with no persons with HIV antibodies there is no AIDS and in countries with many persons with HIV antibodies there is much AIDS. Additionally, the time of occurrence of AIDS in each country is correlated with the time of introduction of HIV into that country; first HIV is introduced, then AIDS appears. [40]

We should note, that if HIV was merely a secondary infection, then this claim of causes would not necessarily occur.

7. "Support for the linkage of HIV infection and AIDS comes as well from the results of public health interventions where interruption of HIV infection almost completely prevented the further appearance of AIDS in blood transfusion recipients. After the introduction of the HIV antibody screening test in the United States, the transmission of HIV in the blood supply in the United States was reduced from as high as 1 in 1,000 infected units in some high risk areas to less than an estimated 1 in 40,000 units countrywide. (The recently recognised cases of virus transmission by blood transfusion are due to donors being missed by current antibody screening tests during the window of seroconversion. There is a period

of about 4 to 8 weeks in which newly HIV-infected persons are capable of transmitting, HIV, but have not yet developed antibodies). As a result of the decrease in blood transfusion - associated transmission of HIV, the incidence of blood transfusion - associated AIDS among U.S. newborns showed a decline.

Thirteen of the cases of blood transfusion-associated seroconversion identified since the start of blood bank screening were recently investigated. In one of these cases, the recipient of one unit of blood was one of a pair of fraternal twins. This baby seroconverted and developed AIDS without any other risk factor. Her twin and her mother received no blood products, developed no HIV antibodies, and remained healthy. The blood donor became HIV seropositive and developed AIDS." [41]

On this basis it is concluded that HIV is the cause of AIDS, and that the received medical view is essentially correct.

3. **Conclusion**

An introduction and summary of the principal argument of this book has now been given. In the next chapter the wider philosophical ramifications of AIDS, and the other global "crises of civilization" are discussed. By this, I am concerned with the relationship between philosophy and social theory (as well as legal theory) as cognitive enterprises, and their relationship with global problems such as AIDS. As the reader will see, each of these disciplines exists at present in a state of epistemological crisis, and as such fail to rise to the profound challenge raised by AIDS and other environmental problems equally as serious for human existence, such as the greenhouse effect, ozone depletion and the destruction of biological diversity. My bold aim now, is to work out a new direction for philosophy and social theory, that will lift them out of their menopausal states, regenerate them, and arm them for the public battles that lie ahead.

NOTES AND REFERENCES

1. P. Conrad, "The Social Meaning of AIDS", Social Policy, Vol. 17, 1986, pp. 51-56. Citation p. 53.

2. R. D'Amico and A.J. Layon, "AIDS and the Politics of Morbidity", Telos, No. 76, 1988, pp. 115-129. Citation p. 129.

3. R. Smith, "Goodbye, Objective Science", New Scientist, Vol. 117, 25 February 1988, p.60.

4. C. Queen, "The Politics of AIDS: A Review Essay", The Insurgent Sociologist, Vol. 14, 1987, pp. 103-124. Citation p. 105.

5. L. Barlow (et al) "The Amazing AIDS Scram", Newstatesman Society, 24 June 1988, pp. 10-13. Citation p. 10.

6. J. Warden, "The Politics of AIDS", British Medical Journal, Vol. 294, 1987, p.455.

7. D. Black, The Plague Years: A Chronicle of AIDS the Epidemic of Our Times, (Picador, London, 1986), p. x.

8. Gene splicers at St. Louis University School of Medicine and Duke University Medical Centre, have used synthetic genes to block the production of proteins that HIV needs to replicate (July 1989). This raises the possibility of blocking HIV replication by flooding the blood-stream with "fake" viral proteins. This also opens up the way for gene therapy, perhaps to genetically engineer an HIV-proof population of white blood cells.

9. The antiviral drug zidovudine AZT works as follows. To reproduce HIV must copy its genetic message from a strand of RNA to a chain of DNA; then with RNA as the template, the viral reverse transcriptase assembles the building blocks for the DNA chain. AZT "appears" to be like thymidine and is incorporated into the chain, but lacks the attachment point for the next "building block" in the sequence, so that the chain is not completed. AZT however has the effect of depressing the bone marrow, resulting in anemia. New drugs DDI and GLQ223 ("Compound Q") may be more effective and less toxic.

10. The factors which make it difficult to construct an effective HIV vaccination include (1) high rate of mutations in the proteins of HIV, (2) long incubation period for the disease; (3) antibodies against one "strain" do not prevent infection against another.

11. An incomplete, unsystematic - but I hope useful reading list on the social ramifications of AIDS includes: R. Weiss (et al), "A National Strategy on AIDS", *Issues in Science and Technology*, Vol. 5, 1989, pp. 52-59; H.B. Kaplan (et al), "The Sociological Study of AIDS: A Critical Review of the Literature and Suggested Research Agenda", *Journal of Health and Social Behavior*, Vol. 28, 1987, pp. 140-157; D. Nelkin, "AIDS and the Social Sciences: Review of Useful Knowledge and Research Needs", *Reviews of Infectious Diseases*, Vol. 9, 1987, pp. 980-986; S. Panem, "Biomedical Miscommunication in the AIDS Crisis", *The Scientist*, Vol. 2 (3), February 8 1988, p. 19, *The AIDS Bureaucracy*, (Harvard University Press, Cambridge, Massachusetts, 1988), "Planning for the Next Health Emergency", *Issues in Science and Technology*, Vol. 4, 1988, pp. 59-64; C. Hunt, "AIDS and Capitalist Medicine", *Monthly Review*, Vol. 40, 1988, pp. 11-25; A.J. Layon and R. D'Amico, "AIDS, Capitalism, and Technology: A Reply to Charles Hunt", *Monthly Review*, Vol. 40, 1988, pp. 31-36; D. Altman, *AIDS in the Mind of America*, (Doubleday, New York, 1987); C. Patton, *Sex and Germs: The Politics of AIDS*, (South End Press, Boston, 1985); S. Kingman, "AIDS Brings Health into Focus", *New Scientist*, Vol. 122, 20 May 1989, pp. 19-24; A. Strauss, "Health Policy and Chronic Illness", *Transaction Social Science and Modern Society*, Vol. 25, No. 1, November/December 1987, pp. 33-39; R.P. Keeling, "Risk Communication about AIDS in Higher Education", *Science, Technology and Human Values*, Vol. 12, 1987, pp. 26-40; D.M. Fox, "AIDS and the American Health Polity: The History and Prospects of a Crisis of Authority", *Milbank Quarterly*, Vol. 64, 1986, pp. 7-33; L. Gostin, "The Future of Communicable Disease Control: Toward a New Concept in Public Health Law", *Milbank Quarterly*, Vol. 64, 1986, pp. 79-96; N.S. Podian and D.P. Francis, "Preventing the Heterosexual Spread of AIDS", *JAMA*, Vol. 260, 1988, p. 1879; C.E. Koop, "Teaching Children About AIDS", *Issues in Science and Technology*, Vol. 4, 1987, pp. 67-70; G. Friedland, "Fear of AIDS", *New York State Journal of Medicine*, May, 1987, pp. 260-261; P.S. Arno and R.G. Hughes, "Local Policy Responses to the AIDS Epidemic: New York and San Francisco", *New York State Journal of Medicine*, May 1987, pp. 264-272; R.O. Valdiserri (et al), "The Effect of Group Education on Improving Attitudes about AIDS Risk Reduction", *New York State Journal of Medicine*, May 1987, pp. 272-278; M.H. Becker and J.G. Joseph, "AIDS and Behavioral Change to Reduce Risk: A Review", *American Journal of Public Health*, Vol. 78, 1988, pp. 394-410; J.R. Allen and J.W. Curran, "Prevention of AIDS and HIV Infection: Needs and Priorities for Epidemiologic Research", *American Journal of Public Health*, Vol. 78, 1988, pp. 381-386; S.C. Joseph (et al), "AIDS Policy and Prevention in New York City", *Bulletin of the New York Academy of Medicine*, Vol. 63, 1987, pp. 659-671; H.V. Fineberg, "Education to

Prevent AIDS: Prospects and Obstacles", *Science*, Vol. 239, 5 February 1988, pp. 592-596; CDC, "Recommendations for Prevention of HIV Transmission in Health-Care Settings", *New York State Journal of Medicine*, January 1988, pp. 25-31; J.E. Ward (et al), "Transmission of Human Immunodeficiency Virus (HIV) by Blood Transfusions Screened as Negative for HIV Antibody", *New England Journal of Medicine*, Vol. 318, 1988, pp. 473-478; A.A. Vass, *AIDS: A Plague in US*, (Venus Academica, St. Ives, 1986); P. Clarke and D.J. Spencer, "Social Barriers to the Control of HIV Infection", in G.P. Wormser (ed.), *AIDS and Other Manifestations of HIV Infection*, (Noyes Publications, New Jersey, 1987), pp. 1071-1081; D.R. Hopkins, "Public Health Measures for Prevention and Control of AIDS", *Public Health Reports*, Vol. 102, 1987, pp. 463-467; A.M. Johnson and D. Miller, "Health Care Planning and Social Policy Issues", *British Medical Bulletin*, Vol. 44, 1988, pp. 203-219; P.R. Abramson, "Sexual Assessment and the Epidemiology of AIDS", *Journal of Sex Research*, Vol. 25, 1988, pp. 323-346; E. Macklin (ed.), *AIDS and Families*, (Howarth Press, New York, 1989); M. Rodway and M. Wright (eds.) *Sociopsychological Aspects of Sexually Transmitted Diseases* (Howarth Press, New York, 1988); E.H. Loewy, "Duties, Fears and Physicians", *Social Science and Medicine*, Vol. 22, 1986, pp. 1363-1366; A. Ron and D.E. Rogers, "New York City's Health Care Crisis: AIDS, The Poor, and Limited Resources", *JAMA*, Vol. 260, 1988, p. 1453; L.H. Kuller and L.A. Kingsley, "The Epidemic of AIDS: A Failure of Public Health Policy", *Milbank Quarterly*, Vol. 64, 1986, pp. 56-78; R. Bayer, "AIDS, Power and Reason", *Milbank Quarterly*, Vol. 64, 1986, pp. 168-182; F.J. Bennett, "AIDS as a Social Phenomenon", *Social Science and Medicine*, Vol. 25, 1987, pp. 529-539; L.C. Shulman and J.E. Mantell, "The AIDS Crisis: A United States Health Care Perspective", *Social Science and Medicine*, Vol. 26, 1988, pp. 979-988; A. Lloyd (ed.), *Proceedings of the Conference - AIDS: Social Policy, Ethics and the Law*, (Monash University, Clayton, 1986); Institute of Medicine, National Academy of Sciences, *Confronting AIDS: Directions for Public Health, Health Care and Research*, (National Academy Press, Washington D.C., 1986); G. Antonio, *The AIDS Cover-Up?* (Ignatious Press, San Francisco, 1987); M.D. Witt (ed.), *AIDS and Patient Mangaement: Legal, Ethical and Social Issues*, (National Health Publishing, Owing Mills, 1986); A.M. Brandt, "AIDS and Metaphor: Toward the Social Meaning of Epidemic Disease", *Social Research*, Vol. 55, 1988, pp. 413-432; G. Kateb, "Moral Dilemmas - An Introduction", *Social Research*, ibid, pp. 455-459; P. Slack, "Responses to Plague in Early Modern Europe: The Implications of Public Health", ibid, pp. 433-453; A. Quinton, "Plagues and Morality", ibid, pp. 477-489; D.A.J. Richards, "Human Rights, Public Health, and the Idea of a Moral Plague", ibid, pp. 491-528; B.S.

Blumberg, "Hepatitis B Virus and the Carrier Problem", ibid, pp. 403-412; W.H. McNeill, _Plagues and Peoples_, (Penguin Books, Harmondsworth, 1976); D.A. Feldman and T.M. Johnson, (eds.), _The Social Dimensions of AIDS_, (Praeger Publishers, New York, 1986); M. Greenly, _Chronicle: The Human Side of AIDS_, (Irvington Publishers, New York, 1986); G. Whitmore, _Someone was Here: Profiles in the AIDS Epidemic_, (New American Library, New York, 1988); G. Hancock and E. Carim, _AIDS: The Deadly Epidemic_, (Victor Gollancz, London, 1986); D. Miller, _Living with AIDS and HIV_, (Macmillan, London, 1987); J.A. Kelly and J. S. St. Lawrence, _The AIDS Health Crisis: Psychological and Social Interventions_, (Plenum Press, New York, 1988); S. Connor and S. Kingman, _The Search for the Virus_, (Penguin, London, 1988); E. Kubler-Ross, _AIDS: The Ultimate Challenge_, (Macmillan, New York, 1987); S. Sontag, _AIDS and its Metaphors_, (Penguin, London, 1989); H. Hayry and M. Hayry, "AIDS Now", _Bioethics_, Vol. 1, 1987, pp. 339-356; E.H. Loewy, "AIDS and the Human Community", _Social Science and Medicine_, Vol. 27, 1988, pp. 297-303; L. Liskin (et al), "AIDS - A Public Health Crisis", _Population Reports_, Vol. XIV, No. 3, July-August 1986, pp. L193-L228; J. Griggs (ed.), _AIDS: Public Policy Dimensions_, (United Hospital Fund of New York, New York, 1987); I.B. Corless and M. Pittman - Lindeman (eds.), _AIDS: Principles, Practices and Politics_, (Hemisphere Publishing Corporation, New York, 1988); K. Siegel (ed.), _AIDS Education: The Public Health Challenge_, (Wiley, New York, 1986); G. Ponsford, "AIDS in the OR: A Surgeon's View", _Canadian Medical Association Journal_, Vol. 137, December 1, 1987, pp. 1036-1039; R.S. Eisenstaedt and T.E. Getzen, "Screening Blood Donors for Human Immunodeficiency Virus Antibody: Cost-Benefit Analysis", _American Journal of Public Health_, Vol. 78, 1988, pp. 450-454; B. Tindall (et al), "The Sydney AIDS Project: Development of Acquired Immunodeficiency Syndrome in a Group of HIV Seropositive Homosexual Men", _Australian and New Zealand Journal of Medicine_, Vol. 18, 1988, pp. 8-15; H.S. Rubenstein, "AIDS and Medical Ethics", _The Lancet_, December 12, 1987, pp. 1401-1402; E.J. Emanuel and L.L. Emanuel, "Is Our AIDS Policy Ethical?", _American Journal of Medicine_, Vol. 83, 1987, pp. 519-520; H.E. Mason, "AIDS: Some Ethical Considerations", _Minnesota Medicine_, Vol. 70, 1987, pp. 194-202; A. Marlet (et al), "The Impact of the "Grim Reaper" National AIDS Education Campaign on the Albion Street (AIDS) Centre and the AIDS Hotline", _Medical Journal of Australia_, Vol. 148, 1988, pp. 282-286; S. Namir (et al), "Coping with AIDS: Psychological and Health Implications", _Journal of Applied Social Psychology_, Vol. 17, 1987, pp. 309-328; L. O'Donnell (et al) "Psychological Responses of Hospital Workers to Acquired Immune Deficiency Syndrome (AIDS)" _Journal of Applied Social Psychology_, Vol. 17, 1987, pp. 269-285;

D.A. Feldman (ed.) <u>AIDS and Social Science</u>, (Prager, New York, 1986); J. Zich and L. Temoshok, "Perceptions of Social Support in Men with AIDS and ARC: Relationships with Distress and Hardiness", <u>Journal of Applied Social Psychology</u>, Vol. 17, 1987, pp. 193-215; K. Schmidt and H. Zoffmann, "AIDS and Social Medicine: Strategies for Research", <u>Scandinavian Journal of Social Medicine</u>, Vol. 15, 1987, pp. 1-2; G.F. Solomon and L. Temoshok, "A Psychoneuroimmunologic Perspective on AIDS Research: Questions, Preliminary Findings, and Suggestions", <u>Journal of Applied Social Psychology</u>, Vol. 17, 1987, pp. 286-308; M.D. Kirby, "AIDS Legislation - Turning Up the Heat?", <u>Journal of Medical Ethics</u>, Vol. 12, 1986, pp. 187-194; J.L. Dolgin, "AIDS: Social Meanings and Legal Ramficiations", <u>Hofstra Law Review</u>, Vol. 14, 1985, pp. 193-209; R.C. Kessler (et al), "Effects of HIV Infection, Perceived Health and Clinical Status on a Cohort at Risk for AIDS", <u>Social Science and Medicine</u>, Vol. 27, 1988, pp. 569-578; A.S. Klovdahl, "Social Networks and the Spread of Infectious Diseases: The AIDS Example", <u>Social Science and Medicine</u>, Vol. 21, 1985, pp. 1203-1216; S.C. McCombie, "The Cultural Impact of the 'AIDS' Test: The American Experience", <u>Social Science and Medicine</u>, Vol. 23, 1986, pp. 455-459; D.A. Feldman, "AIDS and Social Change", <u>Human Organization</u>, Vol. 44, 1985, pp. 343-348; P. Chodoff, "Fear of AIDS", <u>Psychiatry</u>, Vol. 50, 1987, pp. 184-191; J.L. Gerberding (et al), "Risk of Transmitting the Human Immunodeficiency Virus, Cytomegalovirus, and Hepatitis B Virus to Health Care Workers Exposed to Patients with AIDS and AIDS-related Conditions", <u>Journal of Infectious Diseases</u>, Vol. 156, 1987, pp. 1-8; B.F. Farber and M.H. Kaplan, "The AIDS Epidemic: Neglected Issues", <u>Journal of Infectious Diseases</u>, Vol. 155, 1987, pp. 1097-1099; M.F. Rogers and W.W. Williams, "AIDS in Blacks and Hispanics: Implications for Prevention", <u>Issues in Science and Technology</u>, Vol. 3, 1987, pp. 89-94; M.C. Heagarty, "AIDS: A View from the Trenches", <u>Issues in Science and Technology</u>, Vol. 3, 1987, pp.111-117; M.E. Faulstich, "Psychiatric Apects of AIDS", <u>American Journal of Psychiatry</u>, Vol. 144, 1987, pp. 551-556; S. Namir (et al), "Coping with AIDS: Psychological and Health Implications", <u>Journal of Applied Social Psychology</u>, Vol. 17, 1987, pp. 309-328; J.R. Rundell (et al), "Three Cases of AIDS-Related Psychiatric Disorders", <u>American Journal of Psychiatry</u>, Vol. 143, 1986, pp. 777-778; J.L. Martin and C.S. Vance, "Behavioral and Psychosocial Factors in AIDS", <u>American Psychologist</u>, Vol. 39, 1984, pp. 1303-1308; S.F. Morin (et al), "The Psychological Impact of AIDS on Gay Men", <u>American Psychologist</u>, Vol. 39, 1984, pp. 1288-1293; T.J. Coates (et al), "Psychological Research is Essential to Understanding and Treating AIDS", <u>American Psychologist</u>, Vol. 39, 1984, pp. 1309-1314; R.M. Glass, "AIDS and Suicide", <u>JAMA</u>, Vol. 259, 1988, pp. 1369-1370;

P.M. Marzuk (et al), "Increased Risk of Suicide in Persons with AIDS", *JAMA*, Vol. 259, 1988, pp. 1333-1337; I. Warwick (et al), "Constructing Commonsense-Young People's Beliefs about AIDS", *Sociology of Health and Illness*, Vol. 10, 1988, pp. 213-233; N. Ben-Yehuda, "The Sociology of Moral Panics: Toward a New Synthesis", *Sociological Quarterly*, Vol. 27, 1986, pp. 495-513. A special edition of *Daedalus*, Vol. 118, Spring 1989 is devoted to the issue "Living with AIDS" with a moving piece by an AIDS sufferer 'Peter Phoenix', "Alive with AIDS", pp. 85-92.

12. J.E. Harris, "The AIDS Epidemic: Looking into the 1990s", *Technology Review*, Vol. 90 (5), 1987, pp. 58-64.

13. J.M. Mann, "AIDS: A Global Strategy for a Global Challenge", *Impact of Science on Society*, Vol. 38, 1988, pp. 159-167. Citation p. 161.

14. J. Platt, "The Future of AIDS", *The Futurist*, Vol. XXI, November-December 1987, pp. 9-17. Citation p. 16.

15. J. Lederberg, "Pandemic as a Natural Evolutionary Phenomenon", *Social Research*, Vol. 55, 1988, pp. 343-359. Citation pp. 357-358. cf. also L. Thomas, "Science and Health - Possibilities, Probabilities and Limitations", *Social Research*, Vol. 55, 1988, pp. 379-395.

16. A.M. Brandt, "AIDS in Historical Perspective: Four Lessons from the History of Sexually Transmitted Diseases", *American Journal of Public Health*, Vol. 78, 1988, pp. 367-371 and "The Syphilis Epidemic and Its Relation to AIDS", *Science*, Vol. 239, 1988, pp. 375-380:

"AIDS, like syphilis in the past, engenders powerful social conflicts about the meaning, nature, and risks of sexuality; the nature and role of the state in protecting and promoting public health; the significance of individual rights in regard to communal good; and the nature of the doctor - patient relationship and social responsibility. The analogs that AIDS poses to this brief history of syphilis are striking; the pervasive fear of contagion, concerns about casual transmission, the stigmatization of victims, and the conflicts between public health and civil liberties. The response to AIDS will be a function of our own time, our own culture, and our own science. The importance of the history of syphilis is that it reminds us of that range of forces that influence disease, health and social policy". (p.379)

17. A reading guide for the bio-medical aspects of AIDS now follows: D.J. Volsky (et al), "Retroviral Etiology of the Acquired Immune Deficiency Syndrome (AIDS)" *AIDS*

Research, Vol. 2, 1986, pp. 535-548; G. Friedland, "The Acquired Immunodeficiency Syndrome: General Overview", International Journal of Neuroscience, Vol. 32, 1987, pp. 677-686; A.R. Lifson and K.G. Castro, "AIDS Cases with "No Identified Risk", in G.P. Wormser (ed.), AIDS and Other Manifestations of HIV Infection, (Noyes Publications, New Jersey, 1987), pp. 86-95; J.M. Coffin, "Retroviruses: Current Conceptions of Structure and Function", in Wormser ibid, pp. 130-159; F.P. Siegal, "The Immune Deficiency of AIDS", in Wormser ibid, pp. 304-330; B.S. Koppel, "Neurological Complications of HIV Infection: An Overview", ibid pp. 548-578; M.A.A. Cohen, "Psychiatric Aspects of AIDS: A Biopsychosocial Approach", ibid, pp. 579-622; R.E. Stahl, "General Pathology of AIDS", ibid, pp. 838-866; S. Broder (ed.), AIDS: Modern Concepts and Therapeutic Challenges, (Marcel Dekker Inc., New York, 1987); L. Ratner (et al), "Complete Nucleotide Sequences of Functional Clones of the AIDS Virus", AIDS Research and Human Retroviruses, Vol. 3, 1987, pp. 57-69; D.D. Ho and J.C. Kaplan, "Pathogenesis of Human Immunodeficiency Virus Infection and Prospects for Control", Yale Journal of Biology and Medicine, Vol. 60, 1987, pp. 589-600; P. Van de Perre (et al), "The Latex Condom, An Efficient Barrier Against Sexual Transmission of AIDS-Related Viruses", AIDS, Vol. 1, 1987, pp. 49-52; J.J. Burns and J.E. Groopman, "AIDS: Strategic Considerations for Developing Antiviral Drugs", Issues in Science and Technology, Vol. 3, 1987, pp. 102-109; J.L. Fox, "Hurdles to AIDS Vaccines", Bio/Technology, Vol. 6, February 1988, p. 116; L-J. Eales and J.M. Parkin, "Current Concepts in the Immunopathogenesis of AIDS and HIV Infection", British Medical Bulletin, Vol. 44, 1988, pp. 38-55; F. Clavel, "HIV-2, the West African AIDS Virus", AIDS, Vol. 1, 1987, pp. 135-140; H.J.C. Jager and E.J. Ruitenberg, "The Statistical Analysis and Mathematical Modelling of AIDS", AIDS, Vol. 1, 1987, pp. 129-130; G.D. Hsiung, "Perspectives on Retroviruses and the Etiologic Agent of AIDS", Yale Journal of Biology and Medicine, Vol. 60, 1987, pp. 505-514; R.E. Spier, "Modern Approaches to New Vaccines Including Prevention of AIDS", Vaccine, Vol. 6, 1988, pp. 69-70; D. Langley and R.E. Spier, "Is a Vaccine Against AIDS Possible?" Vaccine, Vol. 6, 1988, pp. 3-5; J.E. Osborn, "The AIDS Epidemic: An Overview of the Science", Issues in Science and Technology, Vol. 2, 1986, pp. 40-55; J. Dwyer, The Body at War, (Allen and Unwin, Sydney, 1988); J.A. Kelly and J.S. St. Lawrence, The AIDS Health Crisis, (Plenum Press, New York, 1988); D. Miller, Living with AIDS and HIV, (Macmillan, London, 1987); R.F. Schinazi and A.J. Nahmias (eds.) AIDS in Children, Adolescents and Heterosexual Adults, (Elsevier, New York, 1988); Q. Sattentau, "AIDS: The Search for the Vaccine", New Scientist, Vol. 118, 14 April 1988, pp. 56-60; "Nets cast to Catch the Second Virus", New Scientist, 31 March 1988, p. 24; Q.

Sattentau, "AIDS: Our Defences are Down", New Scientist, 7 April 1988, pp. 49-53; M.S. Saag (et al), "Extensive Variation of Human Immunodeficiency Virus Type - 1 In Vivo", Nature, Vol. 334, 1988, pp. 440-444; A.G. Fisher (et al), "Biologically Diverse Molecular Variants Within a Single HIV-1 Isolate", Nature, Vol. 334, 1988, pp. 444-447; S.L. Buckingham, "The HIV Antibody Test: Psychosocial Issues", Social Casework, Vol. 68, 1987, pp. 387-393; R.W. Price (et al), "The Brain in AIDS: Central Nervous System HIV-1 Infection and AIDS Dementia Complex", Science, Vol. 239, 1988, pp. 586-592; A.S. Fauci, "The Human Immunodeficiency Virus: Infectivity and Mechanisms of Pathogenesis", Science, Vol. 239, 1988, pp. 617-622; A.E. Glatt (et al), "Treatment of Infections Associated with Human Immunodeficiency Virus", New England Journal of Medicine, Vol. 318, 1988, pp. 1439-1448; D.B. Clifford, "AIDS and the Brain", American Family Physician, Vol. 36, 1987, pp. 101-106; B.J. Brew (et al), "Another Retroviral Disease of the Nervous System: Chronic Progressive Myelopathy Due to HTLV-1" New England Journal of Medicine, Vol. 318, 1988, pp. 1195-1197; P.G. Gibson (et al), "Pulmonary Manifestations of the Acquired Immunodeficiency Syndrome", Australian and New Zealand Journal of Medicine, Vol. 17, 1987, pp. 551-556; R.C. Gallo and L. Montagnier, "AIDS in 1988", Scientific American, Vol. 259, No. 4, 1988, pp. 26-32; W.A. Haseltine and F. Wong-Staal, "The Molecular Biology of the AIDS Virus", ibid, pp. 34-42; J.N. Weber and R.A. Weiss, "HIV Infection: The Cellular Picture", ibid, pp. 80-87; R. Yarchoan (et al), "AIDS Therapies", ibid, pp. 88-97; T.J. Matthews and D.P. Bolognesi, "AIDS Vaccines", ibid, pp. 98-105; B. Lorber, "Changing Patterns of Infectious Diseases", American Journal of Medicine, Vol. 84, 1988, pp. 569-578; R.C. Gallo, "The AIDS Virus", Scientific American, Vol. 256, 1987, pp. 38-48; C.A.M. Reitmeijer (et al), "Condoms as Physical and Chemical Barriers Against Human Immunodeficiency Virus", JAMA, Vol. 259, 1988, pp. 1851-1853; S. Dewhurst (et al), "Expression of the T4 Molecule (AIDS virus receptor) by Human Brain-Derived Cells", FEBS Letters, Vol. 213, 1987, pp. 133-137; A.J. Pinching (et al), "AIDS and HIV Infection: New Perspectives", British Medical Bulletin, Vol. 44, 1988, pp. 1-19; J.N. Weber and R.A. Weiss, "The Virology of Human Immunodeficiency Viruses", British Medical Bulletin, Vol. 44, 1988, pp. 20-37, R.S. Janssen (et al), "Neurological Complications of Human Immunodeficiency Virus Infection in Patients with Lymphadenopathy Syndrome", Annals of Neurology, Vol. 23, 1988, pp. 49-55; I. Weissman, "Approaches to an Understanding of Pathogenic Mechanisms in AIDS", Reviews of Infectious Diseases, Vol. 10, 1988, pp. 385-398; G.A. Elder and J.L. Sever, "AIDS and Neurological Disorders: An Overview", Annals of Neurology, Vol. 23, 1988, pp. S4 - S12; J.P. Rushton and A.F. Bogaert, "Population

Differences in Susceptibility to AIDS: An Evolutionary Analysis", <u>Social Science and Medicine</u>, Vol. 28, 1989, pp. 1211-1220; A.R. Lifson, "Do Alternative Modes for Transmission of Human Immunodeficiency Virus Exist?" <u>JAMA</u>, Vol. 259, 1988, pp. 1353-1356; T.A. Peterman (et al), "Risk of Human Immunodeficiency Virus Transmission From Heterosexual Adults with Transfusion-Associated Infections", <u>JAMA</u>, Vol. 259, 1988, pp. 55-58; K.G. Castro (et al), "Investigations of AIDS Patients with No Previously Identified Risk Factors", <u>JAMA</u>, Vol. 259, 1988, pp. 1338-1342; J. Mills, "The AIDS Virus: Prospects for Treatment and Control", <u>Modern Medicine</u>, Vol. 56, 1988, pp. 104-115; "Antibodies Can Disappear from Infected People", <u>New Scientist</u>, Vol. 118, 9 June 1989, p. 41; S. Kingman, "Virus Develops Even with Antibodies Absent", <u>New Scientist</u>, Vol. 118, 26 May 1988, p. 40.

18. P. Cameron, "Corrected Statistical Analysis Suggests Casual Transmission of AIDS in the African Study of the Centers for Disease Control", <u>Psychological Reports</u>, Vol. 60, 1987, pp. 177-178.

19. J.M. Mann (et al), "Prevalence of HTLV-111/LAV in Household Contacts of Patients with Confirmed AIDS and Controls in Kinshasa, Zaire", <u>Journal of the American Medical Association</u>, Vol. 256, 1986, pp. 721-724.

20. Cameron, op.cit., note 18, p. 177.

21. ibid, p. 179. For rebuttal cf. G.H. Friedland (et al), "Lack of Transmission of HTLV-111/LAV to Household Contacts of Patients with AIDS or AIDS Related Complex with Oral Candidiasis", <u>New England Journal of Medicine</u>, Vol. 314, 1986, pp. 344-349.

22. W.H. Masters, V.E. Johnson and R.C. Kolodny, <u>Crisis: Heterosexual Behaviour in the Age of AIDS</u>, (Weidenfeld and Nicolson, London, 1988).

23. NH & MRC Special Unit in AIDS Epidemiology and Clinical Research, AIDS, Cumulative Analysis of Cases in Australia, 16th June 1989.

24. G.L. Engel, "The Need for a New Medical Model: A Challenge for Biomedicine", <u>Science</u>, Vol. 196, 1977, pp. 129-136. R.J. Dubos, "Second Thoughts on the Germ Theory", <u>Scientific American</u>, Vol. 192, May 1955, pp. 31-35.

25. J. McKee, "Holistic Health and the Critique of Western Medicine", <u>Social Science and Medicine</u>, Vol. 26, 1988, pp. 775-784. Citation p. 777. cf. also J.H. Reyner, <u>Psionic Medicine</u>, (Routledge and Kegan Paul, London, 1982); R. Blake, <u>Mind Over Medicine: Can the Mind Kill</u>

or Cure?, (Pan Books, London, 1987); V. Coleman, Mindpower: How to Use Your Mind to Heal Your Body, (Century, London, 1986).

26. L. Pauling, Vitamin C and the Common Cold, (W.H. Freeman and Company, San Francisco, 1970); A. Hoffer and M. Walker, Orthomolecular Nutrition, (Keats Publishing, Connecticut, 1978).

27. V. Herbert, "Medical Practice in a Changing World: What Philosophy and Codes of Practice can Provide Responsible Health Services in the late 20th Century", New Zealand Medical Journal, 25 May, 1988, pp. 309-312. Citation p. 312.

28. I. Brighthope and P. Fitzgerald, You Can Knock Out AIDS with Vitamin C and Immune Nutrients! (Ripon Grove, Australia, 1987); A. Cantwell, AIDS: The Mystery and the Solution, (Aries Rising Press, Los Angeles, 1984); A.R. Cantwell, "The AIDS Epidemic: A Different View", Australasian Health and Healing, Vol. 7, 1988, pp. 19-22; J. Rappenport, "The AIDS - Vaccine Connection: Exploring Alternative Theories of AIDS", Australasian Health and Healing, Vol. 7, 1988, pp. 25-29; R.S. Mendelsohn, "ADIS Linked to Smallpox Vaccine", Australasian Health and Healing, Vol. 7, 1988, pp. 17-18; J. West, Pasteur, Bechamp and AIDS, (The Author, Bundaberg, 1988) and The AIDS Time Bomb, (Veritas Press, Bundaberg, 1988), R.F. Carthcart, "Vitamin C in the Treatment of Acquired Immune Deficiency Syndrome (AIDS), "Medical Hypothesis, Vol. 14, 1984, pp. 423-433.

29. R.P. Doyle, "Orthomolecular Medicine", in The Medical Wars, (William Morrow, New York, 1983), pp. 149-160; J. Fried, Vitamin Politics, (Prometheus Books, New York, 1984).

30. cf. I. Trounce (et al), "Decline in Skeletal Muscle Mitochondrial Respiratory Chain Function: Possible Factor in Ageing", The Lancet, March 25, 1989, pp. 637-639. A.W. Linnane (et al), "Mitochondrial DNA Mutations as an Important Contributor to Ageing and Degenerative Diseases", The Lancet, March 25, 1989, pp. 642-645.

31. "Maverick Threatens to Inject Himself", New Scientist, Vol. 117, 3 March 1987, p. 34.

32. J. Adams, AIDS: The HIV Myth, (Macmillan, London, 1989).

33. D. Campbell, "AIDS: The Duesberg Myth", New Scientist, Vol. 122, 6 May 1989, pp. 42-43. Citation p. 43.

34. P. Duesberg, "Retrovirus as Carcinogens and Pathogens: Expectations and Reality", Cancer Research, Vol. 47, March 1 1987, pp. 1199-1220. Citation p. 1199.

35. P. Duesberg, "HIV is Not the Cause of AIDS", Science, Vol. 241, 29 July 1988, p. 514.

36. ibid.

37. ibid. cf. also P. Duesberg, "Activated Proto-on C Genes: Sufficient or Necessary for Cancer?", Science, Vol. 228, 10 May 1985, pp. 669-677, "Cancer Genes: Rare Recombinants Instead of Activated Oncogenes (A Review)", Proceedings of the national Academy of Sciences, Vol. 84, 1987, pp. 2117-2124; "A Challenge to the AIDS Establisment", Bio/Technology, Vol. 5, November 1987, p. 1244; "AIDS and the 'Innocent' Virus", New Scientist, 28 April 1988, pp. 34-35; J. Lauritsen, "Kangaroo Court Etiology", New York Native, May 9 1988, pp. 14-16, 18-19; H. Rubin, "Is HIV the Causative Factor in AIDS?", Nature, Vol. 334, 21 July 1988, p. 201; W. Booth, "A Rebel Without a Cause for AIDS", Science, Vol. 239, 25 March 1988, pp. 1485-1488; "AIDS: A Medical Blunder?" The Australian, Thursday May 12 1988, p. 11; A. Berken, "Is the Human Immunodeficiency Virus Really the Initiator of Human Immunodeficiency?", New York State Journal of Medicine, February 1988, pp. 85-86.

38. J. Miller, "AIDS Heresy", Discover, Vol. 9, June 1988, pp. 62-64, 66, 68. Citation p. 64.

39. J. Weber, "AIDS and the 'Guilty' Virus", New Scientist, 5 May 1988, pp. 32-33.

40. W. Blattner (et al) "HIV Causes AIDS", Science, Vol. 241, 29 July 1988, p. 515.

41. ibid.

42. B.M. Whyte and D.A. Cooper, "The Surveillance Definition of the Acquired Immunodeficiency Syndrome and the Clinical Classification of Infection with the Human Immunodeficiency Virus Type 1", Medical Journal of Australia, Vol. 149, October 3, 1988, pp. 368-373; CDC, "Revision of the CDC Surveillance Case Definition for Acquired Immunodeficiency Syndrome", Morbidity and Mortality Weekly Report, Vol. 36, August 14, 1987, pp. 1S-15S; J.K. Stehr-Green (et al), "Potential Effect of Revising the CDC Surveillance Case Definition for AIDS", The Lancet, March 8, 1988. pp. 520-521.

2 AIDS, ethics and the limits of philosophy

1   Introduction

2   The Relevance of Philosophy for AIDS Research: Social Relativism, Constructionism, and the Philosophical Crisis of Medicine

3   The Return to Reason : The Moral-Metaphysical Critique of Received Anglo-American Philosophy and Alternatives

4   Ethics, Social Wisdom and the Foundations of Moral Value

5   Conclusion : State of the Argument

1. Introduction

The previous chapter outlined with broad strokes the nature and extent of the AIDS problem. To begin to understand, to analyse and hopefully resolve many of the socio-ethical problems arising from the AIDS pandemic, it is necessary to do some preliminary work in analysis and criticism of the present state of Western philosophy. It is ironic, that at a time when the relevance of philosophy and ethics for modern society has never been greater, the influence of relativism, nihilism, social constructionism and deconstructionism has also never been greater. At a time when philosophers and social theorists should, in the light of the AIDS pandemic and humanity's massive environmental problems, be challenging the standard thought structures of the <u>status quo</u>, we find in the literature something of an inevitable acceptance of the ethical and rational legitimacy of the world order. This trend, in my opinion, is an unfortunate one: philosophers should be the Socratic conscience of their societies, unafraid of received academic opinion, big government and big business. In this chapter I continue the argument developed in my <u>The Progress and Rationality of Philosophy</u> [1], for a new critical philosophy more adequate for the challenge of our times.

A summary of the argument of the chapter now follows. In section 2 I outline some of the challenges posed to the objectivity of medical science and philosophy by some influential contemporary movements such as the strong programme of the sociology of knowledge, social constructionism and deconstructionism. In section 3 I choose a representative relativist and irrationalist - Paul Feyerabend - and subject some of his latest work to critical examination. I then look at the issues of the nature of truth and empirical or inductive justification, areas which have been the breeding ground for relativism. Having sketched a foundation for philosophy, I tend to go on in section 4 to fill out the details of this in a programme that sees the proper role of the philosopher as that of being what I called "the Socratic conscience of society." Central to this task is the cultivation of wisdom and the pursuit of truth and moral value. A theory of moral value and a method of moral reasoning is then developed which will serve as a moral foundation for the investigation of the socio-ethical problems of AIDS, and later in the work, the discussion of the global environmental crisis. It is of course a tall task to develop even a theory of ethics in a chapter, and one which (despite lengthy footnote arguments and documentation) will no doubt require more detailed work. Nevertheless, as I have already said at a time when scepticism about the verisimilitude and worth of philosophy has never been greater - and yet when the social demands for philosophical insight are crucial, a step forward, however small, is well worthwhile. Vision must precede analysis.

2. The Relevance of Philosophy for AIDS Research: Social Relativism, Constructionism, and the Philosophical Crisis of Medicine

Are philosophical, metaphysical and epistemological concerns of relevance to the medical sciences? One argument for the relevance of philosophical and epistemological concerns to medicine has been given by E.K. Ledermann in his excellent text <u>Philosophy and Medicine</u> [2]. Ledermann shows that epistemology lies at the heart of medical research, and that different philosophies of medicine lead to different treatments especially in psychiatry. In particular Ledermann contrasts two competing philosophies of medicine: mechanistic materialism and holism, the former practised by established medicine, the latter by so-called "alternative medicine". He says "The philosophies of mechanistic materialism and holism are theories about the nature of the universe and its features... [They] lead to an interpretation of the patient in terms of individual parts and cause-effect relations, and in terms of wholes and holistic forces respectively". [3] For Ledermann mechanistic materialism and holism are complementary, not contradictory, and he attempts this reconciliation within the framework of a Kantian epistemology. Mechanistic materialism yields "knowledge of efficient causes through the isolation of parts" and holism, "arriving at final causes through relating detailed knowledge to the whole organism". [4] Wholeness implies purposiveness but this purposiveness is purely regulative, being an attribute of the human mind. On this basis Ledermann advances a comprehensive critique of a number of schools of psychiatry and the development of a medical libertarian ethic. Whether his arguments are ultimately correct or not, <u>Philosophy and Medicine</u> shows the relevance of epistemological concerns for modern medicine. [5]

Another illustration of the importance of philosophical considerations to medicine is what we may call the "crisis of Western medicine" tradition, a tradition which calls for a "fundamental reappraisal of medical methodology." David Greaves summarizes the components of the crisis of Western medicine tradition as follows:

"1) The change in disease patterns away from acute treatable illness episodes to chronic intractable conditions, which are only marginally affected by the traditional techniques of medical management already established or being developed by scientific medicine.

2) The failure of increasing levels of expenditure on health care to meet the demands which have been

placed on health services which have partly arisen from these new chronic disease 'epidemics'.

3) A realisation that need for health care is not readily definable as a fixed quantity and that dealing with immediate problems may lead to many more being uncovered.

4) The preceding points have further led to an awareness that a definition of those areas of life which are legitimately medical and should therefore be controlled by health professionals and are appropriately dealt with by their methods of working, is itself problematic.."[6]

Greaves, of the Social Paediatric and Obstetric Research Unit, Glasgow, is critical of modern medicine's ignorance of its philosophical foundations. Following King's 1954 [7] article on the ontology of disease, Greaves also asks whether diseases have a real existence independent of medical inquiry (medical realism) or whether diseases (as individuated processes) are created by medical inquiry (medical Kantianism). Answers to these philosophical questions determines, Greaves rightly claims, whether we accept a conception of diseases as things and a conception of medicine which has the study of these various disease-things as its central focus, or whether an alternative philosophical approach for medicine is adopted where the central focus is upon the sick individual "so his illness is inseperable from him and diseases alone are no longer recognisable". [8] Greaves thus approaches the problem of medical reductionism versus medical holism from a different direction than that taken by Ledermann, but is neverthelss in agreement with him on the intellectual importance of ontological questions in meta-medicine. It is not my aim in this book to discuss at any length metaphysical issues in medicine with respect to AIDS, for this discussion will be reserved for another book. [9] As we shall now see, there are equally as challenging problems confronting us in the field of the epistemology of medicine, concerned with the rationality and objectivity of medicine itself as a cognitive enterprise. This problem is a part of a larger problem of the widespread acceptance of, and influence of cultural and cognitive subjectivism and nihilism. A widespread scepticism and cynicism about scientific rationality itself, must in turn influence the public's perception of modern medicine.

One of the best known writers about the "crisis of Western medicine" tradition, Ivan Illich, can be accurately described as a sceptic of modern medicine. For Illich, the professionals have a tighter control over their "victims" than any Mafia. Illich explores the metaphor of the professionals having a tighter control over people than organised crime by maintaining that gangsters make their profits by force whilst doctors "gain legal power to create the need that, by law, they alone will be allowed to satisfy". [10] The authority of professionals, unlike that of gangsters, comes from claims of the possession of a special knowledge making it an incommunicative authority. Its legitimacy arises from being the sole interpreter, defender and supplier of this knowledge. This, Illich believes is a qualitatively new form of social control. Professionals tell one what one needs, hence defining a person as a client, and then ordain what is right by means of the prescription. Worse, Illich maintains "the medical establishment has become a major threat to health" [11] given the existence of <u>iatrogenesis</u>: physician-caused or generated diseases. [12] In this context Illich is sceptical, along with others, that modern medicine is a <u>progressive</u> science. [13] His best argument for this conclusion is based upon epidemiological data allegedly showing that medicine has had little impact upon the course of epidemics. Tuberculosis, cholera and dysentery had their impact upon the mortality tables and dwindled in social significance before their aetiology was understood and medical treatments by antibiotics and immunization advanced. The most important factor contributing to the decline in mortality by these diseases is increased resistance of people due to better nutrition. [14] Immunization has virtually wiped out paralytic poliomyelitis and reduced the mortality of malaria and sleeping sickness, but Illich claims "for most other infections, medicine can show no comparable results". [15]

It is not my aim here to refute Illich on a point by point basis and nor is it my aim to defend modern medicine as a socially perfect institution - for of course it is not. Illich is no doubt right to point out that professional medicine does exert a form of social control, but then again what institution in the modern world does not? What institution in this modern profit-orientated "bigger is better" world lacks its share of incompetence and coercion? Navarro puts this point well:

> "By focusing their analytical gaze only on medicine, these analysts [crisis of medicine critics] miss the fact that it is not only the practice and institutions of medicine that are in crisis. Other social institutions such as education, welfare, transportation, as well as many political, economic and ideological institutions, are also referred to as being in crisis... Indeed, the whole of our Western world is defined and perceived as in a profound crisis. And these societal crises are not the mere aggregate of the different sectoral crises; rather, the <u>sectoral crises are the sectoral realisations of the overall societal crises</u>. It is precisely the unawareness of this key point that limits most seriously the explanatory value of most current analyses of medicine". [16]

As well, Illich's epidemiological argument could be effectively met by granting that epidemics may have their natural course and that antibiotics and immunization are not fully adequate responses to epidemics - for the reasons of the costs and limits of medical resources (especially for the Third World) as well as the evolving immunity of disease causing organisms, to drugs. Nevertheless all this argument shows is the limits of biochemical medicine divorced from programmes of community and preventative medicine.

Illich's medical scepticism is carried further by B.S. Turner's radical sociology of medicine. [17] Turner points out that it is now common, after Parsons' approach to the sick role [18] to classify human disorders into three distinct categories: sickness, illness and disease. Disease is a biological concept, illness is the individual's subjective awareness of the disorder and sickness refers to the specific social roles that must be played. Turner sees this division as corresponding to a professional division of labour: the physician deals with diseases, the clinical psychiatrist with illness, and clinical sociology with sickness.

The general theory of health and illness in society has three levels of analysis:

1. descriptions of the experience of illness from the perspective of the individual, where disease is seen as an alienated state in which the body is experienced as 'other' or as a thing with phenomenology and symbolic interactionism being of use here;

2. the social construction of disease categories e.g. 'deviance', the 'sick role';

3. social organisation of health-care systems, a macro-sociology, the political economy of illness.

This is a fair contribution, nevertheless Turner wishes to go further and claims that "modern medicine is in fact applied sociology, and sociology is applied medicine". [19] This last claim is based upon the arguments of Foucault. Especially of importance to Turner is Foucault's investigation of knowledge/ power with respect to "the medical struggle around the body historically as the origins of a biopolitics of populations in modern society". [20] Such diseases evolve by discipline over (especially through surveillance and control) the bodies of individuals and populations. [21]

Following Foucault, Turner expresses his epistemology:

> "... we know, or see what our language permits because we can never naively apprehend or know 'reality' outside of language. Like all forms of

human knowledge, scientific discourse is simply a collection of metaphors. Scientific knowledge of the world is a form of narrative (a story) and like all narratives science depends on various conventions of language (a style of writing, for instance). Narrative is a set of events within a language and language is a self-referential system. Nothing occurs outside the language. Therefore, what we know about 'the world' is simply the outcome of the arbitrary conventions we adopt to describe world. Different societies and different historical periods have different conventions and therefore different realities". [22]

Turner denies that Foucault is adopting an idealist position, but not, I believe, very convincingly:

"This epistemology associated with the work of Foucault has radical implications for medical sociology. We can no longer regard 'diseases' as natural events in the world which occur outside the language with which they are described. A disease entity is the product of medical discourses which in turn reflect the dominant mode of thinking (the episteme in Foucault's terminology) within a society. [23]

Diseases are thus seen by Turner as socially constructed products of culture; different types of society have had different conceptions of disease and therapy, which in turn are a product of different cultures and social structures. [24] Turner's best example of the social construction of a disease is RSI or tenosynovitis, which he takes to be an ongoing social process to which a disease label has been pinned. [25]

The radical sociology of medicine [26], based upon the strong programme of the sociology of knowledge [27], has explored the idea that medical knowledge is a social construct with typical relativistic conclusions. I have argued elsewhere that rationalism and the strong programme of the sociology of knowledge can be reconciled without contradiction, because the strong programme of the sociology of knowledge is not necessarily committed to cognitive relativism. [28] This programme advances a causal-explanatory thesis which asserts that true beliefs and theories are open to social explanation, just as false beliefs and theories are. My argument is that in the case of holding some true belief B for sufficient reasons, we do have a satisfactory causal explanation of the subject's acceptance of B following the Davidsonian tradition of taking reasons to be causes. The existence of satisfactory strong social explanation of the acceptance of B would indicate a situation of causal- overdetermination which does not show that B is only "relatively" true. Science is an activity of human rule-following agents, and thus is a social activity. However, it does not logically follow that scientific knowledge is therefore social knowledge anymore than because any social activity involves physical processes, social action is therefore purely physical action and social knowledge merely physical knowledge. Objectivity and rationality could be <u>emergent</u> properties of social activity just as mental properties may be non-reducible emergent properties of (physical) brain processes.

This is not to say that every position associated with the strong programme of the sociology of knowledge and rationalism is consistent, for there must be compromises on both sides. Thus for example Latour and Woolgar in <u>Laboratory Life</u> [29], believe scientific operations are not directed towards an independently existing reality, but directed towards producing 'literary inscriptions' or texts. Scientific argument is an argument about texts, the process of negotiation is called 'agonistic activity' and the context in which it occurs is called the 'agonistic field'. Latour and Woolgar state that

> ".. if reality is the consequence rather than the cause of this construction, this means that a scientist's activity is directed not toward these [agonistic] operations on statements ... The notion of agonistic contrasts significantly with the view that scientists are somehow concerned with 'nature'". [30]

What is ultimately wrong with this position, as I argued in <u>Reductionism and Cultural Being</u> [31] and <u>The Progress and Rationality of Philosophy</u>, is that it is based upon an over-socialized and over-cultured conception of human nature. The sociology of knowledge position assumes that all thought is linguistic, that human nature is purely cultural and that socio-cultural structures are ultimately binding and constitutive of human life. A non-reductionist ecological position on humanity has a different perspective on human nature. It rejects the idea that all thought and reasoning is linguistic, accepting that non-linguistic animals can think and reason. It sees the 'literary inscriptions' or 'texts' beloved of social constructionists and deconstructionists, as only having point if they are attempts to symbolically represent reality. Further it sees sociology as applicable to only a small part of the world and it is highly conscious of the limits and of the sociology of knowledge tradition.

The work of B.S. Turner, which has been summarised here, is more radical than the social constructionism of the strong programme of the sociology of knowledge, and is best described as an application of what is called <u>deconstructionism</u>, <u>post-structuralism</u> or <u>postmodern</u> philosophy to the sociology of medicine. [32] It is difficult, if not impossible, to clearly and precisely summarize the basic tenets of postmodernism or deconstructionism, because the movement itself is very much a revolt against logico-analytical values such as precision and clarity of expression. I. Howe gives us a good example of this temperament:

"We are confronting, then, a new phase in our culture, which in motive ... represents a wish to shake off the bleeding heritage of modernism... The new sensibility is impatient with ideas. It is impatient with literary structure of complexity and coherence, only yesterday the catchwords of our criticism. It wants instead works of literature - though literature may be the wrong word - that will be as absolute as the sun, as unarguable as orgasm, as delicious as a lollipop... It has no taste for that ethical nail-biting of those writers of the left who suffered defeat and would never accept the narcotic of certainty. It is sick of those magnifications of irony that Mann gave us, sick of those visions of entrapment to which Kafka led us, sick of those shufflings of daily horror and grace that Joyce left us. It breathes contempt for rationality, impatience with mind ... It is bored with the past: for the past is a fink". [33]

Douglas Kellner elaborates upon these themes:

"Discussions of postmodernism began in the field of cultural theory as indicators of new forms of 'postmodern' culture in the domains of architecture, literature, painting, and so on, which specified a set of cultural artifacts which allegedly broke with the forms and practices of modernist art. As opposed to the seriousness of 'high modernism', postmodernism exhibited a new insouciance, a new playfulness, and a new eclecticism embodied above all in Andy Warhol's 'pop art' but also manifested in celebrations of Las Vegas architecture, found objects, happenings. Nam June Paik's video installations, underground film, and the novels of Thomas Pynchon. In opposition to the well-wrought, formally sophisticated, and aesthetically demanding modernist art, postmodernist art was fragmentary and eclectic, mixing forms from 'high culture' and 'popular culture', subverting aesthetic boundaries and expanding the domain of art to encompass the images of advertising, the kaleidoscopic mosaics of television, the experiences of the post-holocaust nuclear age, and an always proliferating consumer capitalism. The moral seriousness of high modernism was replaced by irony, pastiche, cynicism, commercialism and in some cases downright nihilism". [34]

Postmodernism thus, is concerned with the irreducible pluralism and relativism of cultures and the impossibility of assessing "knowledge" outside of cultures. [35]

To appreciate how alienated postmodern philosophy and sociology is from the spirit of our times, one need only consider the ramifications of ecopolitical and environmental literature on the greenhouse effect, destruction of the ozone layer, acid rain from industrialism, deforestation, chemical pollution and so on (discussed later in this book) - all of which are the products of massive global industrialization and mechanization. Only a brief glance at industrial smog-filled cities of Japan (and the ruthless destruction of its natural environment, especially its once beautiful coastal regions) [36] would tell us that industrial society is alive and expanding. Postmodernism and postindustrialism, essentialy a Franco-American creation, is seemingly blind to the decline in the global importance of United States capitalism and the emergence of more virile, and perhaps ultimately more environmentally destructive forms of high tech capitalism in the Asia-Pacific region. [37] As I shall argue later in this book, the last thing the world needs now is an extension of the fetish of economic growth for economic growth's sake. Indeed, as we shall see, the postmodernist and deconstructionist has abandoned the Socratic ideal of describing, criticizing and struggling to change the world - at the time when the human race (largely Europe, USA and Japan) has conducted a thoughtless experiment with the life support systems of the planet that may ultimately lead to our extinction. Yet with comfortable affluent smugness, these theorists tell us that no theories can be assessed outside of the context of culture (so that Western culture is not to be criticized), that no objective assessment or criticism of a form of life is possible and that we should presumably face the likely global destruction of the planet with a smile knowing that life and death are only relative, contextual, subjective and ultimately unreal.

Outside of literary and cultural theory, the deconstructive spirit is best seen at work in Richard Rorty's <u>Philosophy and the Mirror of Nature</u>. [38] This work is a historical reconstruction of modern philosophy that argues that mainstream (Western) philosophy is becoming increasingly sterile because the central metaphors of its discourse (such as "our glossy essence" and "mirroring" nature) are themselves sterile. Thus the discipline itself is no more than a great hoax. Rorty concentrates part of his attack upon the doctrine of the correspondence theory of truth, which holds that to know is to represent accurately by theorization that which is outside the mind. For Rorty, there can be no problems of reason that arise as soon as humans think, for philosophy is nothing more than a series of discourses or language games. These language games are accepted by historical accident and are replaced not because of reasoned argument, but in Kuhnian fashion by alternative incommensurable philosophical language games, that in no way "mirror" reality.

In *The Progress and Rationality of Philosophy* I argued that Rorty's criticisms of philosophy self-destruct because his very historical account, if taken to be other than a subjective whim, must presuppose the representation theory of knowledge, because Rorty must refer to historical texts that exist in libraries and not inside his skull. As well, if Rorty is right that the representation theory of knowledge is incorrect, then it not only demolishes (cognitive) philosophy, but also physics and the other natural sciences because they too attempt to theorize about things and processes existing outside of the mind. [39]

This idea of the whole of human intellectual inquiry as a text, of language as primarily literary is carried even further in the work of Jacques Derrida. [40] All that we are presented with is a maze of texts, with perhaps reality itself being one grand text. As D'Amico recognises, postmodernism embraces radical relativism, irrationalism and nihilism [41], for the moment is a radically anti-realist about truth and reference. Now all of this could easily be dismissed by the ordinary people of the world, as another crazy game played by ivory tower middle class academics, and as having no relevance for the real difficulties facing humanity. Confronting a person dying with any of the number of opportunistic diseases that an AIDS infected person may have, with Turner, Rorty and Derrida's talk of "discourse", "conversation", "differance" and the idea that AIDS itself is a social construction, and one produces *absurdity*. [42]

In any case it is doubtful whether the method of deconstruction as practised by Derrida is as challenging to rational philosophy as his supporters believe. For Derrida deconstruction is a "method" for criticizing existing doctrines, showing how arguments often support their negations and for offering a critique of conventional interpretations of texts. This "method" consists in general of two parts: (1) The identification of hierarchical oppositions A and B and their reversal to show that the privileged position of (say) A is "mistaken" as A depends upon B as much as B upon A; (2) Derrida sees a bias in Western philosophy, called the "metaphysics of presence". It uses a preferred concept as a basis for an explanation of another concept in a duality e.g. body/mind, object/subject, society/self, being/non-being. For example, identity depends upon difference because x cannot be identical to itself unless there is a y such that x = y. Identity presupposes difference. Neither concept is fundamental because both are mutually dependent upon each other. Derrida speaks of *differance* here: each term in a hierarchy defers the other, being fundamentally dependent upon the other. Now the example about identity and difference could be questioned on the grounds that for there to be a y in any case presupposes the self-identity of y, and that there is nothing contradictory about supposing that there is only one self-identical object in logical space. All that Derrida shows is that the terms in an oppositional hierarchy cannot be <u>conceptually</u> reduced to one another. His argument does not deal with other methods of preference such as <u>theoretical priority</u> and <u>causal priority</u> - especially in the case of the body/mind duality. Moreover this argument shows nothing of significance about the epistemological grounds of philosophy. Deconstructionism itself because of its obscurity, kitsch and "yuppiness" is itself in need of "deconstruction".

The nihilism of deconstruction is not restricted to abstract philosophy, but is having an impact upon legal theory through the <u>Critical Legal Studies</u> movement. And law surely is a more down-to-earth discipline than philosophy, dealing with concrete problems that directly effects lives, does it not?

There are various arguments advanced by the Critical Legal Studies movement to deconstruct legal theory. The tradition accepts that since Law is concerned with texts and interpretations, it is therefore a branch of literature. [43] With this move criticism flows fast. The idea of a stability of meaning in historical documents is attacked and many writers opt for a radical indeterminacy of meaning in legal texts, maintaining that texts cannot have objective meaning. Another popular argument, often used to deconstruct Constitutional Law is to argue that many values conflict with others (e.g. equality and liberty) and that there is no rational means of resolving this dispute. Thus Critical Legal Studies raises the spectre that there are no rational criteria for making legal decisions and that legal reasoning is indeterminate and contradictory. [44]

As with all deconstructionist theses there is a strong element of a paradox in their claims. It is absurd to suppose that indeterminacy in Western law is so bad as to permit a judge to justify any result she desires. For example, Section 92 of the Australian Constitution cannot be interpreted to mean that trade between the States shall be <u>absolutely unfree</u>, or that there must be no trade at all between the States. The problem of interpretation is about the scope and implications of this freedom - thus the vagueness is specific, not all-encompassing as the Critical Legal theorists would have us believe. [45]

Within the space limits of this chapter I shall attempt to refute the relativism and nihilism associated with the various movements that have been reviewed, without resorting to an author-by-author examination. Here I shall concentrate my critical fire upon one writer who has consistently influenced all of the above movements - Paul Feyerabend. [46] Along with this critique, I summarize my response from my previous books and articles, to the crisis of reason which we have just glimpsed. I shall argue that philosophers and social scientists should abandon their somewhat self-indulgent concern with these sorts of abstract problems and concern themselves <u>exclusively</u> with the global problem of the survival of the human race - how to prevent nuclear war, fatal environmental destruction through the greenhouse effect, acid rain and the destruction of the ozone layer, and in particular the massive health problem of the spread of AIDS. From the critical commonsense position which I shall develop, the writings of the relativists, nihilists and deconstructionists is just idle, practically useless talk. The "sacred" texts of Rorty, Derrida and Foucault can be seen as just a publicly expensive academic language game, that in no way benefits humanity. [47]

3. The Return to Reason: The Moral-Metaphysical Critique of Received Anglo-American Philosophy and Alternatives

In his recent book <u>Farewell to Reason</u> [48] Paul Feyerabend develops his clearest, and perhaps strongest critique of Western rationalism. Feyerabend sees the spread of western values, progress, development, business, science and technology as a threat to both freedom and cultural pluralism. Western forms of life are exported to the detriment of indigenous cultures; variety of culture, true, not superficial multiculturalism within a scientific setting is lost, local adaptation and diversity dwindles. [49] Thus a fog of technological and industrial monotony and sameness descends upon the world. The results for the Third World of Westernization have been the steady increase in hunger, illness and poverty.

Feyerabend sets out with great passion, and I think understandable anger, to criticize the ideals of <u>Reason</u> and <u>Objectivity</u>, which have made Western expansion intellectually respectable. <u>Objectivity</u>, as Feyerabend views it, ascribes validity to a position irrespective of human expectations, attitudes, interests and wishes. Questions of objectivity are brought sharply into focus whenever two or more different cultures confront each other, each having 'absolute' or 'objective' viewpoints. Various reactions to this confrontation include:

1) <u>Persistence</u> - maintaining one's culture, perhaps in the face of opposition.

2) <u>Opportunism</u> - cultural exchange, assimilation.

3) <u>Relativism</u> - customs and practices are valid or true for some societies, invalid or false for others.

Relativism is Feyerabend's solution to the problem of cultural confrontation.

It is Feyerabend's task to show that relativism "is reasonable, humane and more widespread than is commonly assumed". [50] How this can be done once one has bid farewell to reason is unclear, but I shall not press the point. But before detailing Feyerabend's critique of reason and objectivity I shall criticise his claim that rationality is in some way responsible for the plight of the Third World and our social and environmental crises. Feyerabend seems to be claiming that rationality is exclusively a Western export which has exclusively resulted in Third World problems. Others such as Russell have felt that reason has been a very scarce commodity in historical affairs indeed:

> Man is a rational animal - so at least I have been told. Throughout a long life, I have looked diligently for evidence in favour of this statement, but so far I have not had the good fortune to come across it, though I have searched in many countries spread over three continents. On the contrary, I have seen the world plunging continually further into madness. I have seen great nations, formerly leaders of civilization, led astray by preachers of bombastic nonsense. I have seen cruelty, persecution, and superstition increasing by leaps and bounds, until we have almost reached the point where praise of rationality is held to mark a man as an old fogy regretably surviving from a bygone age. All this is depressing, but gloom is a useless emotion. In order to escape from it, I have been driven to study the past with more attention than I had formerly given to it, and have found, as Erasmus found, that folly is perennial and yet the human race has survived. The follies of our own times are easier to bear when they are seen against the background of past follies. [51]

First, the idea that reason and objectivity are exclusively Western exports is absurd: even Buddhism and Islam have their great logicians and dialecticians. Second, Feyerabend's position is utterly mistaken because the driving motor of Western imperialism was <u>not</u> reason, but power, profit and greed. [52] Consequently Feyerabend's moral motivation for his critique of reason is flawed. This is not to say that there is not even an element of truth in his position; indeed it would be more sensible for him to investigate Western exports of technology and industrialism as done by someone such as David Suzuki (who is hardly a relativist), rather than give a blanket criticism of rationality itself. The moral objections which Feyerabend makes about the arrogance of the West - our blind faith in increasing economic growth, our belief that technology can

41

solve every problem - are well taken. But this passionate moralizing, as Suzuki illustrates, presupposes rationality for the critique to achieve its power. Feyerabend is too quick to assume that all rationalists are just apologists for the <u>status quo</u>, and insensitive to the crisis of value of the modern age so well expressed by Komesaroff:

> Science, which promised so much, appears to many to have conspired against us - and then, in the spoils of victory, to have moved also to cut off the possibilities for escape. Certainly, the reverence for the given that in one respect had been so fraught with hope, and indeed so fecund, in another seems to have undermined the very impulses that had given rise to it. The tragic paradox is that the price of the new insights was the enervation of that realm within which classically reflection had taken place on the possibilities for a world that would transcend the given - a world in which the inequities and painful disharmonies of everyday life would be overcome. Today, we must live with the consequences of this ambivalent circumstance and endure the jejune, intractable society that remains, in which the social forms are branded with the all-pervasive stigmata of manipulation and domination and where much of what passes as protest and opposition does little more than affirm and beautify the state of unfreedom. [53]

Feyerabend then advances his position of <u>democratic relativism</u>, which asserts "that different cities (different societies) may look at the world in different ways and regard different things as acceptable". [54] The position can be concisely summarized by the following propositions:

(F1)   Free and democratic societies should give all cultural traditions equal access to funds, education institutions and basic decisions.

(F2)   Democratic societies should give all traditions equal rights.

(F3)   Customs are valid in their restricted domains.

(F4)   The idea of objective truth has limited validity; it rules in some traditions, but not in others.

(F5)   For every statement or theory believed with good reasons to be true, there may exist arguments supporting the opposite or some weaker alternative.

(F6)   For every statement or theory believed to be true with good reasons, there exist arguments showing a conflicting alternative to be at least as good, or even better.

(F7) "There is not a single idea, however absurd and repulsive that has not a sensible aspect and there is not a single view, however plausible and humanitarian that does not encourage and then conceal our stupidity and our criminal tendencies". [55]

Let us deal systematically with the main tenets of democratic relativism, beginning with Feyerabend's epistemological claims. The claim (F4) is that objective truth is limited, and he defends this thesis for the case of scientific truth. He argues that there can be no objectively true set of standards for science, because such standards depend upon metaphysical world view or cosmologies. [56] For example, the Aristotelian world view is one which sees reality as both qualitatively and quantitatively finite. In such a world the demand for explanations with increasingly deeper content is absurd because reality is not infinitely complex. Consequently scientific methodology is alleged by Feyerabend to be metaphysics-dependent. As another example consider Galileo, Cremonini and the discovery of Jovian moons. Cremonini, Libri and Magini refused to look through Galileo's telescope at the alleged moons, because according to their Aristotelianism, these moons simply could not exist. The problem of relativism here seems to be that to simply claim that looking resolves the issue begs the question against Cremonini because the issue is about the standards by which the existence of the Jovian moons can be justified. Is the use of telescopic observation, which is itself highly theory-laden, reliable? In this context Feyerabend quotes with approval Einstein's response to Freundlich's measurements, from Einstein's letter to Max Born:

"Freundlich [whose observations seemed to conflict with the general theory of relativity] does not move me in the slightest. Even if the reflection of light, the perihelion, the lineshift were unknown, the gravitation equations would still be convincing because of the inertial system - the phantom which affects everything but is not itself affected. It is really strange that human beings are normally deaf to the strongest arguments while they are always inclined to overestimate measuring accuracies". [57]

Feyerabend takes this as an example of the notion that scientific theories could be upheld in the face of strong negative evidence and still come out on top in the end. This he takes to be a problem for rationalism.

Now whilst strong criticism can be made of Feyerabend's thesis of theory-ladenness [58], it is not necessary to do this here to defend rationalism, for we can accept Feyerabend's arguments and rationalism without contradiction. It is true, as I have argued in The Progress and Rationality of Philosophy that scientific standards depend upon

43

metaphysical world views; thus many scientific controversies cannot be simply solved by the "look and see" attitude of naive empiricism. There will no doubt be protracted and bloody debates about anomalies that may in the end challenge basic tenets of the field or the anomalies may be resolved by the received position. If in the case of general relativity, increasingly stronger empirical evidence against the theory from a wide range of sources appeared (the evidence being itself theory-laden by highly confirmed theories), then Einstein's remarks would have to be seen as irrational and politically inspired. [59] As it turned out though, this theory which initially faced strong negative evidence, came out on top because it was the evidence which was faulty and not the theory. This was accomplished by further measurement and reasoning. The inability to resolve a dispute by a specific observation, does not in itself disprove the role and importance of observation and measurement in science.

Regarding Feyerabend's cognitive relativism, we should note that there are good reasons for believing the doctrine to be self-referentially incoherent. [60] Consider the claim (F6), that for every statement or theory (ST) which is arguably true, there exists arguments showing that (ST) is at least as good or better. Consider (ST) = (F6). Then (F6) is preferable to (F6) and Feyerabend's theory immediately fails. As well, if (ST) is preferable to (ST), then ((ST)) is preferable to (ST) - that is (ST) is preferable to (ST), a contradiction. In fact (F6) generates an infinity of contradictions and thus is trivial. [61]

The conceptual dilemmas facing cognitive relativism applies to Feyerabend's contribution to social philosophy: the idea of a democratically relativist society. In such a society, citizens use the standards of the traditions to which they belong to, to judge the world. They do this because people have the right to live as they see fit. Feyerabend recognises that there are exceptions to this rule, but the exceptions are dealt with by democratic councils taking democratic relativism as their starting point. But how could even this work in Feyerabend's society, where the more traditions the "better" and where _all_ traditions have equal access to power? Many traditions will desire the limitation of other traditions. Traditions that Feyerabend loves, but probably has never had face-to-face dealings with, are not sympathetic to democratic values - as has been seen to be the case with fundamentalist Islam's response in the "death to Salman Rushdie" affair, and also with certain fundamentalist Christian groups. These traditions want to convert all other traditions to their way, or else eliminate them. And if Feyerabend's irrationalism is accepted, then why not? They are after all, only following their traditions, and if Feyerabend's anti-epistemology is accepted there is nothing special at all about democratic theory - it is just another flawed Western creation.

It is also worth noting that if we do accept the importance of democracy, then the people of a country have the right to decide by democratic means whether they want Feyerabend's relativist society. He writes as if democratic relativism is <u>the big</u> answer for all societies. But it doesn't really matter whether democratic relativism is correct or not. What really counts is the <u>democratic decision</u> process. Feyerabend's political philosophy is therefore mere useless baggage to democratic theory.

Feyerabend's social philosophy is not a major departure from some dogmas about culture widely accepted today as received sociological wisdom. This is the relativistic pluralism that asserts that all traditions are "equal" (morally?) and that it is evil to criticise a cultural tradition. Cultural traditions are assumed by politically influential parts of modern sociology to be basic and defining of the individual. Ethnicity, race and class are raised as more valuable than the dignity and freedom of the living creative individual. The results of this flawed source of plurality is devastating with respect to the freedom and choices of individuals, as Welch recognises:

> "They [the Feyerabendian traditions] are modes of life, according to the social sciences, no less valid than our own. We have our past colonial guilt to expiate. Our former arrogance must be made good by seemly modesty and cultural grovellings.
>
> Our intentions being good, we are baffled by the evil consequences, if we notice them at all. By respecting his culture, we aim to respect the Third World individual. In fact we respect what keeps him in chains - a monstrous embodiment of his own 'cultural identity'. With false kindness, we spare him the exacting requirements of real freedom. The colonial struggles for what is mockingly called freedom, and for its subsequent preservation, have normally involved binding individuals firmly to the collectivity and the ruthless integration of society. The 'I' is submerged in the victorious 'we'. The spirit of the herd (of Herder?) must prevail. One party states are appropriate, inevitable. Thus in the Third World, as Octavio Paz has put it, 'there reigns under various names and disguises a Caligula with a thousand faces.' Reason sleeps, and the Third World is plagued by monsters". [62]

Traditions, including our own industrial profit-guided environmentally destructive Western tradition, are seldom freely chosen by individuals, individuals are born and raised in them. Individuals are constrained by such traditions and often suppressed or forced to become group-chauvinistic with the result that their freedom and self-development may be severely limited. If ethnic and racial categories are taken to be of positive value, rather than as an insignificant veneer, then our interactions with real people in daily life will be distorted by these categories. We will see racial and ethnic qualities (whether good or bad), rather than seeing the person him/herself as a well of value. Cultural traditions are of no value over and above the socially-related individuals in them. Feyerabend's over-cultured view of humanity, when pushed to its logical conclusion becomes a new oppressive absolute. Whilst concentrating upon cultural pluralism, Feyerabend leaves unexamined the social structural sources of domination and conformity. Thus modern Western societies, whilst priding themselves as culturally pluralistic still have social structures which are geared solely around techno-economic values rather than wide programmes of social justice, and which are bureaucratic, centralized, hierarchical and organised in terms of specialisation. This situation, which Bell described as a cultural contradiction of capitalism [63], is praised by many Australian (former radical) academics as a progressive advance. I follow Bell in believing that in this contradiction "one perceives many of the latent social conflicts that have been expressed ideologically as alienation, depersonalization, the attack on authority, and the like". [64] In modern capitalism, one may be as pluralistic as one likes, whilst unemployed, frustrated and alienated.

To give a deeper and ultimately more satisfactory response to Feyerabend and the deconstructionists, I wish now to address two rather abstract problems: the nature of truth and the problem of the ultimate justification of our fundamental principles of reason, such as induction. In attempting this brave task, I shall lay a foundation for a new critical theory of philosophy and ethics.

Let us first consider the perennial dispute between realists and idealists on the nature of truth - or as this question has been debated in American philosophy today around the later work of Putnam - the dispute between metaphysical realism and internal realism. [65] Metaphysical realism is the view that truth should be <u>defined</u> as "correspondence" to a fact of an objective world existing independently of mind and conceptualization. A sentence or a proposition (depending upon whether or not a Platonistic semantics is accepted) is true just in case the "correspondence" relation obtains, and false otherwise. The "correspondence" relation as stated, if not explicated by other vague metaphors such as "mirrors" or "reflects", has usually been explicated by formalising the theory (or body of knowledge) containing the sentence under examination and making use of Tarski's semantical conception of truth and the notion of "satisfaction". [66] The <u>criterion</u> of truth, that is the standard for telling just what sentences are true or not,

46

cannot under pain of circularity be correspondence for the metaphysical realist, and is often taken to be <u>coherence</u>. [67]

The idea of truth as correspondence to fact is no doubt the view of truth held by most non-philosophers. Pressed a little deeper though, about what sorts of facts correspond to negative, hypothetical or counterfactual conditional statements, and the non-philosophers (and probably the philosopher's intuitions as well) become cloudy. Regardless of these technical problems, it is possible to express clearly and simply the essential point underlying metaphysical realist conceptions of truth. For the metaphysical realist, truth is radically non-epistemic: there is a logical gap between truth on the one hand, and reason, knowledge and justification on the other. Ideally coherent theories could in principle be false. [68]

Internalists or coherentists define truth epistemically. A sentence p is true just in case p is implied by science s, accepted through the <u>ideal</u> pursuit (pursuit unlimited by time, resources and possibly pursued by free unexploited beings a la Habermas) of methodology M or epistemic principles EP. Such a view cannot be knocked over immediately by the claim that "truth" is then cut off from <u>experience</u>, and thus from the world, because internalists take coherence to involve coherence with experience. [69]

Russell in <u>The Problems of Philosophy</u> argued that the coherence definition of truth fails because "there is no proof that there can be only one coherent system". [70] Our experience could just as easily be accounted for by a fully coherent deception by an evil demon, or life may be one long coherent dream. This claim, as we saw, is an expression of the metaphysical realist's belief that truth is radically non-epistemic.

The internalist, such as Putnam may respond by claiming that the attempt to define truth independently of epistemic values is essentially sceptical, and ultimately self-refuting. Russell himself recognised this, decades before Putnam; Russell says of the correspondence theory of truth ".... if truth consists in a correspondence of thought with something outside thought, thought can never know when truth has been attained". [71] Since truth is an essential part of knowledge, Russell must conclude that we therefore have no knowledge, that is, scepticism is true. The fact that scepticism is true, cannot be known. But in following Russell's argument we come to know that scepticism is true. Hence scepticism is known, and cannot be known, a contradiction.

The idea that natural scientific theories may be empirically under-determined by <u>all possible</u> observable events [72] raised problems for the correspondence theory of truth, parallel to those problems which Russell thought faced the coherence theory. Consider two rival systems of the world, equally supported by experiential facts, equally simple and logically irreconcilable. In this extreme situation the correspondence theory of truth should tell us that these scientific theories are logically equivalent, since the sentences that are the empirical consequences of each respective theory, <u>ex hypothesi</u> are true by correspondence to empirical facts. But <u>ex hypothesi</u> the two theories are logically inconsistent. In this case the correspondence theory of truth is seen to be inadequate.

What follows from these considerations is a limitation upon both the correspondence and coherence theories of truth. Within a certain range, as Richard Sylvan has shown, both theories are compatible, or coherent. However pushed to their metaphysical limits, both theories fall apart. This means that without a satisfactory theory of truth, at the limit points, shown by consideration of hyper-sceptical hypotheses or when hypotheses or theories are underdetermined by all possible observable evidence, our conception of truth collapses. This is not an argument against the concept of truth <u>per se</u>, which functions well within specific limits, but is rather a limitation result or unsolvability-in-principle result about certain metaphysical speculation and part of an extended plea for philosophy to return to earth. As the reader can see from the notes and references to this chapter, this conclusion strikes off one of the hottest topics in mainstream philosophy, the ultimate truth of realism or anti-realism. The issue is unsolvable in principle. Truth must therefore be accepted as a fundamentally irreducible primitive for all inquiry.

Consider another debate, the problem of the justification of induction, to which considerable forests of trees have been logged. [73] The principle of induction can be defined in various ways. One way is this: if out of n trials, m have resulted in e, then if no other relevant data is available, then the probability of e is m/n, m/n being the past relative frequency of e. In this case the problem is to show that the principle of induction is rational by giving a non-circular defense of it. Why not prefer the counter-inductionist policy: if out of n trials m of them have resulted in e, then the probability of e is 1 - (m/n)? To see the difficulties involved here for the justification of scientific inductive practices, consider the powerfully intuitive formulation of the problem of induction given by Russell in <u>The Problems of Philosophy</u>. How do we know that the sun will rise tomorrow? If you reply by appealing to the laws of motion, then we may ask: how do you know that the laws of motion will operate tomorrow? The only reason we have for supposing this is that the laws have operated hitherto, which of course is the inductive principle itself. Russell says:

> "It has been argued that we have reason to know that the future will resemble the past, because what was the future has constantly become the past, and has always been found to resemble the past, so that we really have experience of the future, namely of times which were formerly future, which we may call past futures. But such an argument really begs the very question at issue. We have experience of past futures, but not of future futures, and the question is: Will future futures resemble past futures? This question is not to be answered by an argument which starts from past futures alone." [74]

The positive acceptance of Hume's problem of induction has formed an essential part of Popper's philosophy of science, which sees science growing by a process of conjectures and refutations. [75] What this position entails is a rejection of <u>justificationism</u>: the position that a justified proposition can be deduced from other justified propositions, unless it is in a set X consisting of necessary truths, statements of experience and <u>a priori</u>, metaphysical and meta-methodological principles. [76] This rejection of justificational rationalism has been endorsed by Radnitzky [77] and Miller:

> "... scientific knowledge is everything that a classical epistemologist says it ought not to be: it is unjustified, untrue, unbelief. From this point of view a logic of induction would not be wanted, even if it were available - for no effort is made, or should be made, to justify even the tiniest fragment of our knowledge". [78]

Most philosophers and other people disagree with Miller for the reasons mentioned by Stephen Priest:

> "... the processes of making present experience intelligible - say in everyday sense perception - can in an important sense be correctly characterized as 'inductive'. This is because the intelligibility of present experience depends upon recognition and recognition means 'understanding an F to be a G'. 'Re-cognising' means 'understanding again' i.e. the understanding of the objects of present experience to be the same sort of objects as those encountered in previous experience". [79]

There are also good reasons for believing that Popper cannot escape an analogue of Hume's problem, as Swann has recently shown. According to Popper's epistemology even though all theories about the world are unjustified, there are still <u>best</u> theories which one should act on. Thus according to Swann, Popper is committed to proposition F: Given a set of competing theories, hold to the "best" theory.

Further Popper does not attempt to justify F, he merely holds onto it until a better theory comes along. However as Swann points out, this argument is merely a form of F, and so begs the question of the satisfactoriness of the theory in question. Another argument leading to the same conclusion is this. To falsify a universal generalization, such as $(\forall x)Fx$, it is necessary to show that there is some object in the domain of $'x'$, say $'a'$, which is not - F. This is to say that the statement Fa is true. There is a problem here which is similar to Popper's problem of the "empirical base", but not exactly. Recall that for Popperians, justificationism is unacceptable. This means that we can't give good reason to believe that Fa is true. Now if Fa is just another conjecture which can't be shown to be true, but can only be falsified, then we must show that Fa is true. This only repeats the basic objection. The only option is to decide by agreement to accept that certain basic statements of science are true, not merely sufficiently tested. Because of the received semantics of deductive logic, we can only falsify a statement $p \rightarrow q$, $\sim q$, $\therefore \sim p$ if our argument is sound. This means that our premises must be truths not mere unfalsified conjectures. To do this though is to let justificationism in by the back door. On Popper's position conventionalistic decisions about the basic statements of science, are thought to be innocuous because basic statements can be further tested. But what is generated then is an infinite regress of dogmatic decisions, that in no way distinguishes Popperianism from irrationalism. The problem is not solved by saying that the basic statements of science are themselves conjectures - that there is no question of trying to give reasons for taking any statement to be true - because of the received semantics of deductive logic which Popperians accept. If on the other hand, if every conceivable empirical statement, including statements about falsification, is a conjecture or a guess, then we can be sure that if Sextus Empiricus was alive today, he would be a Popperian. [80]

   How then can the principle of induction be justified, that is, shown to be rationally believable? First, there are good reasons for rejecting counter-induction. [81] Our task then is to show that there is some non-regressive, non-circular or non-arbitrary reason for accepting the principle of induction. The way in which this can be done is by combining and unifying the two great traditions in the philosophy of science: justification and critical rationalism into a new philosophy of science. One way in which this can be done is by using critical rationalism to show that even though we cannot prove that various fundamental principles such as the intelligibility of the world or the reliability of reason, experience and induction, are in fact true, we can accept these principles as open to criticism and this acceptance is itself sufficient to show rationality and dispel dogmatism. Specifically in the case of the problem of the justification of induction, it is proposed that there is no philosophical proof of the truth of the principle of induction, as it is in fact a <u>fundamental</u> principle. Nevertheless alternatives to this principle can be examined on their merits and criticized. As I pointed out in my discussion of rationality scepticism in <u>Essays on Ultimate Questions</u> and <u>The Progress and Rationality of Philosophy</u> with fundamental principles, principles that only philosophical sceptics question during office hours, we do not accept that the failure to give a positive justification a self-refutation. On the contrary, the inability to be able to give a non-circular justification of a principle that is central to our conceptual scheme, has explanatory power and high epistemic value, and is seriously doubted only by professional sceptics, should be taken as the very criterion of the fundamentality of a principle. The role of scepticism should be to give positive arguments for the falsity, contradictoriness or incoherence of such fundamental principles.

My response then to "criterion" style arguments for rationality scepticism is to deny the sceptic's claim of dogmatism and arbitrariness of stopping at some fundamental point in the process of argumentation. Rationalism's dislike of dogmatism was generated not because of the acceptance of unproven statements, but because dogmatism involved making authoritative and arrogant statements which seemed good, but were in fact bad - particularly morally bad. (The word 'dogma' itself comes via Latin from Greek, from <u>dokein</u>, to seem good). Dogmatism implies a closed mind and a total inability to take criticism seriously. My solution to the problem of rationality scepticism, by definition cannot be dogmatic.

Is the position arbitrary though, that is, subject to personal whim, fantasy and prejudice? Again this is not so, because fundamental principles (such as that the world is intelligible in principle, that human reason is at least partially competent, that knowledge has the potential to promote human well-being) are only doubted by professional sceptics, and even here on essentially <u>negative</u> grounds by constantly placing the burden of proof upon rationalists (e.g. repeating infinitely: "What justifies your belief that x is true).?"

Fundamental principles may be "faiths" but they are not arbitrary, dogmatic or conventional. But why is this? A good answer to this super-ultimate problem of justification in philosophy has been given in a profoundly wise article written by William Davis, a philosopher in the "grand old" tradition. [82] Foundational or fundamental principles in both religion and epistemology involve non-arbitrary faith in Davis' view which is reinforced by three forces: the instinctual, methodological and moral forces. To begin with, these faiths are "natural" in Peirce's sense [83], having an innate psychological appeal, the principles seem right, fitting and intuitively correct. We have from human nature a natural bias which guides us to dismiss certain theories or positions as absurd, no matter how cleverly defended by some philosopher. Hume himself recognized this well enough about scepticism in general, and inductive scepticism in particular; the doctrine even if correct is unnatural and unlivable. Naturalness does not guarantee truth, but a natural hypothesis is more worthy of belief and investigation, as Davis recognizes, than an unnatural one.

The second type of consideration which prevents the descent into nihilism, considered by Davis, is that of <u>methodological</u> considerations. If fundamental principles are assumed to be false without proof or unreliable without evidence, then human life will be much poorer. Davis says:

"If we always assume the worse, or even fail to hope for the best, we will not be inclined to search for and reach out for possible goods that may exist. Without hope in positive goods, the nerve of action is cut. With hope, and to the degree that hope exists - ranging on up to and including various degrees of confidence, men are motivated to search and reach out for goods that are out of immediate sight. Such goods cannot be expected to run up and bite us on the bottom. Men must search to find, even if the finding is often accidental. Hope thus provides a spring of action and does so in degrees up to and including various degrees of confidence. Disappointment is always a possibility, but one has to choose between the possibility and resignation or permanent frustration. Besides, no disappointment need be permanent, since one may always hope for success on the next try. Faith and hope are thus prerequisites to success and discovery". [84]

The third factor inclining people towards the acceptance of fundamental principles is <u>moral value</u>:

"Strangely enough, it is precisely this sense of right and wrong which is the main operative force inclining sincere people to the rejection of various of the other fundamental beliefs. The moral sense is behind the indignation of the skeptic who deplores the wishful and sloppy thinking that he sees on every hand. Even the nihilist, when he is not motivated by contrariness or contempt for the human race, is motivated by the feeling that one ought not accept that for which one has no evidence, that self-indulgent thinking is unworthy, that it is more noble to face the manifestly hard world in a manly if not defiant fashion than to comfort onself with sweet nothings. A really consistent nihilist would say of course that even these values are ungrounded except by way of his personal preference. But he probably still feels them anyway with all the force and authority which define the moral imperative. Even the denial that moral values have any transcendental importance is often made with a passion and urgency and tone of moral indignation that belies the very denial". [85]

To detail these remarks made about truth, reason and the nature of justification in adequate detail, will require a book length treatment. Nevertheless enough material has been presented to defend the position that the trend toward relativism and nihilism in influential sectors of modern philosophy is a mistaken one. I have argued that epistemology ultimately derives its foundation from value theory: the superultimate justification of fundamental epistimological principles depends upon evaluative considerations. In the following section, these remarks are developed further, with the presentation of a theory of moral value and reasoning, necessary for our practical investigations in this book of the social dilemmas raised by the AIDS pandemic.

4. Ethics, Social Wisdom and the Foundations of Moral Value

In this chapter and in my other books I have been highly critical of so-called post modern philosophy with its abandonment of common sense [86] and its ultimate conservativism - its failure to raise basic questions about the social order, to challenge the <u>status quo</u> and propose reasoned alternatives to the existing state of things. In other works I have been critical of the uses and abuses of formal logic in modern philosophy and its creation of a needless smokescreen of symbols that often obscures important issues. Nevertheless there is an important criticism of modern philosophy, the discussion of which can lead us back from abstract epistemology, to more concrete socio-ethical concerns, that relate more directly to the AIDS crisis. To get this train of argument onto the correct logical rails, consider A.B. Palma's thought experiment, about what Socrates would say if he returned from the dead to examine contemporary philosophy (both Anglo-American and Continental):

"Socrates, my friends, would weep. It would only take Socrates a week to weep. He would say between his tears: 'My God, what happened to philosophy? I would have thought that philosophers by now would be at the <u>forefront</u> of their culture - they would stand back and examine thoroughly the truth or falsity of various claims, they would be really concerned about the ultimate nature of reality, they would want to know what constitutes a good man and a good woman. But intellectuals and philosophers in particular, instead of being at the forefront of their culture, ride all <u>sorts</u> of cultural waves, fashionable, ideological, political, psychological, scientific, aesthetic, existential, phenomenological, linguistic, relativistic, semiotical, religious and so on, and they assimilate the language of such waves because, and only because, the language in question appears to them attractive. They don't stop to think that attractive language can sometimes hide inconsistencies and can sometimes hide awkward facts." [87]

Palma is not alone in his belief that modern philosophy has lost its sense of moral direction. To serve as an introduction to my own theory value, I shall briefly (but not I hope too inaccurately) consider a philsopher who has charted an alternative to received philosophical opinion.

Nicolas Maxwell's <u>From Knowledge to Widsom</u> [88] presents a more challenging epistemic and evaluative framework than that developed by Palma. Maxwell argues for nothing short of a comprehensive cognitive revolution in the goals and methods of intellectual inquiry, from a framework concerned with the advancement of <u>knowledge</u> to one concerned with the advancement of personal and social wisdom so that intellectual priority is given to the problem of the global crisis of the modern world rather than knowledge for knowledge's sake or technology for profit's sake. The philosophy of knowledge inherited from the Enlightenment holds that the search for truth is both a fundamental and an intrinsic human value; that is to say obtaining the truth about the world or social processes is prior to social action, and when people act on the basis of true scientific theories (such as true environmental or social theories) inquiry is then of technological or pragmatic value. The intellectual domain of inquiry must always be clean from contamination by social values, political interests, public opinions and moral considerations; if it is not then objective knowledge of fact will be polluted. Intellectual problems are thus to be sharply distinguished from social and political problems. Intellectual problems occur due to internal problems in our theories, such as explanatory incompleteness or inconsistency. Social and political problems arise from difficulties in achieving social and political goals and from problems of living itself. This logical gulf between intellectual problems on the one hand, and social and political problems on the other means that there can very well be scientific progress in a world facing chaos and extinction, that the conditions for the growth of knowledge are not necessarily those conditions needed for human flourishing and for a just, humane and sane society. The philosophy of knowledge in addition may be concisely summarized by the observation that the point of intellectual inquiry is to build theories to express truths about the world and collect data, not to <u>directly</u> serve the human good or to <u>directly</u> try and realise that which is worthwhile in life.

Maxwell's thesis can be dramatically illustrated by the following example. Paul Davies points out in <u>Superforce: The Search for a Grand Unified Theory of Nature</u> [89], that there are plans for building in America (if it is not already built) a new generation of particle accelerators, the basic cost being (U.S.) $2,000 million. [90] No doubt with the effects of inflation, this machine will be the most expensive machine ever built, with the 1989 price tag at (U.S.) $4.4 billion. And already the Superconducting Supercollider is conceptually dated compared to new age plasma particle accelerators. Why do it? Davies attempts to answer this question by first pointing out that "[p]article physics has become something of a national virility symbol. If you do it well, and in spectacular style, it shows that there is nothing much wrong with your science and engineering, or your economy". [91] All this of course is nonsense and unargued nonsense at that. It is quite possible that there could be valuable spin-offs from such a massive investment of tax payer's money. On the other hand, there could be disastrous spin-offs from such research, such as particle weapons, or as yet unimaginably destructive weapons, that may lead to the extinction of the human race. Whichever option you choose to believe in is an act of faith, dictated by your prior acceptance of the philosophy of either technological optimism or technological pessimism. What is not an act of faith, is the realisation that such expenditures have an <u>opportunity cost:</u> $2,000 million spent on a new accelerator is $2,000 million that has to be balanced against other programmes, which are ethically more important than the search for the ultimate building blocks of matter. A small basket of such programmes would include, Third World famine and, programmes for the prevention of disease in the Third World, and on the home front dealing with homeless children and adults, unemployment, environmental destruction and increased funding for AIDS research.

Davies' principal justification for increased spending on particle physics amounts to this: "Abstract enterprises such as particle physics are testimony to the inspiration of the human spirit and, even in a world with many pressing material needs, without that spirit we are lost". [92] Davies' argument misses the point here. The technological critics claim is not that research at any time on abstract physics is totally worthless, but rather in a world that faces for the first time in human history extinction by either a nuclear bang or a polluting whimper, hard choices involving the opportunity costs of competing projects must be made. Alternative projects may also have unexpected spin offs; they may even save lives, and perhaps the human race itself. Maxwell sums up this position nicely:

"That which is intellectually and morally disreputable from the standpoint of a kind of inquiry devoted to promoting cooperative rationality in life becomes wholly honourable from the standpoint of the philosophy of knowledge, it being rather systematic criticism of research priorities that becomes intellectually disreputable. In this way, acceptance of the philosophy of knowledge not only blinds the scientific community to the moral and intellectual scandal inherent in the priorities of current scientific research; it has the further effect of transforming legitimate criticism of the <u>status quo</u> into a dangerous threat to the objectivity, intellectual integrity, and scientific character, of science. Legitimate criticism is ostracized wholesale as irrational and ideological". [93]

The outcome of the attitude that science and technology is beyond moral criticism, is that critics of the philosophy of knowledge paradigm such as Paul Feyerabend, are forced to adopt relativism or irrationalism to combat the excesses of scientism and technologism. Reason falls from grace unfairly, when it should be a vital part of a radical and exciting philosophy of life.

Maxwell defines wisdom as "the capacity to discover and achieve what is desirable and of value in life, both for oneself and for others". [94] The goal of the philosophy of wisdom is thus wiser living in a wiser world. Thus wisdom as far as (social) intellectuals are concerned is achieved by concentrating their research attention exclusively upon the basic problems that matter - AIDS and global disease prevention, world hunger, the environmental crisis, the arms race and economic imperialism. [95] The current passion of academics to support the god of economic growth and increasing material affluence of an elite, becomes highly morally problematic in the light of Socrate's questions: 'what is the good life?' and 'how ought we live?' Maxwell's Socratic programme also cuts through many of the cherished debates in the philosophy of the social sciences concerning rationalism versus romanticism, naturalism, versus anti-naturalism and the structuralist/post-structuralist debate. These debates are internal to the philosophy of knowledge.

The major gap in Maxwell's argument relates to the evaluative basis of his philosophy of wisdom, in particular the satisfactoriness of modern ethical theory. Bernard Williams' <u>Ethics and the Limits of Philosophy</u> [96] and Alasdair MacIntyre's <u>After Virtue</u> [97] are two important works both arguing that the challenges of the modern world cannot be effectively addressed by the ethical theories of today's philosophers, and more importantly we must return to older ideas of ethics characteristic of Ancient Greek philosophy. Williams says for example that "... in some basic aspects the philosophical thought of the ancient world was better off, and asked more fruitful questions, than most modern moral philosophy". [98] In particular "... it was typically less obsessional than modern philosophy, less determined to impose rationality through reductive theory". [99] MacIntyre goes much further than Williams' carefully formulated remarks, proclaiming that we have a choice between <u>Nietzsche's</u> nihilistic deflation of the purpose of modern morality, or go back to "a tradition in which the Aristotelian moral and political texts are canonical". [100] My own position is that even if Williams and MacIntyre are right in their historical arguments, the challenge made by Nietzsche and his followers to the very idea of "moral truth" must be met, and overcome. There are good reasons to believe that MacIntyre has <u>not</u> succeeded in achieving this and it is doubtful whether a consultation of "canonical texts" can answer Nietzsche's nihilism. [101] What is needed is fresh thinking on the issue of the foundations of evaluation and moral theory.

The theory of value which I wish to develop here is a form of <u>objectivism</u>: values are real, action-guiding aspects of the world, independent of individual human desires and wants. This position is to be contrasted with the position of <u>subjectivism</u> which holds that value-judgements do not describe any possible object of knowledge, but are only expressions of attitudes, desires and preferences. For the subjectivist, it is meaningless to characterise the evaluative aspect of a proposition as either true or false. There has been substantial criticism of this sort of subjectivism in ethics, [102] with critics correctly arguing that subjectivism effectively abolishes the possibility of rational practical activity altogether. C.L. Stevenson in <u>Ethics and Language</u> for example says "Any statement about any matter of fact ... may be adduced as a reason for or against any value judgement". [103] If this was so, then it would follow that value theory is trivial. But Stevenson's remarks are wrong even for a subjectivist because if there really is a logical gulf between facts and values, then <u>no</u> statement about any matter of fact may be adduced as a reason for or against any value judgement. This type of subjectivist position has become virtually impossible to maintain with developments within post- empiricist philosophy of science questioning the rigidity of the analytic/synthetic distinction and the theory/fact distinction. As we have seen, given the underdetermination of scientific theories by data, combined with the problem of the justification of induction, epistemic values have been seen to be necessary for theory choice and the justification of scientific theories. This result in itself does not establish objectivism because it is logically possible that relativism or nihilism is "true", but we have already seen that both of these positions are unsatisfactory. The balance of reason therefore exists in favour of objectivism.

What form or direction should an objective theory of value take? One tradition of evaluative reasoning which has its classical genesis in Plato and Aristotle, to St. Thomas Aquinas, the young Marx, - "Natural Law Theory", Brand Blanshard [104], R.B. Perry [105], W.H. Davis [106], R.J. McShea [107], J. Kekes [109], Rodney Allen [110] and others [111] is what we may call <u>the human nature theory of value</u>. In general these theorists hold that there are universally valid prescriptive requirements for the conduct of human beings, based upon the promotion of goods and interests based upon fundamental tendencies of human beings - <u>human nature</u> itself. Human nature is not merely a product of current perceived desires; the sense of 'human nature' required by these theories is that of an underlying essence based upon the inherent potentialities of human beings. Further, human nature not merely sets the <u>necessary</u> conditions for what counts as the good of human beings, but human nature is a <u>sufficient</u> condition for human good - the human good is derivable from human nature.

My mentor, Rodney Allen, a human nature ethical theorist, argues that for there to be moral value in the world, there must be beings who have <u>interests</u>, the satisfaction of which would constitute their well-being or flourishing, the mode of satisfaction being determined by their natures. Not only must there be beings for whom there are states of natural well being, but these beings must be agents, capable of acting to produce the conditions of their well-being. For Allen, agents must act self-consciously and for reasons. Thus "lower" animals and plants definitely cannot be regarded as being of <u>intrinsic</u> value for Allen (unless it was independently argued that <u>all</u> matter has the appropriate mental aspect.) In the light of work on deep ecology [112] this position would seem to be immediately limited because of its explicit human chauvinism. Indeed as J.L. Arbor has argued, it is coherent to speak of even plants having interests in the ordinary sense. [113] Granted this, it is not necessary to claim that all species are of equal value. Theories of value based upon the notion of flourishing can be ecologically deep, but also recognise a hierarchy of value in nature based upon the degree of <u>complexity</u> and organic unity. [114] But more about this shortly.

For humans, Allen claims that the basis of practical reasoning is that the satisfaction of human interests is good, and the frustration of human interests is bad. Values such as health, knowledge, cooperation, freedom, love and so on are the general necessary conditions for the fullest possible satisfaction of human interests. Allen however, also claims that real interests, well-being and value are different facets of each other, so for Allen human nature must also be a sufficient condition for human good. However, human nature is not merely a naked actuality, it also contains potentials or possibilities, so that flourishing exists as Harré - powers [115] that are realised or frustrated to various degrees. But which potentials constitute flourishing? What are the real interests of human beings? Surely just those which are good, in which case the theory is circular. [116] The circle however is not vicious (and we should note that in explicating intensional concepts a circle of interrelations is the norm). The reason for this is that 'well-being' or 'flourishing' are not simply place holders for 'goodness' but there are different modes and levels of flourishing based upon the degree of organic unity or internal relatedness and complexity. Human interests then become the interest in unified development of a complex organic unity.

Gewirth has objected to all types of "natural law" value theories on the grounds that if value is closely linked to facts of nature it would mean that if Nietzsche was correct about the will to power, then the will to power would be the supreme mode of functioning of human beings? [117] Gewirth feels that this is morally counter-intuitive. However "natural law" theories of value are not intended to be logically true, true in all possible worlds, for their concern is with this world where there are already plenty of problems. If Nietzsche was right, then moral theory as we understand it is an illusion. This is a problem for any moral theory because nihilism is a general deconstruction of all value. If modes of flourishing were different from what they are, in some entirely different world, then so would the structure of value. This is an implication of the theory, and cannot itself be taken as an objection. Indeed, unlike other moral theories such as intuitionism, "natural law" value theories do have the virtue of being falsifiable. The position does not exist in a scientific or metaphysical vacuum.

Allen's position does not however constitute a fulfilment of the naturalistic hope to reduce values to facts. It is a consequence of this position that "facts" about human nature used to support claims about human (or natural) flourishing are not "facts" in the traditional empiricist sense, for on this position some factual (i.e. objective truths about the world) are also value-laden. Thus arguments about the validity of Hume's is-ought distinction are largely irrelevant to this position. As well, not all values can be understood in terms of the theory of natures and flourishing. The reason for this, as we saw previously, is that the justification and choice of scientific and metaphysical theories that Allen must use to ground his account of natures and flourishing, themselves ultimately rest on evaluative choices. Thus a complete naturalistic reduction of value to physical facts is impossible.

The "natural law" theories of value are essentially attempts to ontologically ground the notion of value, to show

how value fits into the general metaphysical scheme of things. Such theories are usually silent about **epistemological** and **methodological** questions in value theory. These theories suffer then from a severe limitation. To see this consider the following problem, from William Davis [118].

Suppose that the earth was discovered by a race of alien creatures who were vastly more intelligent and more powerful than ourselves. Just as we humans now farm animals such as cows and pigs, they too decide to farm us for their intellect is so great that they consider the intellect of humans as little beyond that of the cow and pig. They urge our philosophers to accept that their race is a moral one, and that eating humanoid creatures is the way that they are - humanoid creatures are their traditional food and they can no more change their nature than any other predator on earth can. If environmental ethics accepts predation as good in wild nature on earth, then the aliens ask what is wrong with us extending the food chain and preying on you humans? [119] The problem here is how are conflicts about interests to be solved: something A may be good for x by virtue of its nature, and bad for y. A must therefore be both good and not good, a contradiction, if objectivism about moral value is accepted.

The example about the man-eating aliens is fantastic, but it does have important concrete analogues in bioethics. Consider for example the problem of the moral status of the embryo. This bioethical problem is of importance to the debate about embryo experimentation in IVF technology and in particular to the long standing debate about abortion, which in 1989 in both America and Australia still divides the community. For the sake of argument, let us grant that the embryo is at least of some moral standing being part of the life cycle of a person. [120] If we grant this, the moral problem of abortion seems an intractable philosophical problem. [121] Alasdair MacIntyre in <u>After Virtue</u> [122] has stated that the most striking feature of contemporary moral philosophy is the existence of perennial disagreements, where there "seems to be no rational way of securing moral agreement in our culture". [123] In the case of arguments both for and against the morality of abortion, MacIntyre concludes that "... the rival premises are such that we possess no rational way of weighing the claims of one as against another. For each premise employs some quite different normative or evaluative concept from the others, so that the claims made upon us are of quite different kinds". [124] Is the abortion controversy, a typical bioethic problem, then beyond rational resolution, so that <u>a fortiori</u>, all other bioethical problems are beyond rational resolution?

In my book <u>The Progress and Rationality of Philosophy</u> I argued that philosophical plurality and disagreement is an ineliminable facet of intellectual life. However, this fact does not in itself show that all philosophical positions are correct (this sort of radical pluralism is self-referentially inconsistent). Rather it means that the existing philosophical options are to differing extents <u>partial truths</u>. I argued that the objectivity and rationality of all fields of philosophy is assured despite first level disagrees by agreement about the acceptability of certain meta-philosophical methods and arguments and meta-problem solving strategies. These distinctive philosophical arguments can be used to show that certain philosophical positions and theories are limited in explanatory power, inconsistent, incoherence, lead to unsolvable problems or absurdity, are open to counter-examples, lead to a vicious infinite regress, circularity or are question begging and so on. [125] The field of philosophy dealing with the study of such arguments is called <u>dialectics</u> or <u>rhetoric</u>. [126] The study of dialectics was since the time of Socrates and Plato, the most important part of logical studies (and was vital in legal studies) since this subject dealt with the satisfactoriness of actual argument, not merely the validity of certain logical forms. In the twentieth century modern logic is concerned with mathematical forms to the exclusion of dialectics, although in legal circles dialectical or rhetorical reasoning flourishes. I concluded that if philosophy is to be cognitively progressive, it must junk its unhealthy perverted desire to be a branch of mathematics, and take its rightful place alongside law as a rhetorical science.

Dialectics or rhetoric is not particularly disturbed by situations of perennial disputes, indeed it may be characterized as that field of study concerned with perennial disputes and controversy. Thus even if MacIntyre is right about the current impasse in the abortion debate, it does not follow from this that philosophy is therefore helpless in thinking about this problem. Perhaps what is needed is a little less logical machismo, and deeper critical thinking about why this problem is a problem, and what the underlying meta-assumptions of this debate are. [127] An example of this dialectial approach has already been given in this chapter in my claim that inductivism and falsificationism in the philosophy of science can be reconciled. Carl Wellmen sums up this response accurately:

> "The fact of existing disagreement on some ethical argument need not undermine its claim to validity, for it might be possible to reach agreement by further rational criticism. It might, for example, be possible to establish the validity of one argument by a second-order argument referring to it. Or someone might come to feel the validity of an ethical argument after having its point explained to him. Conversely, those who begin by disagreeing about the logical status of an argument might come to agree on its invalidity after someone

has revealed an ambiguity in its language or has presented an analogous argument that is clearly invalid. Disagreement about the validity of an ethical argument before it has been critically discussed and carefully rethought, or even after prolonged criticism and reflection, does not show that agreement will not emerge from continuing the process of challenge and response. No actual disagreement at any given point in time rules out the ideal agreement projected at the ideal limit of reasoning through indefinite time". [128]

Having said this, let us return to the example of the abortion question. If it is correct that unwanted pregnancies and the decision to have an abortion may place women in seemingly rationally insoluble moral dilemmas, then we must look with a critical eye at the society which leads women into these dilemmas. The abortion issue is particularly acute in a society which has commodified, objectified and exaggerated the value of sexuality without providing women with reliable and personally safe forms of contraception, being freely and cheaply available. Any sociologist worth her salt would tell you that this is simply asking for moral and social problems to develop. Further, even if this so-called naturally good sexuality is consummated in marriage, the state's total contribution to the well-being of children is less than adequate and abortion may be necessary for the family's survival. If the woman is unfortunate enough not to have financial support from a male partner, then she may be eligible for a single partner's benefit. Yet in accepting such mere subsistence she is then subject to periodical investigation into her personal life, with the prospects of the cessation of benefits standing in front of any love relationship which she may establish with a man. In short, the prospects of bringing an unwanted pregnancy to term are discouraging for women, to say the least. Abortions however are not fun; "no woman in her right mind enjoys an abortion" is a phrase that can be heard if one chooses to listen to women's experience. Abortions are in general, both physically and emotionally painful, even as a means of contraception rather than the outcome of a life or death struggle to save a woman's life. [129] Both alternatives therefore have their disutility.

In particular the abortion problem arises in a social order which is not only sexist and sexually irresponsible, but one where short-term profits are seen as the most valuable things in the universe, where the all-consuming passion of members of society is fast money. In this context abortion is a social disaster to the same extent as environmental destruction, youth homelessness and drug abuse. Its ultimate solution is not by purely philosophical speculation, but by social transformation.

Moral philosophy does not present a complete and ultimately satisfactory solution to the abortion dilemma. What is ultimately needed is a social order where this problem does not arise or when it does, it does not present so many people with traumatic dilemmas. Thus we may take the abortion problem as a <u>reductio ad absurdum</u> of the satisfactoriness of the received social order. The abortion example illustrates an important point about the conduct of contemporary moral philosophy. Moral problems do not exist in a social vacuum, and the solution to what at first glance seems a purely logical problem, may in many cases require changing the rules of the social game.

The remarks made about the abortion controversy, apply <u>mutatis mutandis</u> to another bioethical debate which has divided the Australian community in particular, the IVF programmes and associated reproductive technologies and their social costs. Let us ignore the fact that we have here a set of technologies which raises substantial moral and legal problems. [130] Bartels has estimated that the costs to the Australian Government for 1980-1984 for in-vitro fertilization to be $3.2 million with $4.4 million for the years 1985-1986. [131] Stanely points out that when the hidden costs of pregnancy complications and neonatal intensive care for premature and multiple births are taken into account this figure will be much greater. [132] For example, the cost of neonatal intensive care for 107 very low birthweight babies was 1.6 million. Stanley points out that whilst these vast amounts of money are spent on IVF "studies of the causes of infertility or its primary prevention in Australia is neglected - a gross imbalance." [133] A recent World Health Organisation Report (unreleased at the time of writing) [134] questioned the benefits of IVF with respect to its costs; babies produced by IVF may cost up to $64,000 (Aust) and possibly more for the same reasons listed by Stanley. The success rate for IVF has been considered poor [135] in Australia for 1987 at 8.8 percent.

P. Singer and D. Wells in <u>The Reproduction Revolution</u> [136] consider the question of the philosophical justification of IVF costs in more detail than has occurred in the strictly medical literature. They recognize that private payment for IVF goes only part of the way of meeting the cost objection to IVF because medical students are educated, at public expense, and because of the time it takes to train to be a doctor, the supply of doctors cannot respond quickly to demand. There is thus a potential problem that IVF may divert doctors from areas where they are needed more. To decide the importance of IVF, Singer and Wells decide how severe a disability infertility is, and what its priority is. There are two perspectives from which a priority ranking may be viewed. The first is in terms of current expenditure. Here Singer and Wells rank IVF as less important than kidney dialysis, but at least as important as post-operative cosmetic surgery. As we have seen the worth of IVF is being questioned even here. However there is another way of deciding priorities and this is in terms of a rational ideal for health care. Singer and Wells say:

> "In an ideal world, each dollar of medical expenditure would be used to maximum effect to eliminate illness and disability wherever it occurs. Thus we would not have a situation in which millions of children die from malnutrition (and from the diseases that afflict the malnourished because they are too weak to resist) while major hospitals develop coronary care units that are marvels of technology but of uncertain value in saving lives. There can be little doubt that more lives would be saved by providing adequate food and a very basic level of health care for those who need it than by providing the latest electronic equipment for heart-attack victims. This kind of redistribution, however, would require the wealthy nations to share more equally with the poorer nations, and this is something that the wealthy nations have so far been unwilling to do.
>
> Even if we limit our attention to a single nation such as Australia, similar irrationalities in the use of medical resources are not hard to find. Once again, the large sums spent on the most sophisticated forms of intensive care would be difficult to justify when compared with the relatively small amounts required to make real inroads into infant mortality, blindness, and infectious disease among Aborigines". [137]

Their response to this powerful objection, is that there are institutional barriers to an ideally rational ordering of medical expenditure and that applying this sort of standard is too exacting and stringent. Presumably then the loss of Aboriginal life is not sufficient to count as an argument for a fairer ordering of medical expenditure. Yet surely, sending money to deal with infectious diseases amongst Aborigines is morally superior to sending the same scarce health dollars to assist infertile middle class women to have babies, because infertility qua infertility does not kill one, whilst many infectious diseases do.

Neither Singer nor Wells recognises the fact that once their flimsy conservative defense of IVF technology is swept away, it is quite reasonable to begin to ask questions outside of the narrow self-imposed limits of moral philosophy, such as: 'does society _really_ benefit from this research?'; does it address _fundamental_ social and scientific problems?' and 'is the cost worth it, or is the money best spent elsewhere on socially more important projects?' These are the sorts of questions which a philosophy of wisdom must ask.

5. Conclusion: State of the Argument

The aim of this chapter has been to sketch with broad sweeps, a theory of, and direction for philosophy, and particularly for moral theory. Much of the chapter has dealt with foundational issues in both philosophy and ethics, but not because of any intrinsic interest of these topics in themselves. Rather it has been to respond to the widespread scepticism that exists today about the verisimilitude and worth of philosophy as a cognitive enterprise. In this respect the argument of this chapter complements the argument of <u>The Progress and Rationality of Philosophy</u>. However, this chapter has also departed substantially with mainstream philosophy in its support of the philosophy of wisdom over the philosophy of knowledge. This approach was illustrated with respect to two bioethical problems the abortion issue and the IVF programme. I maintain that the most interesting work in ethics, is that which tries to find ways around heated social debates, or bulldozes straight through the problem, rather than attempting neat analytical reforms. It is the argument of this book, that the philosophical dilemmas raised by AIDS (and the environmental crisis) cannot be resolved without radical changes in the structure of modern society.

NOTES AND REFERENCES

1. J.W. Smith, *The Progress and Rationality of Philosophy*, (Gower, Aldershot, 1988).

2. E.K. Ledermann, *Philosophy and Medicine*, Revised edition, (Gower, Aldershot, 1986) and "Personal Freedom and Psycho-therapeutic Straitjackets: A Contribution to a Medical Libertarian Ethic", *Explorations in Knowledge*, Vol. 4, No. 1, 1987, pp. 1-9.

3. ibid p. 43 (*Philosophy and Medicine*).

4. ibid p. 56.

5. My principal objection to Ledermann's Kantian foundation for medicine is that he fails to resolve the reductionism versus holism problem in medicine, because he cannot explain <u>why</u> the human mind should see purpose in the world, if purposeness is not objective, but only regulative. Why is it that our cognitive faculties require teleological judgements? Surely only because there are teleological processes in nature.

6. D. Greaves, "What is Medicine?: Towards a Philosophical Approach", *Journal of Medical Ethics*, Vol. 5, 1979, pp. 29-32; cf. also V. Navarro, *Crisis, Health, and Medicine: A Social Critique*, (Tavistock, New York, 1986).

7. L.S. King, "What is Disease?", *Philosophy of Science*, Vol. 21, 1954, pp. 193-203.

8. Greaves, op.cit., note 6, p. 31.

9. cf. J.W. Smith and K.N. White, "The Concepts of Health, Illness, Sickness and Disease", *Darshana International*, Vol. 24, 1984, pp. 35-42.

10. I. Illich (et al.) *Disabling Professions*, (Marion Boyars, London, 1977), pp. 11-39. Citation p. 16.

11. I. Illich, *Limits to Medicine/Medical Nemesis: The Expropriation of Health*, (Marion Boyars, London, 1976).

12. cf. R.F. Morgan (ed.) *The Iatrogenics Handbook*, (IPI Publishing, Toronto, 1983); S. Rice, *Some Doctors Make You Sick: The Scandal of Medical Incompetence*, (Angus and Robertson, N.S.W, 1988).

13. cf. R. Dubos, *The Mirage of Health*, (Anchor Books, New York, 1959); T. McKeown and G. McLachlan (eds.) *Medical History and Medical Care*, (Oxford University Press, New

York, 1971); R. Carlson, <u>The End of Medicine</u>, (Wiley Interscience, New York, 1975).

14. R. and J. Dubos, <u>The White Plague: Tuberculosis, Man and Society</u>, (Little Brown, Boston, 1953); C.E. Rosenberg, <u>The Cholera Years</u>, (University of Chicago Press, Chicago, 1962); W.J. van Zijl, "Studies on Diarrheal Disease in Seven Countries", <u>Bulletin of the World Health Organisation</u>, Vol. 35, 1966, pp. 249-261.

15. Illich, op.cit., note 11, p. 23.

16. Navarro, op.cit., 6, p. 2.

17. B.S. Turner, <u>The Body and Society</u>, (Basil Blackwell, Oxford, 1984) and <u>Medical Power and Social Knowledge</u>, (Sage Publications, London, 1987).

18. T. Parsons, <u>The Social System</u>, (Routledge and Kegan Paul, London, 1951).

19. Turner, <u>Medical Power and Social Knowledge</u>, op.cit., note 17, p. 5.

20. ibid p. 10.

21. On Foucault cf. M. Cousins and A. Hussain, <u>Michel Foucault,</u> (St. Martin's Press, New York, 1984); H.L. Dreyfus and P. Rabinow, <u>Michel Foucault: Beyond Structuralism and Hermeneutics</u>, (Harvester Press, Brighton, 1982); C. Lemert and G. Gillan, <u>Michel Foucault, Social Theory and Transgression</u>, (Columbia University Press, New York, 1982); B. Smart, <u>Foucault</u> (Tavistock, Chichester, 1985).

22. Turner, op.cit., note 19, p.11.

23. ibid p. 11.

24. cf. P.N. Unschuld, <u>Medicine in China, A History of Ideas</u>, (University of California Press, Berkeley, 1985) and <u>Medicine in China, A History of Pharmaceutics</u>, (University of California Press, Berkely, 1986).

25. On RSI cf. D. Ferguson, "The 'New' Industrial Epidemic", <u>Medical Journal of Australia</u>, Vol. 140, 1984, pp. 318-319; E. Willis, "RSI as a Social Process", <u>Community Health Studies</u>, Vol. 10, 1986, pp. 210-219.

26. On the radical sociology of medicine cf. K. White, "Towards a Sociology of Medical History", <u>Explorations in Knowledge</u>, Vol. 5, 1988, pp. 33-47 and "The Sociology of Knowledge and Medical Sociology: A Synthesis", <u>Explorations in Knowledge</u>, Vol. 6, 1989, pp. 31-65; M.R. Bury, "Social Constructionism and the Development of

Medical Sociology", <u>Sociology of Health and Illness</u>, Vol. 8, 1986, pp. 137-169; D. Armstrong, "The Invention of Infant Mortality", <u>Sociology of Health and Illness</u>, Vol. 8, 1986, pp. 211-232; M.J. Bloor, "Social Control in the Therapeutic Community: Re-examination of a Critical Case", <u>Sociology of Health and Illness</u>, Vol. 8, 1986, pp. 305-324; D. King, "Social Constructionism and Medical Knowledge: The Case of Transsexualism", <u>Sociology of Health and Illness</u>, Vol. 9, 1987, pp. 351-377; M. Nicolson and C. McLaughlin, " Social Constructionism and Medical Sociology: A Reply to M.R. Bury", <u>Sociology of Health and Illness</u>, Vol. 9, 1987, pp. 107-126; R. Pill, "Models and Management: The Case of 'Cystitis' in Women", <u>Sociology of Health and Illness</u>, Vol. 9, 1987, pp. 265-285; M.R. Bury, "Social Constructionism and Medical Sociology: A Rejoinder to Nicolson and McLaughlin", <u>Sociology of Health and Illness</u>, Vol. 9, 1987, pp. 439-441; A. Radley and R. Green, "Illness as Adjustment: A Methodology and Conceptual Framework", <u>Sociology of Health and Illness</u>, Vol. 9, 1987, pp. 179-207; I. Lowy, "Ludwik Fleck on the Social Construction of Medical Knowledge", <u>Sociology of Health and Illness</u>, Vol. 10, 1988, pp. 133-155; M. Nicolson and C. McLaughlin, "Social Constructionism and Medical Sociology: A Study of the Vascular Theory of Multiple Sclerosis", <u>Sociology of Health and Illness</u>, Vol. 10. 1988, pp. 234-261.

27. On the strong programme of the sociology of knowledge cf. D. Bloor, "The Strengths of the Strong Programme", <u>Philosophy of the Social Sciences</u>, Vol. 11, 1981, pp. 199-213; J. Wettersten, "The Sociology of Knowledge vs. the Sociology of Science: A Conundrum and An Alternative", <u>Philosophy of Social Sciences</u>, Vol. 13, 1983, pp. 325-333; R.C. Jennings, "Truth, Rationality and the Sociology of Science", <u>British Journal for the Philosophy of Science</u>, Vol. 35, 1984, pp. 201-211; P. Tibbetts, "The Sociology of Scientific Knowledge: The Constructivist Thesis and Relativism", <u>Philosophy of the Social Sciences</u>, Vol. 16, 1986, pp. 39-57; C. Radford, "Must Knowledge - or 'Knowledge' - be Socially Constructed?", <u>Philosophy of the Social Sciences</u>, Vol. 15, 1985, pp. 15-33; R.A. Morrow, "The Sociology of Knowledge Dispute Revisited: Implications of a Failed Theoretical Debate", <u>Philosophy of the Social Sciences</u>, Vol. 15, 1985, pp. 507-511; W. Schmaus, "Reasons, Causes and the 'Strong Programme' in the Sociology of Knowledge". <u>Philosophy of the Social Sciences</u>, Vol. 15, 1985, pp. 189-196; A. Chalmers, "The Sociology of Knowledge and the Epistemological Status of Science", <u>Thesis Eleven</u>, No. 21, 1988, pp. 82-102.

28. J.W. Smith, "Rationalism and the Strong Programme of the Sociology of Knowledge: Reconciliation Without Tears", <u>Philosophical Papers</u>, Vol. 21, 1983, pp. 1-31;

"Primitive Classification and the Sociology of Knowledge: A Reply to Bloor", <u>Studies in History and Philosophy of Science</u>, Vol. 15, 1984, pp. 237-243 and <u>The Progress and Rationality of Philosophy</u>, op.cit., note 1.

29. B. Latour and S. Woolgar, <u>Laboratory Life: The Social Construction of Scientific Facts</u>, (Sage, California, 1979).

30. ibid p. 237.

31. J.W. Smith, <u>Reductionism and Cultural Being</u>, (Martinus Nijhoff, The Hague, 1984).

32. This footnote is a comprehensive reading guide to the many theories about, and criticisms of, poststructuralism and deconstructionalism.

S.K. White, "Poststructuralism and Political Reflection", <u>Political Theory</u>, Vol. 16, 1988, pp. 186-208; T.L. Dumm, "The Politics of Post-Modern Aesthetics: Habermas Contra Foucault", <u>Political Theory</u>, Vol. 16, 1988,, pp. 209-228; A. Kroker and D. Cook, <u>The Postmodern Scene: Excremental Culture and Hyper-Aesthetics</u>, (Macmillan, London, 1988); J. Fekete (ed.), <u>Life After Postmodernism</u>, (Macmillan, London, 1988); H.I. Silverman and D. Welton (eds.), <u>Postmodernism and Continental Philosophy</u>, (State University of New York Press, Albany, 1988); (Special Issue on Postmodernism); <u>Theory, Culture and Society</u>, Vol. 5, Nos 2-3, June 1988. M.C. Taylor (ed.) <u>Deconstruction in Context: Literature and Philosophy</u>, (University of Chicago Press, Chicago, 1986); F.R. Kellogg, "Holmes, Pragmatism, and the Deconstruction of Utilitarianism", <u>Transactions of the Charles S. Peirce Society</u>, Vol. 23, Winter, 1987, pp. 99-120; D. Loy, "The <u>Cloture</u> of Deconstruction: A Mahayana Critique of Derrida", <u>International Philosophical Quarterly</u>, Vol. 27, 1987, pp. 59-80; A. Sandor, "Metaphor or Diaphor: On the Difference Particular to Language", <u>Diogenes</u>, No. 134, 1986, pp. 106-128; R. Roderick, "Reading Derrida Politically (Contra Rorty)", <u>Praxis International</u>, Vol. 6, January 1987, pp. 442-449; R. Bontekoe, "A Fusion of Horizons: Gadamer and Schleiermacher", <u>International Philosophical Quarterly</u>, Vol. 27, March 1987, pp. 3-16; G. Olivier, "Art and Transformation", <u>South African Journal of Philosophy</u>, Vol. 6, February, 1987, pp. 16-23; F.J. Ambrosio, "Gadamer, Plato and the Discipline of Dialogue", <u>International Philosophical Quarterly</u>, Vol. 27, March 1987, pp. 17-32; P. Giurlanda, "Habermas' Critique of Gadamer: Does It Stand Up?", <u>International Philosophical Quarterly</u>, Vol. 27, March 1987, pp. 33-41; T. Serequeberhan, "Heidegger and Gadamer: Thinking as "Meditative" and as "Effective - Historical

Consciousness", *Man and World*, Vol. 20, 1987, pp. 41-64; R.J. Dostal, " The World Never Lost: The Hermeneutics of Trust", *Philosophy and Phenomenological Research*, Vol. 47, March 1987, pp. 413 - 434; F.R. Dallmayr, "Democracy and Post-Modernism", *Human Studies*, Vol. 10, 1987, pp. 143-170; M.C. Moore, "Ethical Discourse and Foucault's Conception of Ethics", *Human Studies,* Vol. 10, 1987, pp. 81-95; B.C. Flyn, "Foucault and the Body Politic", *Man and World*, Vol. 20, 1987, pp. 65-84; R. Paden, "Foucault's Anti-humanism", *Human Studies*, Vol. 10, 1987, pp. 123-141; G.J. Hinkle, "Foucault's Power/Knowledge and American Sociological Theorizing", *Human Studies*, Vol. 10, 1987, pp. 35-59; S.F. Schneck, "Michel Foucault on Power/Discourse, Theory and Practice", *Human Studies*, Vol. 10, 1987, pp. 15-33; M.A. Paternek, "Norms and Normalization: Michel Foucault's Overextended Panoptic Machine", *Human Studies*, Vol. 10, 1987, pp. 97-121; T. Keenan, "The "Paradox" of Knowledge and Power: Reading Foucault on a Bias", *Political Theory*, Vol. 15, February 1987, pp. 5-37; G. Horowitz, "The Foucaultian Impasse: No Sex, No Self, No Revolution", *Political Theory*, Vol. 15, February 1987, pp. 61-80; A.E. Hooke, "The Order of Others: Is Foucault's Antihumanism, Against Human Action?", *Political Theory*, Vol. 15, February 1987, pp. 38-60; A. Megill, "The Reception of Foucault by Historians", *Journal of the History of Ideas*, Vol. 48, 1987, pp. 117-142; C.U.M. Smith, ""Clever Beats who Inverted Knowing": Nietzsche's Evolutionary Biology of Knowledge", *Biology and Philosophy*, Vol. 2, January 1987, pp. 65-91; J. Taminiaux, "Art and Truth in Schopenhauer and Nietzsche", *Man and World*, Vol. 20, 1987, pp. 81-102; R.E. Allinson, "Having Your Cake and Eating it too: Evaluation and trans-evaluation in Chuang Tzu and Nietzsche", *Journal of Chinese Philosophy*, Vol. 13, December 1986, pp. 429-443; J.C. Weinscheimer, *Gadamer's Hermeneutics: A Reading of 'Truth and Method'* (Yale University Press, New Haven, 1985); B.D. Smith, "Distanciation and Textual Interpretation", *Lavel Theologique et Philosophique*, Vol. 43, June 1987, pp. 205-216; J.P. Hogan, "Hermeneutics and the Logic of Question and Answer: Collingwood and Gadamer", *Heythrop Journal*, Vol. 28, July 1987, pp. 263-284; K. Kierans, "On the Limits of Contemporary Reflection on Freedom: An Analysis of Marxist and Existential Responses to Hegel", *Dionysius*, Vol. 10, 1986, pp. 85-128; J. Geneva (ed.), *Power, Gender, Values*, (Academic, Alberta, 1987); H. White, *The Content of the Form: Narrative Discourse and Historical Representation*, (John Hopkins Press, Baltimore, 1987); J. Bennett, *Unthinking Faith and Enlightenment: Nature and the State in a Post-Hegelian Era*, (New York University Press, New York, 1987); G. Gillan, "Foucault's Philosophy", *Philosophy and Social Criticism*, Vol. 12, 1987, pp. 145-155; P.L. McLaren, "Ideology, Science and the Politics of Marxian

Orthodoxy...", *Educational Theory*, Vol. 37, 1987, pp. 301-326; K. Racevskis, "Michel Foucault, Rameau's Nephew and the Question of Identity", *Philosophy and Social Criticism*, Vol. 12, 1987, pp. 132-144; J.W. Bernauer, "Michel Foucault's Ecstatic Thinking", *Philosophy and Social Criticism*, Vol. 12, 1987, pp. 156-193; D. Marshall (ed.) *Literature as Philosophy/Philosophy as Literature*, (University of Iowa Press, Iowa City, 1987); S.R. Yarbrough, "Differance, Deference, and the Question of Proper Reading, Man and World", Vol. 20, August 1987, pp. 257-282; F.R. Dallmayr, *Critical Encounters: Between Philosophy and Politics,* (Notre Dame University Press, Notre Dame, 1987); S. Knapp and W. B. Michaels, "Against Theory II: Hermeneutics and Deconstruction", *Critical Inquiry*, Vol. 14, Autumn 1987, pp. 49-68; B.P. Dauenhauer, *At the Nexus of Philosophy and History*, (University of Georgia Press, Athens, 1987); A. Nehamas, *Nietzsche: Life as Literature*, (Harvard University Press, Cambridge, 1985); J.A. Bernstein, *Nietzsche's Moral Philosophy*, (F. Dickinson University Press, Cranbury, 1987); G.T. Martin, "A Critique of Nietzsche's Metaphysical Scepticism", *International Studies in Philosophy*, Vol. 19, Summer 1987, pp. 51-59; M. Clark, "Deconstructing *The Birth of Tragedy*", *International Studies in Philosophy*, Vol. 19, Summer 1987, pp. 67-75; D.W. Conway, "Nietzsche's Internal Critique of Foundationalism", *International Studies in Philosophy*, Vol. 19, Summer 1987, pp. 103-110; S.G. Crowell, "Nietzsche's View of Truth", *International Studies in Philosophy*, Vol. 19, Summer 1987, pp. 3-18; A. White, "Nietzschean Nihilism: A Typology", *International Studies in Philosophy*, Vol. 19, Summer 1987, pp. 29-44; G.C.F. Bearn, "Reply to Martin's "A Critique of Nietzsche's Metaphysical Scepticism"", *International Studies in Philosophy*, Vol. 19, Summer 1987, pp. 61-65; D.B. Bergoffen, "Seducing Historicism", *International Studies in Philosophy*, Vol. 19, Summer 1987, pp. 85-98; M. Midgley, "Can Specialization Damage Your Health?" *International Journal of Moral and Social Studies*, Vol. 2, Spring 1987, pp. 3-9; R. Bernasconi, "Bridging the Abyss: Heidegger and Gadamer", *Research in Phenomenology*, Vol. 16, 1986, pp. 1-24; B.R. Wachterhauser, "Interpreting Texts: Objectivity of Participation", *Man and World*, Vol. 19, 1986, pp. 439-457; T.R. Martland, "Quine's "Half-Entities" and Gadamer's Too", *Man and World*, Vol. 19, 1986, pp. 361-373; J. Margolis (ed.), *Rationality, Relativism and the Human Sciences*, (Martinus Nijhoff, Dordrech, 1986); J. Sawicki, "Foucault and Feminism: Towards a Politics of Difference", *Hypatia*, Vol. 1, Fall 1986, pp. 23-36; D. Ingram, "Foucault and the Frankfurt School: A Discourse on Nietzsche, Power and Knowledge", *Praxis International*, Vol. 6, October 1986, pp. 311-327; S. Ijsseling, "Foucault with Heidegger", *Man and World*, Vol. 19, 1986, pp. 413-424; J. Sallis, *Delimitations:*

Phenomenology and the End of Metaphysics, (Indiania University Press, Bloomington, 1986); I.E. Harvey, Derrida and the Economy of "Difference", (Indiana University Press, Bloomington, 1986); H. Lawson, Reflexivity: The Post-Modern Predicament, (Open Court, La Salle, 1985); R. Gasche, The Tain of the Mirror: Derrida and the Philosophy of Reflection, (Harvard University Press, Cambridge, 1986); J. Margolis, "Deconstruction: A Cautionary Tale", Journal of Aesthetic Education, Vol. 20, Winter 1986, pp. 91-94; F. Wilson, "Hume and Derrida on Language and Meaning", Hume Studies, Vol. 12, November 1986, pp. 99-121; G. Nicholson, "Deconstruction or Dialogue", Man and World, Vol. 19, 1986, pp. 263-274; C.F. Reeves, "Deconstruction, Language, Motive: Rortian Pragmatism and the Uses of "Literature"," Journal of Aesthetics and Art Criticism, Vol. 44, 1986, pp. 351-356; J.D. Caputo, "Telling Left From Right: Hermeneutics, Deconstruction and the Work of Art", Journal of Philosophy, Vol. 83, 1986, pp. 678-685, and "Heidegger and Derrida: Cold Hermeneutics", Journal of the British Society for Phenomenology, Vol. 17, 1986, pp. 252-274; J. Risser, "Nietzsche's View of Philosophical Style" : Comments", International Studies in Philosophy, Vol. 18, 1986, pp. 83-86; J.G. Murphy, "Meaningfulness and the Doctrine of Eternal Return", International Studies in Philosophy, Vol. 18, 1986, pp. 61-66; D.C. Shaw, "Nietzsche as Sophist: A Polemic", International Philosophical Quarterly, Vol. 26, 1986, pp. 331-339; M. Tanner, "Nietzsche Beyond Good and Evil", Philosophy, Vol. 20, 1986 (Supp), pp. 197-216; M. Clark, "Nietzsche's Perspectivist Rhetoric", International Studies in Philosophy, Vol. 18, 1986, pp. 35-43; A. Moles, "Nietzsche's Critique of Causality: Does this Entail his Rejection of Metaphysics?" International Studies in Philosophy, Vol. 18, 1986, pp. 17-27; K. Higgins, "Nietzsche's View of Philosophical Style", International Studies in Philosophy, Vol. 18, 1986, pp. 62-81; I. Soll, "The Hopelessness of Hedonism and the Will to Power", International Studies in Philosophy, Vol. 18, 1986, pp. 97-112; A. Close, "Centering the De-Centerers: Foucault and Las Meninas," Philosophy and Literature, Vol. 11, 1987, pp. 21-36; J. Salis (ed.) Deconstruction and Philosophy: The Texts of Jacques Derrida, (University of Chicago Press, Chicago, 1987); T. Clark, "Heidegger, Derrida and the Greek Limits of Philosophy", Philosophy and Literature, Vol. 11, 1987, pp. 75-91; S. Haulgate, Hegel, Nietzsche and the Criticism of Metaphysics, (Cambridge University Press, Cambridge, 1986); D.W. Goldberg, "A Dionysian Epistemology", Kinesis, Vol. 16, 1987, pp. 22-40; E.I. Okhamafe, "Deconstruction and Humanism, Part I: Economy of Gaiety and Gravity in Nietzsche", Auslegung, Vol. 13, 1987, pp. 152-174; C.W. Harvey, "Nietzsche on Knowledge and Interpretation", Dialogos, Vol. 22, 1987, pp. 65-76;

R. Nola, "Nietzsche's Theory of Truth and Belief", *Philosophy and Phenomenological Research*, Vol. 47, 1987, pp. 525-582; G.A. Pfeifer, "The Ubermensch and Eternal Recurrence", *Dialogue* (PST), Vol. 29, 1987, pp. 45-49; J. Llewelyn, *Beyond Metaphysics: The Hermeneutic Circle in Contemporary Continental Philosophy*, (Humanities Press, Atlantic Highlands, 1985); J.C. Weinsheimer, *Gadamer's Hermeneutics: A Reading of Truth and Method*, (Yale University Press, New Haven, 1985); H.J. Silverman (ed.), *Hermeneutics and Deconstruction*, (SUNY Press, Albany, 1985); R. Detsch, "A Non-Subjectivist Concept of Play - Gadamer and Heidegger versus Rilke and Nietzsche", *Philosophy Today*, Vol. 29, 1985, pp. 156-172; F.J. Ambrosio, "Dawn and Dusk: Gadamer and Heidegger on Truth", *Man and World*, Vol. 19, 1986, pp. 21-53, and "Gadamer and the Ontology of Language: What Remains Unsaid?", *Journal of the British Society for Phenomenology*, Vol. 17, 1986, pp. 124-142; D.J. Rothberg, "Gadamer, Rorty, Hermeneutics and Truth: A Response to G. Warnke's "Hermeneutics and the Social Sciences: A Gadamerian Critique of Rorty"," *Inquiry*, Vol. 29, 1986, pp. 355-361; C. Norris, *Contest of Faculties: Philosophy and Theory After Deconstruction*, (Methuen, London, 1985); J.Minson, *Genealogies of Morals: Nietzsche, Foucault, Donzelot and the Eccentricity of Ethics*, (St. Martin's Press, New York, 1985); S.D. Ross, "Belonging to a Philosophic Discourse", *Philosophy and Rhetoric*, Vol. 19, 1986, pp. 166-177; H. Sluga, "Foucault, The Author and the Discourse", *Inquiry*, Vol. 28, 1985, pp. 403-415; S. Ross, "Foucault's Radical Politics", *Praxis International*, Vol. 5, 1985, pp. 131-144; R. Paden, "Locating Foucault - Archeology vs. Structuralism", *Philosophy and Social Criticism*, Vol. 11, 1986, pp. 19-37; N. Fraser, "Michel Foucault: A Young Conservative?" *Ethics*, Vol. 96, 1985, pp. 165-184; T.R. Flynn, "Truth and Subjectivation in the Later Foucault", *Journal of Philosophy*, Vol. 82, 1985, pp. 531-540; A. Megill, *Prophets of Extremity: Nietzsche, Heidegger, Foucault, Derrida*, (University of California Press, Berkeley, 1985); R.P. Blum, "Deconstruction and Creation", *Philosophy and Phenomenological Research*, Vol. 46, 1985, pp. 293-306; D. Carrier, "Derrida as Philosopher", *Metaphilosophy*, Vol. 16, 1985, pp. 221-234; D. Novitz, "Metaphor, Derrida and Davidson", *Journal of Aesthetics and Art Criticism*, Vol. 44, 1985, pp. 101-114; R.L. Howey, "Nietzsche and the "New" French Philosophers", *International Studies in Philosophy*, Vol. 17, 1985, pp. 83-93; J.R. Boly, "Nihilism Aside: Derrida's Debate Over Intentional Models", *Philosophy and Literature*, Vol. 9, 1985, pp. 152-165; T.J. Stapleton, "Philosophy and Finitude: Husserl, Derrida and the End of Philosophy", *Philosophy Today*, Vol. 30, 1986, pp. 3-15; D. Novitz, "The Rage for Deconstruction", *Monist*, Vol. 69, 1986, pp. 39-55; D. Cook, "Translation as a Reading", *British*

Journal or Aesthetics, Vol. 26, 1986, pp. 143-149; P. Tibbetts, "The Sociology of Scientific Knowledge: The Constructivist Thesis and Relativism", Philosophy of the Social Sciences, Vol. 16, 1986, pp. 39-57; M. Kerlin, "Truth and Social Construction of Reality", Proceedings of the American Catholic Philosophical Association, Vol. 59, 1985, pp. 289-298; P.A. Chambige, "Comment: Nietzsche and the 'New' French Philosophers", International Studies in Philosophy, Vol. 17, 1985, pp. 95-98; H. Veatch, "Deconstruction in Philosophy", Review of Metaphysics, Vol. 39, 1985, pp. 303-320; G.C.F. Bearn, "Nietzsche, Feyerabend and the Voices of Relativism:, Metaphilosophy, Vol. 17, 1986, pp. 135-152; R.M. Stewart, "Nietzsche's Perspectivism and the Autonomy of the Master Type", Nous, Vol. 20, 1986, pp. 371-389; L.K. Schmidt, The Epistemology of Hans-Georg Gadamer, (Lang, New York, 1985); A.R. How, "A Case of Creative Misreading: Habermas's Evolution of Gadamer's Hermeneutics", Journal of British Society for Phenomenology, Vol. 16, 1985, pp. 132-144; S. Hekman, "Action as Text: Gadamer's Hermeneutics and the Social Scientific Analysis of Action", Journal for the Theory of Social Behaviour, Vol. 14, 1984, pp. 333-354; L.D. Derksen, "Language and the Transformation of Philosophy", Philosophia Reformata, Vol. 49, 1984, pp. 134-149; J. Wallulis, "Philosophical Hermeneutics and the Conflict of Ontologies", International Philosophical Quarterly, Vol. 24, 1984, pp. 283-302; J. Risser, "Practical Reason, Hermeneutics and Social Life", Proceedings of the American Catholic Philosophical Association, Vol. 58, 1984, pp. 84-92; A.M. Hjort, "The Conditions of Dialogue: Approaches to the Habermas-Gadamer Debate", Eidos, Vol. 4, 1985, pp. 11-37; H.L. Dreyfus and P. Rabinow, Michel Foucault: Beyond Structuralism and Hermeneutics, (University of Chicago Press, Chicago, 1983); B. Cooper Michel Foucault, An Introduction to the Study of his Thought, (Mellen Press, New York, 1981); F.R. Dallmayr, Polis and Praxis, (MIT Press, Cambridge 1985); G. Shapiro (ed.), Hermeneutics, (University of Massachusetts Press, Amherst, 1984); C. Taylor, "Connolly, Foucault and Truth", Political Theory, Vol. 13, August 1985, pp. 377-386; D.R. Hiley, "Foucault and the Question of Enlightenment", Philosophy and Social Criticism, Vol. 11, 1985, pp. 63-84. T.E. Wartenberg, "Foucault's Archaeological Method: A Response to Hacking and Rorty", Philosophical Forum (Boston), Vol. 15, 1984, pp. 345-364; W.E. Connolly, "Michel Foucault: An Exchange: Taylor, Foucault and Otherness", Political Theory, Vol. 13, 1985, pp. 365-376; P. Kemp, "Death and the Machine: From Jules Verne to Derrida and Beyond", Philosophy and Social Criticism, Vol. 10, 1984, pp. 75-96; J. Sallis, "Heidegger/Derrida", Journal of Philosophy, Vol. 81, 1984, pp. 594-601; C.A. Pressler, "Redoubled: The Bridging of Derrida and Heidegger", Human Studies, Vol.

7, 1984, pp. 325-342; B.G. Chang, "The Eclipse of Being: Heidegger and Derrida", *International Philosophical Quarterly*, Vol. 25, 1985, pp. 113-138; H.J. Silverman, "The Limits of Logocentrism (on the way to Grammatology)", *Man and World*, Vol. 17, 1984, pp. 347-360; C.D. Eckhardt, "A Commonsensical Protest Against Deconstruction, or how the Real World at last became a Fable", *Thought*, Vol. 60, 1985, pp. 310-321; R. Eldridge, "Deconstruction and its Alternatives", *Man and World*, Vol. 18, 1985, pp. 147-170; S. Tyman, "Heidegger and the Deconstruction of Foundations", *International Philosophical Quarterly*, Vol. 24, 1984, pp. 347-372; S. Fuller, "Is There a Language - Game that even the Deconstructionist can Play?", *Philosophy and Literature*, Vol. 19, 1985, pp. 104-109; A.D. Schrift, "Language, Metaphor, Rhetoric: Nietzsche's Deconstruction of Epistemology", *Journal of the History of Philosophy*, Vol. 23, 1985, pp. 371-396; W. Kendrick, "Literary Criticism: The State of the Art", *Thought*, Vol. 59, 1984, pp. 514-526; D. Bloor, "A Sociology Theory of Ojectivity", *Philosophy*, Vol. 17, 1984 (Supp.) pp. 229-246; L.M. Hinman, "Comments on Mittelman's "Perspectivism, Becoming and Truth in Nietzsche", *International Studies in Philosophy*, Vol. 16, 1984, pp. 23-26; W.J. Zanardi, "Comments: Aims and Forms of Discourse Regarding Nietzsche's Truth-telling", *International Studies in Philosophy*, Vol. 16, 1984, pp. 53-56; G.J. Stack, "Eternal Recurrence Again", *Philosophy Today*, Vol. 28, 1984, pp. 242-264; M. Warren, "Nietzsche and Political Philosophy", *Political Theory*, Vol. 13, 1985, pp. 188-212; M.G. Hallman, "Nietzsche and Pragmatism", *Kinesis*, Vol. 14, 1985, pp. 63-78; J. McBridge, "Nietzsche's Existential Ethic", *Philosophical Studies* (Ireland) Vol. 30, 1984, pp. 73-82; W. Mittelman, "Perspectivism, Becoming, and Truth in Nietzsche", *International Studies in Philosophy*, Vol. 16, 1984, pp. 3-22; T.B. Strong, "Reflections on Perspectivism in Nietzsche", *Political Theory*, Vol. 13, 1985, pp. 164-182; A.F. Lingis, "The Truth Imperative", *Auslegung*, Vol. 11, 1984, pp. 317-339; T.B. Ommen, "Bultmann and Gadamer: The Role of Faith in Theological Hermeneutics", *Thought*, Vol. 59, 1984, pp. 348-359; D. Jenner, "Hermeneutic Philosophy: History as the Singular Ground of Thought", *Cogito*, Vol. 1, 1983, pp. 88-108; P.A. Johnson, "The Task of the Philosopher: Kierkegaard/ Heidegger/Gadamer", *Philosophy Today*, Vol. 28, 1984, pp. 3-19; K. Racevskis, *Michel Foucault and the Subversion of Intellect* (Cornell University Press, Ithaca, 1983); D.R. Hiley, "Foucault and the Analysis of Power : Political Engagement without Liberal Hope or Comfort", *Praxis International*, Vol. 4, 1984, pp. 192-207; A.J. Cascardi, "Skepticism and Deconstruction", *Philosophy and Literature*, Vol. 8, 1984, pp. 1-4; J.T. Wilcox, "A Note on Correspondence and Pragmatism in Nietzsche", *International Studies in Philosophy*, Vol 12, 1980, pp.

77-80; R. Small, "Eternal Recurrence", <u>Canadian Journal of Philosophy</u>, Vol. 13, 1983, pp. 585-606; R. Schact, "Nietzsche on Philosophy, Interpretation and Truth", <u>Nous</u>, Vol. 18, 1984, pp. 75-85; P.J. Kain, "Nietzsche, Skepticism and Eternal Recurrence", <u>Canadian Journal of Philosophy</u>, Vol. 12, 1983, pp. 365-388; N. Davey, "Nietzsche's Doctrine of Perspectivism", <u>Journal of the British Society for Phenomenology</u>, Vol. 14, 1983, pp. 240-257; E.G. Newman, "Truth as Art - Art as Truth", <u>International Studies in Philosophy</u>, Vol. 15, 1983, pp. 25-33; R.L. Maddox, "Hermeneutic Circle - Vicious or Victorious", <u>Philosophy Today</u>, Vol. 27, 1983, pp. 66-76; M. Philp, "Foucault on Power: A Problem in Radical Translation?" <u>Political Theory</u>, Vol. 11, 1983, pp. 29-51; C. Norris, <u>Deconstruction: Theory and Practice</u>, (Methuen, London, 1982); J. Culler, <u>On Deconstruction: Theory and Criticisms After Structuralism</u>, (Cornell University Press, Ithaca, 1982); D.W. Hamlyn, "Schopenhauer on the Will in Nature", <u>Midwest Studies in Philosophy</u>, Vol. 8, 1983, pp. 457-468; H. Neumann, "Nietzsche, The Superman, the Will to Power and Eternal Return", <u>Ultimate Reality and Meaning</u>, Vol. 5, 1982, pp. 280-295; G.J. Stack, "Nietzsche's Analysis of Causality", <u>Idealistic Studies</u>, Vol. 12, 1982, pp. 260-275; and "Nietzsche's Myth of the Will to Power", <u>Dialogos</u>, Vol. 17, 1982, pp. 27-50; K. Jenking, "The Dogma of Nietzsche's Zarathustra", <u>Journal of Philosophy of Education</u>, Vol. 16, 1982, pp. 251-254; E.G. Newman, "The Meta-Moralism of Nietzsche", <u>Journal of Value Inquiry</u>, Vol. 16, 1982, pp. 207-222; D.B. Bergoffen, "Why a Genealogy of Moral?" <u>Man and World</u>, Vol. 16, 1983, pp. 129-138; R.J. Bernstein, "From Hermeneutics to Praxis", <u>Review of Metaphysics</u>, Vol. 35, 1982, pp. 823-846; N. Fraser, "Foucault on Modern Power: Empirical Insights and Normative Confusions", <u>Praxis</u>, Vol. 1, 1981, pp. 272-287; J. Bernauer, "Foucault's Political Analysis", <u>International Philosophical Quarterly</u>, Vol. 22, 1982, pp. 87-96; C.E. Scott, "History and Truth", <u>Man and World</u>, Vol. 15, 1982, pp. 55-56; R. Rorty, "Method, Science and Social Hope", <u>Canadian Journal of Philosophy</u>, Vol. 16, 1981, pp. 569-588; R. Rorty, "From Epistemology to Hermeneutics", <u>Acta Philosophica Fennica</u>, Vol. 30, 1978, pp. 11-30; L. Shiner, "Reading Foucault: Anti-method and the Genealogy of Power - Knowledge", <u>History and Theory</u>, Vol. 21, 1982, pp. 382-398; B. Flynn, "Sexuality, Knowledge and Power in the Thought of Michel Foucault", <u>Philosophy and Social Criticism</u>, Vol. 8, 1981, pp. 329-348; B. Barnes, "On the Conventional Character of Knowledge and Cognition", <u>Philosophy of the Social Sciences</u>, Vol. 11, 1981, pp. 303-334; M. Clark, <u>Michel Foucault: An Annotated Bibliography: Tool Kit for a New Age</u>, (Garland Publishing Inc., New York, 1983); G.J. Stack, "Nietzsche and the Correspondence Theory of Truth", <u>Dialogos</u>, Vol. 16, 1981, pp. 93-118; S. Miri, "The Exceptional Man and

Nietzsche", *Indian Philosophical Quarterly*, Vol. 9, 1981, pp. 1-6; K.S. Walters, "The Ontological Basis of Nietzsche's Perspectivism", *Dialogue* (PST), Vol. 24, 1982, pp. 35-46; J.S. Hans, "Hermeneutics, Play, Deconstruction", *Philosophy Today*, Vol. 24, 1980, pp. 299-317; M. Ermarth, "The Transformation of Hermeneutics", *Monist*, Vol. 64, 1981, pp. 175-194; R.S. Gall, "Between Tradition and Critique", *Auslegung*, Vol. 8, 1981, pp. 5-18; M. Sprinker, "The Use and Abuse of Foucault", *Humanities in Society*, Vol. 3, 1980, pp. 1-22; D. Wood, "Derrida and the Paradoxes of Reflection", *Journal of the British Society for Phenomenology*, Vol. 11, 1980, pp. 225-238, and "Style and Strategy at the Limits of Philosophy", *Monist*, Vol. 63, 1980, pp. 494-511; R.D. Cumming, "The Odd Couple: Heidegger and Derrida", *Review of Metaphysics*, Vol. 34, 1981, pp. 487-522; G.J. Stack, "Nietzsche and Perspectival Interpretation", *Philosophy Today*, Vol. 25, 1981, pp. 221-241; J.E. Atwell, "Nietzsche's Perspectivism", *Southern Journal of Philosophy*, Vol. 19, 1981, pp. 157-170; L. Dupre, "Secularism and the Crisis of our Culture", *Thought*, Vol. 51, 1976, pp. 271-281; P.L. Brown, "Epistemology and Method: Althusser, Foucault, Derrida", *Cultural Hermeneutics*, Vol. 3, 1975, pp. 147-162.

33. I. Howe, "The New York Intellectuals", cited from R. Wolin, "Modernism vs. Postmodernism", *Telos*, No. 62, Winter 1984-85, pp. 9-29. Citation p. 20.

34. D. Kellner, "Postmodernism as Social Theory: Some Challenges and Problems", *Theory, Culture and Society*, Vol. 5, 1988, pp. 239-269. Citation p. 239.

35. Z. Bauman, "Is There a Post Modern Sociology?" *Theory, Culture and Society*, Vol. 5, 1988, pp. 217-237.

36. cf. G. McCormack, "Some Comments on the MFP (Multifunctionalpolis) Project", Department of Asian Studies, The University of Adelaide.

37. On Japan as a counter-example to the modernism literature cf. C. Deutschmann, "The Japanese Type of Organization as a Challenge to the Sociological Theory of Modernisation", *Thesis Eleven*, No. 17, 1987, pp. 40-58; J.P. Arnason, "The Modern Constellation and the Japanese Enigma, *Thesis Eleven*, No. 17, 1987, pp. 4-39.

38. R. Rorty, *Philosophy and the Mirror of Nature*, (Princeton University Press, Princeton, 1979).

39. cf. C.J Berry, *Human Nature*, (Macmillan, London, 1986), pp. 126-131; On the self-refuting nature of Foucault's programme cf. J.G. Merquior, Foucault, (University of California Press, Berkeley, 1985), p. 147.

40. J. Derrida, Speech and Phenomena, translation D. Allison, (Northwestern University Press, Evaston, 1973), Of Grammatology, translation G.C. Spivak, (John Hopkins, Baltimore, 1976), Writing and Difference, translation A. Bass, (University of Chicago Press, Chicago, 1978); Spurs, Nietzsche's Styles, translation B. Harlow, (University of Chicago Press, Chicago, 1979), Positions, translation A. Bass (Univerity of Chicago Press, Chicago, 1981), Margins of Philosophy, translation A. Bass (University of Chicago Press, Chicago, 1982).

41. R. D'Amico, "Going Relativist", Telos, No. 67, 1986, pp. 135-145. Citation p. 136.

42. R. Rorty, Consequences of Pragmatism, (Harvester Press, Sussex, 1982), p. 210 gives us a sample of his conservatism and deep anti-humanism in his claim that capitalist society is the "best polity actualised so far". Ignoring the question of how a "nihilist" such as Rorty can speak of "best", we should note that "best polity" is "irrelevant to most of the problems of the population of the planet". As C.J. Berry, Human Nature, (op.cit., note 39) p. 130 points out that this means that the problems of the world for Rorty are beyond solution. This conservatism (or self-indulgent despair) perhaps more than anything else, makes deconstructionism a sterile, immoral and repulsive doctrine that deserves political opposition.

    It is interesting to note, in the context of the conservatism and immorality of some of the so-called "great sociologists", recent material documenting Talcott Parsons role in bringing Nazi collaborators to the U.S cf. J. Wiener, "Talcott Parsons' Role in Bringing Nazi Sympathizers to the U.S", The Nation, March 6, 1989 (cover story). The debate about Heidegger's collaboration with the Nazi's has raged for many years. Now many postmodernists have drawn upon Parsons' work, and many more, such as Rorty, upon Heidegger's. This same tradition rejects the validity of the genetic fallacy, that the truth of a doctrine is distinct from cultural causation. Thus this movement is left with an obvious dilemma.

43. The claim that law is merely a branch of literature because it *exclusively* deals with interpretations, can be challenged. There are of course great problems of meaning in legal texts, but a lot of legal argument is argument about *facts* as anyone who has spent any time in court can tell you. There *is* a commonsense distinction between interpretation and fact that is maintained in law, but is challenged by the sceptical arguments of post-empiricist philosophy of science.

44. On Critical Legal Studies and the deconstructionist turn in legal theory cf. J. Stick, "Can Nihilism be Pragmatic?" <u>Harvard Law Review</u>, Vol. 100, 1986, pp. 332-401; S. Levison, "Law as Literature", <u>Texas Law Review</u>, Vol. 60, 1982, pp. 371-403; G. Graff, "Keep off the Grass", "Drop Dead", and Other Indeterminacies: A Reply to Stanford Levinson", <u>Texas Law Review</u>, Vol. 60, 1982, pp. 405-413; J.B. White, "Law as Language: Reading Law and Reading Literature", <u>Texas Law Review</u>, Vol. 60, 1982, pp. 415-445; W.E. Nelson, "Standards of Criticism", <u>Texas Law Review</u>, Vol. 60, 1982, pp. 447-493; S. Fish, "Interpretation and the Pluralist Vision", <u>Texas Law Review</u>, Vol. 60, 1982, pp. 495-505; M. Hancher, "Dead Letters: Wills and Poems", <u>Texas Law Review</u>, Vol. 60, 1982, pp. 507-525; R. Dworkin, "Law as Interpretation", <u>Texas Law Review</u>, Vol. 60, 1982, pp. 527-550; S. Fish, "Working on the Chain Gang: Interpretation in Law and Literature", <u>Texas Law Review</u>, Vol. 60, 1982, pp. 551-567; G.E. White, "The Text, Interpretation, and Critical Standards", <u>Texas Law Review</u>, Vol. 60, 1982, pp. 569-586; E. Sparer, "Fundamental Human Rights, Legal Entitlements, and the Social Struggle: A Friendly Critique of the Critical Legal Studies Movement", <u>Stanford Law Review</u>, Vol. 36, 1984, pp. 509-574; D.M. Trubek, "Where the Action Is: Critical Legal Studies and Empiricism", <u>Stanford Law Review</u>, Vol. 36, 1984, pp. 575-622; M. Tushnet, "Critical Legal Studies and Constitutional Law: An Essay in Deconstruction", <u>Stanford Law Review</u>, Vol.36, 1984, pp. 623-647; G.E. White, "The Inevitability of Critical Legal Studies", <u>Stanford Law Review</u>, Vol. 36, 1984, pp. 649-672; M.G. Kelman, "Trashing", <u>Stanford Law Review</u>, Vol. 36, 1984, pp. 293-348; L.A. Kornhauser, "The Great Image of Authority", <u>Stanford Law Review</u>, Vol. 36, 1984, pp. 349-389; L.B. Schwartz, "With Gun and Camera Through Darkest CLS - Land", <u>Stanford Law Review</u>, Vol. 36, 1984, pp. 413-464; O.M. Fiss, "Objectivity and Interpretation", <u>Stanford Law Review</u>, Vol. 34, 1982, pp. 739-763; P. Brest, "Interpretation and Interest", <u>Stanford Law Review</u>, Vol. 34, 1982, pp. 765-773; S. Stark, "Why Lawyers Can't Write", <u>Harvard Law Review</u>, Vol. 97, 1984, pp. 1389-1393; S.L. Carter, "Constitutional Adjudication and the Indeterminate Text: A Preliminary Defense of an Imperfect Muddle", <u>Yale Law Journal</u>, Vol. 94, 1985, pp. 821-872; C. Dalton, "An Essay in the Deconstruction of Contract Doctrine", <u>Yale Law Journal</u>, Vol. 94, 1985, pp. 997-1114; C.M. Yablon, "Law and Metaphysics", <u>Yale Law Journal</u>, Vol. 96, 1987, pp. 613-636; S. Fish, "Dennis Martinez and the Uses of Theory", <u>Yale Law Journal</u>, Vol. 96, 1987, pp. 1773-1800; J. Slick, "Can Nihilism be Pragmatic?", <u>Harvard Law Review</u>, Vol. 100, 1986, pp. 332-401; J.W. Singer, "The Player and the Cards: Nihilism and Legal Theory", <u>Yale Law Journal</u>, Vol. 94, 1984, pp. 1-70; L.B. Solum, "On the Indeterminacy Crisis: Critiquing Critical Dogma",

University of Chicago law Review, Vol. 54, 1987, pp. 462-503; D. Kairys, "Law and Politics", George Washington Law Review, Vol. 52, 1984, pp. 243-262; K. Hegland, "Goodbye to Deconstruction", Southern California Law Review, Vol. 58, 1985, pp. 1203-1221; J.M. Balkin, "Deconstructive Practice and Legal Theory", Yale Law Journal, Vol. 96, 1987, pp. 743-786.

45. cf. D. Solomon, "The High Court's Revolution", The Weekend Australian, January 7-8, 1989, p. 23. This article deals with a reinterpretation of Section 92 of the Australian Constitution that provides that "trade, commerce and intercourse among the States ... shall be absolutely free". In the past this statement was interpreted to mean that if a proposed law imposed a restriction or liability with respect to trade, commerce or intercourse, the law was invalid unless there was some other overriding importance to the law, such as health. The High Court received in 1987 a joint submission from the Commonwealth and the States, asking that the past history of interpretations of Section 92 be put aside, and a new more relevant interpretation be given. The interpretation of Section 92 that came from the High Court was that Section 92 prohibited legislation that was framed in a protectionist spirit, imposing discriminatory burdens. This in effect meant that the traditional goal of the Labour movement, abandoned by the Hawke Government (cf. G. Maddox, The Hawke Government and the Labour Tradition, Penguin, Victoria, 1989) of the "socialisation of industry, production, distribution and exchange to the extent necessary to eliminate exploitation and other antisocial features in those fields", (p.23) could be attained. This example illustrates the point that legal documents, such as the Constitution, can be reinterpreted to give Governments powers that were not envisaged when the original document was written. The key legal epistemological question is: is this reinterpretation justified by reason, or is it mere legal opinion produced by changing times?

46. That Feyerabend is a satisfactory representative of relativism and deconstructionism cf. C.C.F. Bearn, "Nietzsche, Feyerabend and the Voices of Relativism", Metaphilosophy, Vol. 17, 1986, pp. 135-152.

47. It is not my intention to claim that all of Foucault's work is useless (treated as a contribution to the sociology of prisons, madness, sexuality and so on). It is the deconstructionist reading of Foucault which is problematic.

48. P.K. Feyerabend, Farewell to Reason, (Verso, London 1987); cf. also Science in a Free Society, (New Left

Books, London 1978); Against Method, (New Left Books, London 1975).

49. Feyerabend, Farewell to Reason, ibid pp. 2-3.

50. ibid p. 13 emphasis added.

51. B. Russell, "An Outline of Intellectual Rubbish", in R.E. Egner and L.E. Denonn (eds.) The Basic Writings of Bertrand Russell (George Allen and Unwin, London, 1961), pp. 73-99. Citation p. 73.

52. C.K. Wilber (ed.) The Political Economy of Development and Underdevelopment, (Random House, New York, 1973).

53. P.A. Komesaroff, Objectivity, Science and Society: Interpreting Nature and Society in the Age of the Crisis of Science, (Routledge and Kegan Paul, London, 1986), pp. 3-4.

54. Feyerabend op.cit., note 49, p. 59.

55. P.K. Feyerabend, "Dialogue on Method", in G. Radnitzky and G. Anderson (eds), The Structure and Development of Science, (D. Reidel, Dordrecht, 1979), pp. 63-131. Citation, p.64.

56. This argument against rationalism and objectivism is substantially better than an earlier argument used by Feyerabend, that these positions are wrong because many leading nineteenth century scientists denied the existence of a general scientific method, believing that scientists should use standards appropriate to the subject matter under review, rather than mechanically using some general scientific method. This does not lead to an end of the philosophy of science. It merely means that the appropriate standards in say the philosophy of physics, will differ from those in say sociology. It will mean an end to positivist and materialist dreams of the "unity of science".

57. Quoted from Feyerabend op.cit., note 49, p. 146.

58. cf. R. Routley, Exploring Meinong's Jungle and Beyond, (Australian National University, Canberra, 1980), pp. 813-831; M. Hesse, Revolutions and Reconstructions in the Philosophy of Science, (Harvester Press, Sussex, 1980), pp. 94-99; R.W. Miller, Fact and Method, (Princeton University Press, Princeton, 1987).

59. cf. P. Sturrock, "Brave New Heresies", New Scientist, Vol. 120, No. 1644/1645, 1988, pp. 49-51.

60. cf. J.W. Smith, "Meiland and the Self-Refutation of Protagorean Relativism", Grazer Philosophische Studien,

Vol. 23, 1985, pp. 119-128 and H. Siegel, *Relativism Refuted: A Critique of Contemporary Epistemological Relativism*, (D. Reidel, Dordrech, 1987). The self refutation argument is that if epistemological or cognitive relativism (CR) is true, then CR is itself relative to alternative standards of evaluation and there is no neutral standard of evaluation. Thus if according to some standard, anti-relativism, where CR is judged to be false, then if CR is true according to that set of standards, then CR is false. Hence CR is self-refuting. The standard relativist reply is that the argument is question-begging because it presupposes that truth is absolute or framework independent rather than framework relative. cf. J.W. Meiland, "Is Protagorean Relativism Self-Refuting?", *Grazer Philosophische Studien*, Vol. 9, 1979, pp. 51-68. I argued in reply to Meiland, that the self-refutation argument against relativism does not presuppose an absolute conception of truth. According to relativism, anti-relativism is relatively true by its own standard and framework. But if this is so, then according to anti-relativism, relativism is not even true-relatively, because from the anti-relativist's perspective, relativism is false-absolutely. Hence relativism if relatively-true, is absolutely-false. The doctrine is therefore paradoxical.

61. On the cognitive relativism debate cf. L. Foster, "Strong Relativism Revisted", *Philosophy and Phenomenological Research*, Vol. XLIX, 1988, pp. 145-155; C. Swoyer, "True For", in M. Krausz and J. Meiland (eds.), *Relativism: Cognitive and Moral*, (University of Notre Dame Press, Notre Dame, 1982), pp. 84-108; C.B. McCullagh, "The Intelligibility of Cognitive Relativism", *Monist*, Vol. 67, 1984, pp. 327-340; E. Beach, "The Paradox of Cognitive Relativism Revisted: A Reply to Jack W. Meiland, *Metaphilosophy*, Vol. 15, 1984, pp. 1-15; J.W. Smith, "Meiland and the Self-Refutation of Protagorean Relativism", *Grazer Philosophische Studien*, Vol. 23, 1985, pp. 119-128; R.B. Brandt, "Relativism Refuted?" *Monist*, Vol. 67, pp. 297-307; G. Doppelt, "Kuhn's Epistemological Relativism: An Interpretation and Defense", *Inquiry*, Vol. 21, 1978, pp. 33-86, and "A Reply to Siegel on Kuhnian Relativism", *Inquiry*, Vol. 23, 1980, pp. 117-123; H. Field, "Realism and Relativism", *Journal of Philosophy*, Vol. LXXIX, 1982, pp. 553-567; J.N. Jordan, "Protagoras and Relativism: Criticisms Bad and Good", *Southwestern Journal of Philosophy*, Vol. 2, 1971, pp. 7-29; J.W. Meiland, "Cognitive Relativism: Popper and the Argument from Language", *Philosophical Forum*, Vol. 4, 1973, pp. 406-421' "Concepts of Relative Truth", *Monist*, Vol. 60, 1977, pp. 568-582, "Is Protagorean Relativism Self-Refuting", *Grazer Philosophische Studien*, Vol. 9, 1979, pp. 51-68; and "On the Paradox of Cognitive Relativism",

Metaphilosophy, Vol. 11, 1980, pp. 115-126; W.V. Quine, "Relativism and Absolutism", *Monist*, Vol. 67, 1984, pp. 293-296; M. Hollis and S. Lukes (eds.) *Rationality and Relativism*, (Basil Blackwell, Oxford, 1982).

62. C. Welch, "Beware of Cultures", *The Spectator*, 3 December 1988, pp. 36-37. Citation p. 37; S. Steele, "The Recoloring of Campus Life: Student Racism, Academic Pluralism and the End of a Dream", *Harper's*, Vol. 278, February 1989, pp. 47-55.

63. D. Bell, *The Cultural Contradictions of Capitalism*, (Heinemann, London, 1976).

64. ibid p. 14.

65. H. Putnam, *The Many Faces of Realism*, (Open Court, La Salle, 1987), *Realism and Reason, Philosophical Papers*, Vol. 3, (Cambridge University Press, Cambridge 1983), *Reason, Truth and History*, (Cambridge University Press, Cambridge 1981); P.A. Frech (et al, eds.) *Midwest Studies in Philosophy Volume XII, Realism and Antirealism*, (University of Minnesota Press, Minneapolis, 1988); J.F. Rosenberg, "Comparing the Incommensurable: Another Look at Convergent Realism", *Philosophical Studies*, Vol. 54, 1988, pp. 163-193; G. Iseminger, "Putnam's Miraculous Argument", *Analysis*, Vol. 48, 1988, pp. 190-195; B. Ellis, "Internal Realism", *Synthese*, Vol. 76, 1988, pp. 409-434; R. Bertolet, "Putnam on the *A priori*", *Philosophia*, Vol. 18, 1988, pp. 253-263; A.C. Genova, "Fantastic Realisms and Global Scepticism", *Philosophical Quarterly*, Vol. 38, 1988, pp. 205-213; J. Heil "The Epistemic Route to Anti-Realism", *Australasian Journal of Philosophy*, Vol. 66, 1988, pp. 161-173, and "Are We Brains in a Vat? Top Philosopher Says 'No'", *Canadian Journal of Philosophy*, Vol. 17, 1987, pp. 427-436; N. Rescher, *Scientific Realism: A Critical Reappraisal*, (D. Reidel, Dordrecht, 1987); C. Hansen, "Putnam's Indeterminacy Argument: The Skolemization of Absolutely Everything", *Philosophical Studies*, Vol. 51, 1987, pp. 77-99; P. Tichy, "Putnam on Brains in a Vat", *Philosophia*, Vol. 16, 1986, pp. 137-146; F.B. Farrell, "Putnam and the Vat-People", *Philosophia*, Vol. 16, 1986, pp. 147-160; M. Kinghan, "The External World Sceptic Escapes Again", *Philosophia*, Vol. 16, 1986, pp. 161-174; W. Demopoulos, "The Rejection of Truth - Conditional Semantics by Putnam and Dummett", *Philosopical Topics*, Vol. 13, 1985, pp. 135-153; J. Stephens and L-M. Russow, "Brains in Vats and the Internalist Perspective", *Australasian Journal of Philosophy*, Vol. 63, 1985, pp. 205-212; N. Melchert, "Why Constructive Empiricism Collapses into Scientific Realism", *Australasian Journal of Philosophy*, Vol. 63, 1985, pp. 213-215; M. Devitt, *Realism and Truth*, (Basil Blackwell, Oxford 1984); J. McIntyre, "Putnam's Brains",

Anaysis, Vol. 44, 1984, pp. 59-61; D. Lewis, "Putnam's Paradox", *Australasian Journal of Philosophy*, Vol. 62, 1984, pp. 221-236; C.Z. Elgin, "Lawlikeness and the End of Science", *Philosophy of Science*, Vol. 47, 1980, pp. 56-68; G.H. Merrill, "The Model-Theoretic Argument Against Realism", *Philosophy of Science*, Vol. 47, 1980, pp. 69-81; R. Nole, "'Paradigms Lost, or the World Regained' - An Excursion into Realism and Idealism in Science", *Synthese*, Vol. 45, 1980, pp. 317-350.

66. A Tarski, *Logic, Semantics, Metamathematics*, (Oxford University Press, Oxford, 1956).

67. On coherence cf. F.H. Bradley, *Essays on Truth and Reality*, (Clarendon Press, Oxford, 1914); B. Blanshard, "Reply to Nicholas Rescher: "Blanshard and the Coherence Theory of Truth"," in P.A. Schilpp (ed.) *The Philosophy of Brand Blanshard*, (Open Court, La Salle, 1980), pp. 588-600; L. BonJour, *The Structure of Empirical Knowledge*, (Harvard University Press, Cambridge, Massachusetts, 1985); S. Blackburn, *Spreading the Word*, (Clarendon Press, Oxford, 1986); P.K. Moser, "Internalism and Coherentism: A Dilemma", *Analysis*, Vol. 48, 1988, pp. 161-163; for a defense of a coherence *definition* of truth, that is, coherence as optimal coherence with a perfected data base cf. N. Rescher, "Truth as Ideal Coherence", in *Forbidden Knowledge*, (D. Reidel, Dordrech, 1987), pp. 17-27.

68. It is not the case, as Putnam argues in *The Many Faces of Realism* (op.cit note 65, p. 19) that the metaphysical realist's idea of a single world runs into difficulties because we humans do not have any *neutral* description of the contents of the world. The metaphysical realist need not deny that the notions of *object* and *existence* have a multitude of different uses. What the metaphysical realist does claim is that once a meaning for these notions is fixed, then the *truth* of statements containing these notions is best understood according to the metaphysical realist theory of truth. No one is claiming that there is a use of 'exists' inherent in the world itself.

69. cf. R. Sylvan, "Establishing the Correspondence Theory of Truth and Rendering it Coherent", in J.T.L. Srzednick (ed.) *Stephan Korner - Philosophical Analysis and Reconstruction* (Martinus Nijhoff, Dordrecht, 1987), pp. 75-82, and "On Making a Coherence Theory of Truth True", (Typescript).

70. B. Russell, *The Problems of Philosophy*, (Oxford University Press, London, 1971), p.71. More recently C.A. Hooker, *A Realistic Theory of Science*, (State University of New York Press, Albany, 1987), p.277, objects to the coherence theory of truth on the grounds

that the statement (H) and its negation asserting the adequacy of the methods used to investigate truth in the coherence definition itself, cannot be true. Now to escape this, coherence theorists must accept that there are intuitive basic truths. They should also ask the correspondence theorists what fact does this sentence correspond to: (J) the correspondence theory of truth is itself true.

71. Russell, ibid p.71.

72. W.V. Quine, "On Empirically Equivalent Systems of the World", <u>Erkenntnis</u>, Vol. 9, 1975, pp. 313-328.

73. A.J. Swann, "Popper on Induction", <u>British Journal for the Philosophy of Science</u>, Vol. 39, 1988, pp. 367-373; B. Ellis, "Solving the Problem of Induction Using a Values-Based Epistemology", <u>British Journal for the Philosophy of Science</u>, Vol. 39, 1988, pp. 141-160; N. Stemmer, "Hume's Two Assumptions", <u>Dialectica</u>, Vol. 42, 1988, pp. 93-103; M. P. Levine, "Madden's Account of Necessity in Causation", <u>Philosophia</u>, Vol. 18, 1988, pp. 75-96; J. Blachowicz, "Discovery as Correction", <u>Synthese</u>, Vol. 71, 1987, pp. 235-321; P. Weiss, "Induction: Its Nature, Justification, and Presuppositions", <u>Journal of Speculative Philosophy</u>, Vol. 1, 1987, pp. 16-19; G.T. Ferrari, "The Resolution of Hume's Problem and New Russellian Antinomies of Induction, Determinism and Relativism", <u>Philosophy Research Archives</u>, Vol. 12, 1986-87, pp. 471-517; D.C. Stove, <u>The Rationality of Induction</u>, (Clarendon Press, Oxford, 1986); J.W. Roxbee Cox, "Induction and Disjunction", <u>Philosophical Papers</u>, Vol. XV, 1986, pp. 89-95; K. Halbasch, <u>Philosophy: A Tough-Minded Contemporary Approach</u>, (Prometheus Press, Buffalo, 1987); F.J. Clendinnen, "Induction, Indifference and Guessing", <u>Australasian Journal of Philosophy</u>, Vol. 64, 1986, pp. 340-344; P.J.R. Millican, "Natural Necessity and Induction", <u>Philosophy</u>, Vol. 61, 1986, pp. 395-403; R.P. Amico, "On the Vindication of Deduction and Induction", <u>Australasian Journal of Philosophy</u>, Vol. 64, 1986, pp. 322-330; B. Rundle, "Induction and Justification", <u>American Philosophical Quarterly</u>, Vol. 23, 1986, pp. 115-123; T.A. Young, <u>Completing Berkeley's Project: Classical vs. Modern Philosophy</u>, (University of America Press, Lanham, 1985); R.N. Boyd, "The Logician's Dilemma: Deductive Logic, Inductive Inference and Logical Empiricism", <u>Erkenntnis</u>, Vol. 22, 1985, pp. 197-252; J. Earman, "Concepts of Projectibility and the Problem of Induction", <u>Nous</u>, Vol. 19, 1985, pp. 521-535; J.R. Brown, "Explaining the Success of Science", <u>Ratio</u>, Vol. XXVII, 1985, pp. 49-66; K.F. Machina, "Induction and Deduction Revisited", <u>Nous</u>, Vol. 19, 1985, pp. 571-578; R.H. Schlagel, "A Reasonable Reply to Hume's Scepticism", <u>British Journal for the Philosophy of</u>

Science, Vol. 35, 1984, pp. 359-374; A. Naess, *A Sceptical Dialogue on Induction*, (Humanities Press, Atlantic Highlands, 1984); J.L. Pollock, "A Solution to the Problem of Induction", *Nous*, Vol. 18, 1984, pp. 423-462; G.N. Schlesinger, *Metaphysics: Methods and Problems*, (Basil Blackwell, Oxford, 1983); K. Gemes, "A Refutation of Inductive Scepticism", *Australasian Journal of Philosophy*, Vol. 61, 1983, pp. 434-438; N. Rescher, *Induction*, (Basil Blackwell, Oxford, 1980).

74. Russell op.cit., note 70, pp. 35-36.

75. K.R. Popper, *Objective Knowledge*, (Clarendon Press, Oxford, 1979), p.1.

76. K.R. Popper, *The Open Society and Its Enemies*, (Routledge and Kegan Paul, London, 1966), p. 230 and A.J. Swann, "Popper on Induction", op.cit., note 73, both claim that narrow rationalism cannot itself be deduced from the set X of fundamental truths. However both Popper and Swann create a strawman by failing to make the set X comprehensive. I shall deal with the problem of the super-ultimate justification of rationalism in the text.

77. G. Radnitzky, "From Justifying a Theory to Comparing Theories and Selecting Questions: Popper's Alternative to Foundationalism and Scepticism", *Revue Internationale De Philosophie*, Vol. 34, 1980, pp. 179-228. Radnitzky's following remarks show how difficult it is for Popperians to fully abandon justificationism: "we cannot say more about the truth-value of a *particular* sentence than that "good reasons" are avaialble for the conjecture that the sentence is true or false..." (p.202). If justificationism was really rejected, then so too would talk of "good reasons".

78. D. Miller, "Falsification versus Inductionism", in L.J. Cohen and M. Hesse (eds.) *Applications of Inductive Logic*, (Clarendon Press, Oxford, 1980), pp. 109-129.

79. S. Priest, "A Short Justification of Induction", *Explorations in Knowledge*, Vol. 2, 1985, pp. 39-43, citation p. 41; B.S. Gower, "A Short Justification of Counter-Induction", *Explorations in Knowledge*, Vol. 4, 1987, pp. 41-42.

80. For further criticisms of falsification cf. M. Bunge, "The GST Challenge to the Classical Philosophies of Science", *International Journal of General Systems*, Vol. 4, 1977, pp. 29-37.

81. A. Ofsti, "Some Problems of Counter-Inductive Policy as Opposed to Inductive", *Inquiry*, Vol. 5, 1962, pp. 267-283.

82. W.H. Davis, "The Meaning of Life", <u>Metaphilosophy</u>, Vol. 18, 1987, pp. 288-305.

83. cf. C. Hartshorne and P. Weiss (eds.) <u>Collected Papers of Charles Sanders Peirce</u>, (The Belknap Press of Harvard University Press, Cambridge, 1960).

84. Davis, op.cit., note 82, p. 298.

85. ibid pp. 299-300.

86. G.N. Schlesinger, "Is It True What Cicero Said About Philosophers?", <u>Metaphilosophy</u>, Vol. 19, 1988, pp. 288-293; K. Campbell, "Philosophy and Commonsense", <u>Philosophy</u>, Vol. 63, 1988, pp. 161-174.

87. A.B. Palma, "Intellectual Robotry", <u>Philosophy</u>, Vol. 61, 1986, pp. 491-501. Citation pp. 500-501.

88. N. Maxwell, <u>From Knowledge to Wisdom: A Revolution in the Aims and Methods of Science</u>, (Basil Blackwell, Oxford, 1987).

89. P. Davies, <u>Superforce: The Search for a Grand Unified Theory of Nature,</u> (Unwin Paperbacks, London, 1987); J.M. Dawson, "Plasma Particle Accelerators", <u>Scientific American</u>, Vol. 260, March 1989, pp. 34-41.

90. ibid p. 98.

91. ibid p. 98.

92. ibid p. 100.

93. Maxwell op.cit., note 88, p. 56.

94. ibid p. 66.

95. T. Dendy (ed.) <u>Greenhouse '88: Planning for Climatic Change</u>, (Department of Environment and Planning, Adelaide, 1989); L.R. Brown (et al), <u>State of the World 1988</u>, (W.W. Norton, New York, 1988); M. Tobias (ed.), <u>Deep Ecology</u>, (Avant Books, California, 1988); I.M. Mintzer, <u>A Matter of Degree</u>, (World Resources Institute, Washington D.C., 1987); World Commission on Environment and Development, <u>Our Common Future</u>, (Oxford University Press, New York, 1987); M. Bookchin, <u>The Modern Crisis</u>, (Black Rose Books, Montreal, 1987); J. Bellini, <u>High Tech Holocaust</u>, (Greenhouse Publications, Victoria, 1986); International Task Force, <u>Tropic Forests: A Call for Action, Part I: The Plan</u> (World Resources Institute, Washington D.C., 1985); J. McCormick and J. Tinker (eds.) <u>Acid Earth: The Global Threat of Acid Pollution</u>, (Earthscan, London, 1985); M. Redclift, <u>Development and the Environmental Crisis</u>, (Methuen, London, 1984); R.

Bahro, <u>Socialism and Survival</u>, (Heretic Books, London, 1982); W.R. Catton, <u>Overshoot: The Ecological Basis of Revolutionary Change</u>, (University of Illinois Press, Urbana, 1982); J. Rifkin and T. Howard, <u>Entropy: A New World View</u>, (Viking Press, New York, 1980); E.F. Renshaw, <u>The End of Growth: Adjusting to a No-Growth Economy</u>, (Duxbury Press, Massachusetts, 1976).

96. B. Williams, <u>Ethics and the Limits of Philosophy</u>, (Fontana, London, 1985). The title of this chapter is taken from Williams' book; Williams' thesis though is not explicitly about the limits of philosophy which we have discussed, but the limits of morality, particularly the limits of applicability of the concept of moral obligation.

97. A. MacIntyre, <u>After Virtue: A Study in Moral Theory</u>, 2nd edition, (Duckworth, London, 1985).

98. Williams, op.cit., note 96, p. 195.

99. ibid p. 195.

100. MacIntyre, op.cit., note 97, p. 239.

101. cf. R.J. Bernstein, "Nietzsche or Aristotle? Reflections on Alasdair MacIntyre's <u>After Virtue</u>", in <u>Philosophical Profiles: Essays in a Pragmatic Mode</u>, (University of Pennsylvania Press, Philadelphia, 1986).

102. B. Blanshard, <u>Reason and Goodness</u>, (George Allen and Unwin, London, 1961) and R. Allen, "The Idea of a Value-Free Social Science", <u>Journal of Value Inquiry</u>, Vol. 9, 1975, pp. 95-117.

103. C.L. Stevenson, <u>Ethics and Language</u>, (Yale University Press, New Haven, 1944), p. 114.

104. Blanshard, op.cit., note 102.

105. R.B. Perry, <u>General Theory of Value</u>, (Harvard University Press, Cambridge, Massachusetts, 1926).

106. W.H. Davis, "Transcendental Needs", <u>Philosophy Today</u>, Vol. 20, 1976, pp. 184-193.

107. R.J. McShea, "Human Nature Ethical Theory", <u>Philosophy and Phenomenological Research</u>, Vol. 39, 1979, pp. 386-401.

108. D. Walhout, "Human Nature and Value Theory", <u>The Thomist</u>, Vol. 44, 1980, pp. 278-297.

109. J. Kekes, "Human Nature and Moral Theories", <u>Inquiry</u>, Vol. 28, 1985, pp. 231-245.

110. R. Allen, op.cit., note 102 and "Materialism, Marxism and Moral Philosophy", (Typescript, Philosophy Department, Flinders University).

111. cf. G. Harman, "Human Flourishing, Ethics and Liberty", Philosophy and Public Affairs, Vol. 12, 1983, pp. 307-322.

112. The literature on deep ecology and environmental ethics is vast. A selective and somewhat unorganised reading guide now follows: H. Rolston III, Philosophy Gone Wild: Essays in Environmental Ethics, (Promethus Books, New York, 1986); R. Attfield, The Ethics of Environmental Concern, (Columbia University Press, New York, 1983) and A Theory of Value and Obligation, (Croom Helm, London, 1987); J.B. Callicott, "Non-Anthropocentric Value Theory and Environmental Ethics", American Philosophical Quarterly, Vol. 21, 1984, pp. 299-309; R. Disch (ed.) The Ecological Conscience, (Prentice-Hall, Englewood Cliffs, 1970); A. Leopold, A Sand County Almanac, (Oxford University Press, New York, 1968); E. Partridge (ed.) Responsibilities to Future Generation, (Prometheus Books, New York, 1981); A. Weston, "Beyond Intrinsic Value: Pragmatism in Environmental Ethics", Environmental Ethics, Vol.7, 1985, pp. 321-339; V.R. Potter, "Evolving Ethical Concepts", Bioscience, Vol. 27, 1977, pp. 251-253; P.G. Muscari, "Is Man the Paragon of Animals?" Journal of Value Inquiry, Vol. 20, 1986, pp. 303-308; D. Pepper, "Determinism, Idealism and the Politics of Environmentalism - A Viewpoint", International Journal of Environmental Studies, Vol. 26, 1985, pp. 11-19; P.E. O'Sullivan, "Environmental Science and Environmental Philosophy - Part I Environmental Science and Environmentalism", International Journal of Environmental Studies, Vol. 28, 1986, pp. 97-107 and Part 2 "Environmental Science and the Coming Social Paradigm", International Journal of Environmental Studies, Vol. 28, 1987, pp. 257-267; C.J. Hughes, "Gaia: A Natural Scientist's Ethic for the Future", Ecologist, Vol. 15, 1985, pp. 92-95; A. Jones, "From Fragmentation to Wholeness: A Green View of Science and Society (Part II)", Ecologist, Vol. 18, 1988, pp. 30-34; J. Biehl, "Ecofeminisism and Deep Ecology: Unresolvable Conflict?", Our Generation, Vol. 19, 1988, pp. 19-31; R. Attfield, "Biocentrism, Moral Standing and Moral Significance", Philosphica, Vol. 39, 1987, pp. 47-58; D. Scherer, "Anthropocentrism, Atomism and Environmental Ethics" in D. Scherer and T. Attig (eds.) Ethics and the Environment, (Prentice-Hall, New Jersey, 1983), pp. 73-81; P.D. Murphy, "Sex-Typing the Planet: Gaia Imagery and the Problem of Subverting Patriarchy", Environmental Ethics, Vol. 10, 1988, pp. 155-168; C.D. Stone, "Moral Pluralism and the Course of Environmental Ethics", Environmental Ethics, Vol. 10, 1988, pp. 139-154; M.E.

Zimmerman, "Quantum Theory, Intrinsic Value, and Pantheism", *Environmental Ethics*, Vol. 10, 1988, pp. 3-30; D. Lamb, "Animal Rights and Liberation Movements", *Environmental Ethics*, Vol. 4, 1982, pp. 215-233; A. McLaughlin, "Images and Ethics of Naure", *Environmental Ethics*, Vol. 7, 1985, pp. 293-319; H.W. Wood, "Modern Pantheism as an Approach to Environmental Ethics", *Environmental Ethics*, Vol. 7, 1985, pp. 151-163; R. and V. Routley, "Human Chauvinism and Environmental Ethics", in D.S. Mannison, M.A. McRobbie and R. Routley (eds.) *Environmental Philosophy*, (Australian National University, Canberra, 1980), pp. 96-189.

113. J.L. Arbor, "Animal Chauvinism, Plant-Regarding Ethics and the Torture of Trees", *Australasian Journal of Philosophy*, Vol. 64, 1986, pp. 335-339.

114. On organic unity cf. R. Nozick, *Philosophical Explanations*, (Clarendon Press, Oxford, 1981), Chapter 5.

115. cf. J.W. Smith, "A Reply to Frankel's Criticism of Harre's Theory of Causality", *Philosophy of Science*, Vol. 49, 1982, pp. 282-289.

116. A. Gewirth, *Human Rights*, (University of Chicago Press, Chicago, 1982), p. 111.

117. A. Gewirth, "The Ontological Basis of Natural Law: A Critique and Alternative", *American Journal of Jurisprudence*, Vol. 29, 1984, pp. 95-121.

118. W.H. Davis, "Man-Eating Aliens", *Journal of Value Inquiry*, Vol. 10, 1976, pp. 178-185.

119. On the ethics of predation cf. H. Rolston III, *Environmental Ethics*, (Temple University Press, Philadelphia, 1988) and S.F. Sapontzis, "Predation", *Ethics and Animals*, Vol. 5, 1984, pp. 27-38.

120. On the moral status of the embryo with respect to the IVF technology debate cf. S. Holm, "New Danish Law: Human Life Begins at Conception", *Journal of Medical Ethics*, Vol. 14, 1988, pp. 77-78; R. Gillon, "Pregnancy, Obstetrics and the Moral Status of the Fetus", *Journal of Medical Ethics*, Vol. 14, 1988, pp. 3-4; R.M. Hare, "Possible People", *Bioethics*, Vol. 2, 1988, pp. 279-293; H. Kuhse, "A Report from Australia: When a Human Life has Not Yet Begun: According to the Law", *Bioethics*, Vol. 2, 1988, pp. 334-342; M. Lockwood, "Hare on Potentiality: A Rejoinder", *Bioethics*, Vol. 2, 1988, pp. 343-352; M. Lockwood, "Warnock versus Powell (and Harradine): When does Potentiality Count?" *Bioethics*, Vol. 2, 1988, pp. 187-213; R.M. Hare, "When Does Potentiality Count? A Comment on Lockwood", *Bioethics*,

Vol. 2, 1988, pp. 214-226; S. Buckle, "Arguing from Potential", *Bioethics*, Vol. 2, 1988, pp. 227-253; P. Singer and K. Dawson, "IVF Technology and the Argument from Potential", *Philosophy and Public Affairs*, Vol. 17, 1988, pp. 87-104; J. Bigelow and R. Pargetter, "Morality, Potential Persons and Abortion", *American Philosophical Quarterly*, Vol. 25, 1988, pp. 173-181; J. Stone, "Why Potentiality Matters", *Canadian Journal of Philosophy*, Vol. 17, 1987, pp. 815-830.

The thesis that the embryo is a *potential* person, and of some (debatable) moral standing, can I believe be defended against recent criticisms. Whilst it would take a separate essay to do this, here I shall briefly run through the arguments. P. Singer and D. Wells, *The Reproduction Revolution: New Ways of Making Babies*, (Oxford University Press, Oxford, 1984), p. 91 maintain that everything that can be said about the potential of the embryo can be said about the potential of the separate egg and sperm, and since it is not wrong to destroy the gametes, it is not wrong to destroy the embryo. This argument can be criticised along the following line: just as water molecules have *emergent* properties that hydrogen and oxygen do not separately have (or choose any other example of holistic properties, even from quantum mechanics), the embryo has emerged genetic properties uncombined gametes do not have. It is Singer's biological reductionism which is problematic cf. J.W. Smith, B.C. Goodwin and G. Webster, "Neo-Darwinism and Constructional Biology", *Explorations in Knowledge*, Vol. 4, No. 1, 1987, pp. 29-40.

Eric Russert Kraemer "Abortion and Cloning", *Southern Journal of Philosophy*, Vol. 21, 1983, pp. 537-545 has called that certain class of body cells that could be used for human cloning C cells. The existence of C cells would pose a major problem for those who believe that it is wrong to kill an entity which marked the beginning of a human body. It seems to follow that if it is wrong to kill the zygote, then it is wrong to kill a C cell "[f]or C cells are such that they, given the proper chemical environment and a certain amount of luck, could also turn into full-fledged humans. In this they are surely closely analogous to zygotes which also require a proper chemical environment and a certain amount of luck in order to become fully developed human beings" (p. 539). It is absurd to grant a right to life to C cells - for this would make even shaving a morally dangerous practice - hence the pro-abortionist claims, that the Zygote does not have a right to life.

The above argument is, despite its ingenuity, invalid. The anti-abortionist claims that it is morally wrong to kill that entity, which marks the beginning of the human body. Traditionally this entity has been called a zygote, formed by the fusion of the sperm and ovum.

Cloning shows that this is not the only possible way to begin human life. An unfertilized egg cell can have its nucleus removed by microsurgery or irradiation and have the nucleus of a body cell of the person replaced in the egg. The egg cell now develops in the normal manner. However, all that this shows is that the idea of a zygote is in need of revision. One could claim that both a cloned cell and the zygote have the same moral status, but a C cell and the cloned cell, and the sperm and ovum and the zygote respectively do not.

The reason one can claim this is as follows. If the foetus is a potential person, it doesn't follow that the sperm-ovum pair is a potential person, if it is a potential foetus. If this was so, then nothing prevents one from taking the DNA constituents of sperm and ova to the potential persons as well, as well as the molecular constituents of DNA and so on in infinite regression. This destroys the uselessness of the concept of potentiality, and since good reasons have been given by Harre, Madden and Bhaskar for accepting the concept of potentiality and emergent powers, we can reject this argument. An unfertilized egg and sperm do not have the capacity to develop into a foetus. They do have the capacity to carry genetic material, and in the case of the sperm, to move. The zygote however does have the capacity to develop into a person as a result of its continuous growth and development. It does this in a suitable maternal environment as the result of the actions of its genetic and morphological mechanisms, in the absence of intervening mechanisms such as diseases which may cause spontaneous abortions. The cloned cell, like the zygote has this same power, but an ordinary body cell does not.

This interpretation of the morality of cloning also enables us to refute an argument given by M. Tooley, Abortion and Infanticide, (Clarendon Press, Oxford, 1983). Tooley's criticism of giving moral standing to potential persons is based upon his use of the moral symmetry principle. Stated roughly, this principle asserts that there is no moral difference between on the one hand, interfering with a causally interrelated collection of states of affairs so that they give rise to a special state of affairs, and on the other hand, intentionally refraining from producing states of affairs so interrelated that they constitute a collection that could give rise to that special state of affairs. On this basis Tooley asks, if it is wrong to kill, why is it not equally wrong to abstain from procreative sex - the consequence is the same - there will not be a person who might otherwise have had a worthwhle life? However, the consequence of killing is the death of an <u>actually</u> existing organism, whilst the consequence of abstaining from sex is the prevention of the development of a <u>potential</u> person. Consider this counter example: it would be wrong to destroy a hybrid organism such as a chimp-human. However it is not wrong to prevent the hybrid from coming into existence in the first place, and given human racial intolerance and exploitation, it is clearly a good thing. Hybridization of higher organisms may be morally wrong, even though hybrids once they exist, may have a right to life. The moral symmetry principle is false. cf. R. Routley, <u>In Defense of Cannibalism I. Types of Admissible and Inadmissible Cannibalism</u>, (Discussion Papers in Environmental Philosophy, Australian National University, Canberra), p.31.

121. R.S. Pfeiffer, "Abortion Policy and the Argument from Uncertainty", <u>Social Theory and Practice</u>, Vol. 11, 1985, pp. 371-386; D.S. Levin, "Abortion, Personhood, and Vagueness", <u>Journal of Value Inquiry</u>, Vol. 19, 1985, pp. 197-209; J. Baker, "Philosophy and the Morality of Abortion", <u>Journal of Applied Philosophy</u>, Vol. 2, 1985, pp. 261-270; D.S. Levin, "Thomson and the Current State of the Abortion Controversy", <u>Journal of Applied Philosophy</u>, Vol. 2, 1985, pp. 121-125; C. Overall, "New Reproductive Technology: Some Implications for the Abortion Issue", <u>Journal of Value Inquiry</u>, Vol. 19, 1985, pp. 279-292; E.R. Winkler, "Abortion and Victimisability", <u>Journal of Applied Philosophy</u>, Vol. 1, 1984, pp. 305-318; N. Davis, "Abortion and Self-Defense", <u>Philosophy and Public Affairs</u>, Vol. 13, 1984, pp. 175-207; J.F. Smith, "Rights-Conflict, Pregnancy and Abortion", in C.C. Gould (ed.) <u>Beyond Domination: New Perspectives on Women and Philosophy</u>, (Rowman and Allanheld, Totowa, 1984), pp. 265-273; S.A. Ketchum, "The Moral Status of the Bodies of Persons", <u>Social Theory and Practice</u>, Vol. 10, 1984, pp. 25-38; B.W. Harrison, <u>Our Right to Choose: Towards a New Ethic of Abortion</u>, (Beacon Press, Boston, 1983); A.S. Moraczewski, "Human Personhood: A Study in Person-alised Biology", in W.B. Bondeson (et al., eds.) <u>Abortion and the Status of the Fetus</u>, (D. Reidel, Dordrecht, 1983), pp. 301-311; R. Puccetti, "The Life of a Person" ibid, pp. 169-182; L. Glantz, "Is the Fetus a Person? A Lawyer's View", ibid, pp. 107-117; H.T. Engelhardt, "Viability and the use of the Fetus", ibid, pp. 183-208; H.M. Smith, "Intercourse and Moral Responsibility for the Fetus", ibid, pp. 229-245; C. Whitbeck, "The Moral Implications of Regarding Women as People: New Perspectives on Pregnancy and Personhood", ibid, pp. 247-272; P.E. Devine, "Abortion, Contraception, Infanticide", <u>Philosophy</u>, Vol. 58, 1983, pp. 513-520; P.A. Roth, "Personhood, Property Rights and the Permissibility of Abortion", <u>Law and Philosophy</u>, Vol. 2,

1983, pp. 163-191; S.L. Ross, "Abortion and the Death of the Fetus, "Philosophy and Public Affairs, Vol. 11, 1982, pp. 232-245; S.F. Sapontzis, "A Critique of Personhood", Ethics, Vol. 91, 1981, pp. 607-618; G. Sher, "Subsidized Abortion: Moral Rights and Moral Compromise", Philosophy and Public Affairs, Vol. 10, 1981, pp. 361-372; M.R. Wicclair, "The Abortion Controversy and the Claim that This Body is Mine", Social Theory and Practice, Vol. 7, 1981, pp. 337-346; A. Zaitchik, "Viability and the Morality of Abortion", Philosophy and Public Affairs, Vol. 10, 1981, pp. 18-26; A.D. Farr, "The Marquis de Sade and Induced Abortion", Journal of Medical Ethics, Vol. 6, 1980, pp. 7-10; A.G.M. Campbell and R.S. Duff, "Deciding the Care of Severely Malformed or Dying Infants", Journal of Medical Ethics, Vol. 5, 1979, pp. 65-67; E.F. Paul, "Self-Ownership, Abortion and Infanticide", Journal of Medical Ethics, Vol. 5, 1979, pp. 133-138; R. Weiss, "The Perils of Personhood", Ethics, Vol. 89, 1978, pp. 66-75; P.E. Devine, "Fetuses and 'Human Vegetables'", in The Ethics of Homicide, (Cornell University Press, Ithaca, 1978), pp. 74-105; G. Sher, "Hare, Abortion and the Golden Rule", Philosophy and Public Affairs, Vol. 6, 1977, pp. 185-190; J.M. Humber, "Abortion, Fetal Research and the Law", Social Theory and Practice, Vol. 4, 1977, pp. 127-147; M.D. Bayles, "Harm to the Unconceived", Philosophy and Public Affairs, Vol. 5, 1976, pp. 292-304; D. Van De Veer, "Justifying 'Wholesale Slaughter'", Canadian Journal of Philosophy, Vol. 5, 1975, pp. 245-258; P. Ramsey, "The Morality of Abortion", in J. Rachels (ed.) Moral Problems, (Harper and Row, New York, 1975), pp. 37-58; R. M. Herbenick, "Remarks on Abortion, Abandonment, and Adoption Opportunities", Philosophy and Public Affairs, Vol. 5, 1975, pp. 98-104; R. Werner, "Abortion: The Moral Status of the Unborn", Social Theory and Practice, Vol. 3, 1975, pp. 201-222; R.J. Gerber, "Abortion: Parameters for Decision", Ethics, Vol. 82, 1972, pp. 137-154; R.B. Brandt, "The Morality of Abortion", Monist, Vol. 56, 1972, pp. 503-526; D. Gerber, "Abortion: The Uptake Argument", Ethics, Vol. 83, 1972-73, pp. 80-83; B.A. Brody, "Abortion and the Sanctity of Human Life", American Philosophical Quarterly, Vol. 10, 1973, pp. 133-140; J.B. Nelson, "The Humanity in Abortion", in Human Medicine, (Augsburg Publishing House, Minneapolis, 1973), pp. 31-58; J. Margolis, "Abortion", Ethics, Vol. 84, 1973-74, pp. 51-61; T. H. Engelhardt, "The Ontology of Abortion", Ethics, Vol. 84, 1973-74, pp. 217-234; J. Feinberg (ed.) The Problem of Abortion, (Wadsworth, Belmont, 1973); J. Finnis, "The Rights and Wrongs of Abortion: A Reply to Judith Thomson", Philosophy and Public Affairs, Vol. 2, 1973, pp. 117-145; J.J. Thomson, "Rights and Deaths", Philosophy and Public Affairs, Vol. 2, 1973, pp. 146-159; R. Wertheimer, "Understanding the Abortion Argument", Philosophy and Public Affairs, Vol.

1, 1971, pp. 67-95; G.G. Grisez, Abortion: The Myths, The Realities, and the Arguments, (Corpus Books, New York, 1970); D. Callahan, Abortion: Law, Choice and Morality, (Macmillan, London, 1970).

122. MacIntrye, op.cit., note 97.

123. ibid p. 6.

124. ibid p. 8.

125. J.H. Fetzer (ed.) Principles of Philosophical Thinking, (Rowman and Allanheld, New Jersey, 1984).

126. M Meyer (ed.) From Metaphysics to Rhetoric (Kluwer, Dordrecht, 1989).

127. On the limits of received ethic reasoning cf. V. Luizzi, "Problems with Solutions to Contemporary Moral Problems", Journal of Value Inquiry, Vol. 18, 1984, pp. 169-180; P. Abbott, "Philosophers and the Abortion Question", Political Theory, Vol. 6, 1978, pp. 313-335.

128. C. Wellman, "Ethical Disagreement and Objective Truth", American Philosophical Quarterly, Vol. 12, 1975, pp. 211-221. Citation p. 215.

129. S. Finkbine, "The Lesser of the Two Evils", in A.F. Guttmaker (ed.), The Case for Legalized Abortion Now, (Diablo Press, Berkeley, 1967), pp. 15-25.

130. Literature on the scientificity and morality of IVF and the reproduction technologies include S. Dodds and K. Jones, "Surrogacy and Autonomy", Bioethics, Vol. 3, 1989, pp. 1-17; L.M. Purdy, "Surrogate Mothering: Exploitation or Empowerment?", Bioethics, Vol. 3, 1989, pp. 18-34; G. Sheridan, "Arrogant Science Threatens to Realise a Brave New World", The Weekend Australian, February 4-5, 1989; A. Yates and J. Ferguson, "Brain-Dead Surrogacy Outcry", The News, (Adelaide), Friday June 24, 1988, p.1 (Dr. Paul Gerber felt that the use of the brain-dead for surrogacy was a "magnificent use of a corpse"!); "'Quality tested' IVF Babies Forecast", The Advertiser, (Adelaide) Saturday, April 16, 1988, p.3; R.A. Belliotti, "Marxism, Feminism and Surrogate Motherhood", Social Theory and Practice, Vol. 14, 1988, pp. 389-417; S. Downie, Babymaking: The Technology and Ethics, (Bodley Head, London, 1988); B. Brecher, "Surrogacy and Its Consequences: Some Misgivings", Explorations in Knowledge, Vol. 5, 1988, pp. 17-25; P. Chesler, "What is a Mother?", Ms, May 1988, pp. 36-39; M. Thom, "Dilemmas of the New Birth Technologies", Ms, May 1988, pp. 70-72, 74-76; P. Kasimba, "Regulating IVF Human Embryo Experimentation: The Search for a Legal Basis", Australian Law Journal, Vol. 62, 1988, pp. 128-

138; L. Grey, "Reproduction Technology: Cataloguing the Criticisms: A Legal View", <u>Ohio Medicine</u>, Vol. 84, 1988, pp. 203-205; P. Horn, "Reproduction Technology: Cataloguing the Criticisms: An Ethical View", <u>Ohio Medicine</u>, Vol. 84, 1988, pp. 197-199; R.J. Neuhaus, "Renting Women, Buying Babies and Class Struggles", <u>Transaction Social Science and Modern Society</u>, Vol. 25, 1988, pp. 8-10; B.S. Heyl, "Commercial Contracts and Human Connectedness", ibid, pp. 11-16; M.B. Morris, "Reproductive Technology and Restraints", ibid, pp. 16-21; B.K. Rothman, "Cheap Labor: Sex, Class, Race - and Surrogacy", ibid, pp. 21-23; V.A. Zelizer, "From Baby Farms to Baby M", ibid, pp. 23-28; R.J. Neuhaus, "Power, Money and High-Minded Intentions", ibid, pp. 28-29; E.C. Wood and P. Singer, "Whither Surrogacy?", <u>Medical Journal of Australia</u>, Vol. 149, 1988, pp. 426-430; M. Stanworth (ed.) <u>Reproductive Technologies: Gender, Motherhood and Medicine</u>, (Polity Press, Oxford, 1987); C. Overall, <u>Ethics and Human Reproduction</u>, (Allen and Unwin, London, 1987); M.N. Coleman, "Embryo Transplant, Parental Conflict, and Reproductive Freedom: A Prospective Analysis of Issues and Arguments Created by Forthcoming Technology", <u>Hofstra Law Review</u>, Vol. 15, 1987, pp. 609-630; British Medical Association, Report of the Board of Science and Education, <u>Surrogate Motherhood</u>, (British Medical Association, London, 1987); T.S. Bradley, "Prohibiting Payments to Surrogate Mothers: Love's Labor Lost and the Constitutional Right of Privacy", <u>John Marshall Law Review</u>, Vol. 20, 1987, pp. 715-745; K. Dawson, "Fertilization and Moral Status: A Scientific Perspective", <u>Journal of Medical Ethics</u>, Vol. 13, 1987, pp. 173-178; A.M. Capron, "Alternative Birth Technologies: Legal Challenges", <u>U.C. Davis Law Review</u>, Vol. 20, 1987, pp. 679-704; M. Gallagher, "Womb to Let", <u>National Review</u>, April 24, 1987, pp. 27-30; D. Morgan, "Legislation: Who to Be or Not to Be: The Surrogacy Story", <u>Modern Law Review</u>, Vol. 49, 1986, pp. 358-368; M.D. Kirby, "Human Rights - The Challenge of the New Technology", <u>Australian Law Journal</u>, Vol. 60, 1986, pp. 170-181; A.E. Stumpf, "Redefining Mother: A Legal Matrix for New Reproductive Technologies", <u>Yale Law Journal</u>, Vol. 96, 1986, pp. 187-208; J. Waugh, "Breeding Money", <u>Business Review Weekly</u>, May 9 1986, pp. 52-53, 55-57, 59; G. Corea, <u>The Mother Machine</u>, (Harper and Row, New York, 1985); L. Skene, "Moral and Legal Issues in the New Biotechnology", <u>Australian Law Journal</u>, Vol. 59, 1985, pp. 379-392; E. Page, "Donation, Surrogacy and Adoption", <u>Journal of Applied Philosophy</u>, Vol. 2, 1985, pp. 161-172; D. Parker, "Surrogate Mothering: An Overview", <u>Family Law</u>, Vol. 14, 1984, pp. 140-144; R. Arditti (ed. et al), <u>Test-Tube Women</u>, (Pandora Press, London, 1984); J.R.S. Prichard, "A Market for Babies", <u>University of Toronto Law Journal</u>, Vol. 34, 1984, pp. 341-357; H.B. Holmes, B.B. Hoskins and M. Gross (eds.) <u>The Custom Made Child? Woman-Centred</u>

Perspectives, (Humana Press, New Jersey, 1981); M. La Bar, "The Pros and Cons of Human Cloning", Thought, Vol. 59, 1984, pp. 319-333; W.A.W. Walters and P. Singer (eds.) Test-Tube Babies, (Oxford University Press, Melbourne, 1982).

131. D. Bartels, "Government Expenditure on IVF Programs: An Exploratory Study", Prometheus, Vol. 5, 1987, pp. 304-324.

132. F.J. Stanley, "In-Vitro Fertilization - A Gift for the Infertile or a Cycle of Despair", Medical Journal of Australia, Vol. 148, 1988, pp. 425-426.

133. ibid p. 426.

134. J. Allender, "WHO warns IVF a $64,000 Risk", The Australian, Tuesday May 16, 1989, p. 8.

135. G. Vines, "Poor Success Rate for Test-Tube Baby Techniques", New Scientist, 19 May 1988, p. 26; S. Fishel and J. Webster, "IVF and Associated Techniques: Whom Can We Believe?", The Lancet, August 1, 1987, p.273 and F.J. Stanley, op.cit., note 132.

136. Singer and Wells, op.cit., note 120.

137. ibid p. 64.

3 Public policy and AIDS: paradoxes of social choice

1   Introduction

2   AIDS, Public Policy and Legal Paternalism

      (1) Quarantines

      (2) Prostitution

      (3) Testing for AIDS

      (4) Prisons

      (5) Schools and the Workplace

3   Homosexuality and AIDS

4   Homosexuality, Sexual Perversion and the Metaphysics of Anal Sex

5   Homosexuality and Conservative Christianity

"AIDS is a very serious medical problem. However, it is more than merely a medical problem, it is first and foremost a <u>social and psychological</u> one which has serious consequences both at the level of individual suffering and at the wider societal level of <u>human rights, equality as well as the quality and value of human life</u>, all of which are under threat at present. Consequently, any action to combat the spread of the disease and helping those affected by it must include more than medical considerations alone...

This grave human, social and medical crisis, threatening the well-being and human rights of many more people than are at risk of contracting AIDS, [requires] urgent, open, honest and trusting co-operation between all those parties who have the capacities, resources and responsibility to contain the crisis and reduce suffering". [1]

1. Introduction

In this chapter various philosophical problems in AIDS public policy will be discussed. The problems in general are concerned with a conflict, or perhaps more accurately a contradiction between individual freedom and social responsibility. This problem in itself, is the most basic problem of sociological and political theory and various responses to it have shaped the way we live our lives and think about our wider role as social agents. It is not my aim here to attempt to solve the grand general metaphysical problem of the social sciences and construct a political theory that allows us to mechanically solve every major socio-political problem about AIDS that rests upon the individual freedom/social responsibility dilemma. This type of approach, is I will argue below with respect to the subject of "legal paternalism", bound to be unsatisfactory. Nevertheless I believe that philosophers can contribute to the public policy debate about AIDS, by the use of cunning and wit, to show paths around problems rather than leading us through them. In this chapter I shall illustrate the philosophical methodology and approach to problem solving discussed previously with respect to public policy issues related to the broad theme of legal paternalism and highly controversial discrimination issues regarding homosexuality. My general argument is that whilst there are some methodologically conservative measures that must be adopted immediately, a satisfactory response to the AIDS epidemic must involve a public debate and (hopefully) democratic reform of many problematic institutions in society.

2. AIDS, Public Policy, and Legal Paternalism

One of the most important philosophical objections to various public policy proposals for limiting the spread of AIDS - such as closing gay bars and bath houses and even for the provision of quarantines for (presumably) HIV positive people - is that these measures are an unjustifiable <u>paternalistic</u> intrusion into the life styles of rational consenting adults. Others disagree, believing that the State does have the right to regulate such behaviour for the good of all. The issue of <u>paternalism</u> was raised by John Stuart Mill in "On Liberty" [2] and there is an enormous secondary literature debating this issue. [3] Mill maintained the following:

> "The object of this essay is to assert one very simple principle, as entitled to govern absolutely the dealings of society with the individual in the way of compulsion and control, whether the means used be physical force in the form of legal penalties, or in the moral coercion of public opinion. That principle is, that the sole end for which mankind are warrented, individually or collectively, in inferfering with the liberty of action of any of their number, is self protection. THat the only purpose for which power can be rightfully exercised, over any member of a civilized community, against his will, is to prevent harm to others. His own good, either physical or moral, is not a sufficient warrent. He cannot rightfully be compelled to do or forbear because it will be better for him to do so, because it will make him happier, because, in the opinions of others, to do so would be wise, or even right. These are good reasons for remonstrating with him, or reasing with him, or persuading him, or entreating him, but not for compelling him, or visiting him with any evil in case he do otherwise. To justify that the conduct from which it is desired to deter him, must be calculated to produce evil to someone else. The only part of the conduct for anyone, for which he is amenable to society, is that which concerns others. In the part which merely concerns himself, his independence is, of right, absolute. Over himself, over his own body and mind, the individual is sovereign." [4]

This area, Mill saw as a sphere of action in which society has only indirect interest. It includes conscience, freedom of thought and feeling, feeling of opinion and speech on all subjects, the liberty to form our life plans as we see fit, the freedom of individuals to unite for any purpose not involving harm to others: "the only freedom which deserves the name, is that of pursuing our own good in our own way, so long as we do not attempt to deprive others of theirs, or impede their efforts to obtain it". [5] To support this Mill claims to argue on the basis of <u>utility</u> rather than from the idea of abstract rights. As such, it is clear on utilitarian grounds that Mill cannot make his case, for in a complex interrelated society, the sort of liberty which Mill is concerned with, is very limited in any case. Mill himself was sensitive of the objection that his position was one of "selfish indifference", and admitted that what one does to onseself may influence the interests of others. But if so, such behaviour is no longer self-regarding! The problem with Mill's response is that there are social costs of the free asocial pursuit of interests as Pellegrino notes with respect to health:

> These costs are imposed involuntarily on the whole society. They are of sufficient magnitude to warrant some restraints on the freedoms of smokers, drunken drivers, drug users and drinkers, for example, to injure themselves and their fellow citizens and thus to divert resources that might otherwise be used for more desirable social purposes. Financial disincentives, selectively higher insurance premiums, higher taxes on tobacco and alcohol, enforced speed limits, mandatory helmets for motorcyclists or seat belts and seat restraints for children could be defended morally. Education of all segments of society, especially the young, warnings about the hazards of these practices, or social coercion by making the smoker, for example, a social pariah in polite society, in public places and restaurants - these are not unreasonable restraints or invasions of privacy given the weight of the burden they place on the whole of society. Those who become ill because of their own deleterious life-style must be cared for in any society that claims to be human and humane. To care for them costs those who are innocent. Unrestrained freedom to indulge in unhealthy behavior is a constraint on the freedoms and lives of those who do not share the same damaging life-styles. [6]

It is always possible to argue for paternalistic coercion, regardless of the correctness of Mill's position (which Mill himself did not get around to justifying on utilitarian terms, despite his introductory promise). As well, Mill's main argument against legal paternalism was based upon the value of individual spontaneity; Cohen [7] has pointed out that if a government could restrict citizens' conduct to prevent self-inflicted harms, without compromising their individuality, then this form of paternalism would escape Mill's main objection. In overview, there is general agreement among philosophers that paternalism is almost sometimes justified.

On the other hand paternalism in many cases can lead to evil consequences, depriving people of the democratic right, to choose and decide for themselves. [8] Paternalism taken to its extreme leads to a situation where governments adopt social and cultural policies which are objectionable to the majority of citizens of a country, because of the influence of intellectual or business elites, and refuse to budge. The democratic process is treated with contempt, as are the views of the ordinary people. This entire issue is made more complex by deeper politico-philosophical questions that are raised by anarchists about the justification of the state itself. [9] Even so, a parallel moral problem will still exist for anarchism insofar as there will be times in the life of any community where social interests and the ends of individual free action conflict.

The situation regarding the philosophy of paternalism would appear to be that paternalism is sometimes justified, and sometimes not. The attempt to draw an adequate general distinction between justifiable and unjustifiable paternalism has not been successful. There is a good, general reason for this. The relationships between individuals in modern society is complex, diverse and mutli-dimensional. How then could any set of simple rules adequately deal with such complex relationships? For example, in speaking of the multi-dimensionality of social relationships, I refer to the various qualitatively different spheres of social action through which individuals interact - health, sport, government, industry, science, culture, sex and so on. How could any simple moral rule adequately deal with such diversity? It would be certain to be subjected to counter-examples and incompleteness. Thus we are forced in the end to consider paternalistic intervention on a case by case basis, rather than attempting to deal with complex moral dimensions by neat, but ultimately inadequate formulations.

David Conway in his paper "AIDS and Legal Paternalism" [10] is I believe a step in the right direction with respect to the issue of paternalism and AIDS. Conway seeks non-paternalistic reasons for activities such as closing bath houses or quarantining carriers of the AIDS virus, even though everyone who might get the disease consents to do so. These reasons, _if_ they exist at all, will depend upon whether or not society will face harmful consequences if for example the bath houses were not closed. However having said that Conway then qualifies his position out of existence:

> "But the fact that the closings and quarantines are not in principle illegitimate does not mean that they are warranted overall. For whatever non-paternalistic reasons there may be for closing baths and quarantining carriers, there may be stronger reasons against such actions. For instance, it might be wise to leave the baths open because they serve as locations for educating gays

on sexual safety. And quarantining all carriers of the AIDS virus - which, some say, could be as many as two million people - would most likely be completely unworkable even if it were somehow desirable.

There are difficult issues of substance here. My aim has not been to argue that they should be resolved in any particular way. It has been to show that even if AIDS is spread exclusively through consensual acts there can be non-paternalistic grounds for closing the baths or quarantining the carriers. Without question there is a great deal of plausibility in the claim that it is no one's business but Smith's if he freely chooses to frequent the baths or even to have a homosexual relationship with a known carrier. But in spite of the plausibility of this position, it is altogether too simple. The hard social issues posed by AIDS cannot be so easily disposed of by appeal to an anti-paternalistic principle. [11]

What the community is hoping to obtain from philosophers though is precisely an answer to the very questions that Conway avoids. However, if I am right in believing that the problem of the conflict between individual freedom and social responsibility can only be dealt with on a case-by-case basis, rather than solved completely by one grand moral distinction, it does not follow that there are no general public policy principles at all which can be used to conceive of a rational and just philosophical foundation for a public policy with respect to AIDS. It may be possible to find a way "around" many complex moral problems, to use the cunning of reason to avoid full-blown moral conflict. I will argue that a proper understanding of the empirical data about AIDS, along with some intuitively plausible decision-theoretical principles enables us to side step many of the moral dilemmas of public policy formation with respect to AIDS.

(1) <u>QUARANTINES</u> The issue of quarantining of HIV infected individuals, has been raised repeatedly in the Australian AIDS debate not only by anxious members of the public as well as by certain medical practitioners. In the United States, the state of Virginia planned a quarantine programme to isolate AIDS patients who still continue to have sex. [12] In March 1986, an article in the influential <u>American Spectator</u> said:

"From what we know now, the only alternative available until cures or vaccines, or, both, are developed is to prevent the spread of the disease by making it physically impossible. This implies strict quarantine as has always been used in the past when serious - not necessarily lethal - infections have been spreading". [13]

103

The argument relied upon by the supporters of quarantines is as follows. Quarantines in medical usage involve the restriction of the movements of an infected person who has a specific infectious disease, or a person who may have been exposed to such a disease, to avoid their contact and transmission of the disease to the wider population, for either the time of infectiveness or successful treatment or the longest general incubation period for the disease - after which if there is a negative result, the person can leave isolation. The paradigm case of justifiable quarantines are those cases where someone has contracted a disease such as smallpox which is easily spread by casual contact. Consideration of historical data, summarized by Wendy Parmet [14] indicates that the property of a disease which motivates public health authorities to conduct mass quarantines and isolation is not whether a disease is <u>lethal</u>, but whether it is <u>contagious</u>. For example under most American State statutes venereal disease classifications would allow state interventions such as quarantine and isolation because such diseases are regarded as high contagious - albeit, not from casual non-sexual contact. AIDS however, has been classified as a communicable or reportable disease, but not as a venereal or sexually transmitted disease. [15] Along with the aspect of contagion, there is general agreement that quarantines only make medical sense if there is a precisely identifiable population of people can be clearly identified as being infectious. A writer in the <u>Harvard Law Review</u> for 1986 argued that quarantines cannot meet even the most basic prerequisites for the control of AIDS:

> "Medical uncertainty prevents quarantine from being a constitutional alternative for controlling AIDS. Physicians are not yet able to determine when an AIDS carrier is infectious, and no cure or vaccine is available. Furthermore, tests now available to detect antibodies produce a significant number of falsely positive results, creating problems of over inclusiveness. Given these gaps in medical knowledge, a quarantine of AIDS carriers could require the lifelong confinement of a healthy individual who does not even carry the virus. Such a law would undoubtedly deter many carriers from seeking tests on treatment and would be neither an effective nor a constitutional means of protecting the public from disease". [16]

This author believes that even more narrowly defined quarantines will be unsatisfactory:

> "A quarantine aimed at AIDS carriers who are considered unable or unwilling to refrain from sexual contacts or from sharing intravenous needles may appear, on its face, to be targeted sufficiently narrowly. Nonetheless, even these quarantines should not be upheld. It would be

virtually impossible to identify the dangerous individuals in a pool of one million carriers of the virus. Determinations would necessarily be based on predictions of future behavior that either could not be substantiated, or could not be made with sufficient certainty to meet the tests of close fit and least restrictive means; an individual could face indefinite confinement simply because of assumptions about what he might do in the future. Such an individual would be considered not merely ill, but lacking in self-control, prone to engage in unacceptable behavior, and a danger to society. Under such a regulation, an individual who did not commit a crime could be involuntarily confined and permanently stigmatized without receiving the safeguards of a criminal trial". [17]

Gastin and Curran [18] list a number of objections to AIDS-quarantines. First, only a small portion of the population who are HIV seropositive engage in unsafe sex or share contaminated needles. A quarantine would confine individuals who are non-dangerous, and this violates any reasonable conception of natural justice. Second, even to isolate the seropositive population would involve massive quantities of the health budget, with continuous compulsory testing. Third, even if this could be done, the sheer number of people who are seropositive would make any quarantine unmanageable. (This applies <u>a fortiori</u> to the case of Africa). Any such quarantine would have to be for life, for no effective "cure" for AIDS exists. The expense in running a quarantine would be a great drain upon the financial resources of society, for it must be run as a prison, with the use of armed force to prevent escapes. Any such prospect is morally appalling, and is a sad reflection of the level of compassion of a society, that would construct such a programme. It would involve authoritarianism and state violence in its most ugly form, for any such quarantine will involve infringement of the individual liberties of a large number of people who pose no danger to society at all. Further excellent discussions of the ineffectiveness and inadequacy of the concept of an AIDS quarantine include Musto [19], Gleason [20], Ford and Quam [21], and Elsberry [22].

The most plausible argument for an AIDS quarantine, involves restricting its scope to those who refuse, once having been identified as being HIV antibody positive, continue to engage in unsafe sex with multiple partners, prostitution, or the sharing of "dirty" IV needles. Dr. Vernon Mark of the Harvard Medical School has proposed quarantining "carriers of AIDS who persist in spreading it by 'irresponsible' behaviour" on an island in the middle of Massachusetts Bay, that was once used as a leper colony. [23] The limited AIDS quarantine proposal for "Typhoid Marys" escapes the objections made to the comprehensive AIDS quarantine proposals made above. Nevertheless, even here there are strong objections to any such quarantine. It is clear that dealing with the AIDS epidemic effectively requires establishing trust between public health officials and members of the high risk groups. It is also clear that with a highly politicized disease such as AIDS and with the perceived discrimination attached to any form of quarantine, public health officials should use such measures only if it is better than doing nothing at all. A preferable option is to use the criminal law to punish deliberate malicious offenders - such as HIV antibody positive people who deliberately attempt to contaminate blood supplies.

Even here there are many complications. How for example is society to deal with prostitutes with AIDS who continue to practice? I believe that the issue of prostitution has not been examined in the depth which it deserves, and I shall deal with this issue in the next subsection. My position is that even here, quarantines do not go to the heart of the matter. Whilst it may be true that prostitution has always and will always be present in human societies, the problem which prostitution raises for modern society, which on paper at least recognises the equal rights of women, is - why should prostitutes be treated as criminals and stigmatized by society (including, as one prostitute put it in an interview with me, by "all those educated ladies, who look down on us") when their clients are not? - and why does such an activity exist in an age presumably enlightened about women's rights? My conclusion shall be that this presumption is false, and than the widespread existence of prostitution, sufficient to create a booming "sex industry" is a symptom of a strongly sexist and exploitative society.

(2) <u>PROSTITUTION</u>. Prostitutes, as depicted by American movies, are psychopathic nymphomaniacs with a razor taped to their inner thigh, and a small calibre semi-automatic pistol kept inside high heeled boots. But let us consider real life here. Marianne is a 25 year old prostitute who became HIV positive, after being thrown out of a methadone programme because of her stormy temper. Desperate for a "fix" she picked up a syringe laying in one of the streets of Kings Cross and contracted AIDS. When she was 14 she was raped by her father; she left home after this and went to Melbourne where a "friend" introduced her to heroin. Once she was addicted, she found that to support her habit, it was necessary to work as a prostitute, and she went to Kings Cross where she was making $500 a night. She became pregnant to another heroin addict and gave birth to her son, John. It was after the birth of her son, that she became infected with the AIDS virus. When her mother found out that Marianne was HIV antibody positive, she sought and won custody of her grandchild and refuses to allow Marianne to see her son. Marianne says "My mother has told me that when I die she will break my tombstone and spit on my grave". A friend who she told about her antibody status, publicized the fact with the local community's response of threats of violence and broken

windows. "They call me the 'AIDS germ' and they say they are going to get the pest control van to come out and spray me". To help pay the bills, Marianne still works occasionally as a prostitute, although she does not tell her clients that she has AIDS, she makes them wear a condom. [24] Sometimes they don't - when for example they rape her.

Whether we view Marianne as subject for punishment, or a victim who should receive compassion and help depends ultimately upon our philosophical conception of prostitution: is prostitution a commercial venture like any other within capitalist society, or is prostitution essentially the economic exploitation and sexual abuse of women (and to a lesser degree gay men) by men (heterosexual male prostitutes to serve women are very rare if not entirely a male fantasy). [25] Carole Pateman in her important contribution to feminist theory, The Sexual Contact [26] points out that prostitution, whilst once viewed by the bulk of feminists as a part of patriarchal exploitation, is now defended by many feminist contradctorians, who see prostitution as a job, and the prostitute as a worker. The prostitute contracts out part of her property (and male prostitutes from the standpoint of contracts are no different from female prostitutes) in a market for a certain time and for certain uses, in exchange for money. If sex is just one more commodity among so many others, then what could possibly be wrong in selling it on the market as a commodity? [27] Viewed in this light, Marianne would be seen as much like the car salesperson, who sells a car with known defective brakes, or someone who sells a food product with known hidden toxins.

Pateman by contrast sees that the _real_ problem of prostitution is not a problem about women, but one about _men_. Why do men wish to buy or hire womens bodies through sexual contracts? Why should sex be commodified in this way? It cannot be merely an instance of free-love because free-love involves mutual sexual attraction and mutual sexual pleasure without the exchange of money as direct payment for the act itself - and certainly without a rigidly fixed time limit for orgasm. Pateman's answer is that "prostitution is part of the exercise of the law of male sex - right, one of the ways in which men are ensured access to women's bodies". [28] There is no mystery why women become prostitutes in Pateman's opinion - they do it for money, often to support their families, not because of any excitement or enjoyment of the activity. Prostitution is a means for usually poor, homeless and "uneducated" (by the standares of technocratic society) women to obtain large sums of money fast. This is especially so, as in the case of Marianne cited earlier, if drug addiction is involved. Indeed pimps on the lookout for new girls, may try to get them hooked on heroin, so that they are very easily controlled. The undeniable elements of economic coercion, the constant dangers of disease and physical injury and subordination establish a clear distinction between prostituion and other occupations. As Pateman powerfully puts it:

> "When women's bodies are on sale as commodities in the capitalist market, the terms of the original contract cannot be forgotten; the law of male sex-right is publicly affirmed, and men gain public acknowledgement as women's sexual masters - that is what is wrong with prostitution". [29]

Laurie Shrage [30] agrees that prostitution constitutes a degrading and unsatisfactory form of sexual conduct which "epitomizes and perpetuates pernicious patriarchial beliefs and values and, therefore, is both damaging to the women who sell sex and as an organised social practice, to all women in our society". [31] The action of the prostitute and her client legitimize the belief that women can benefit from patriarchy. It follows then that prostitution would be remedied, at least as far as fallible human beings can present a remedy to anything, by a concentrated attempt to change the patriarchal foundation of our social institutions and practices, in the family, the work place and in the political arena, rather than attempting some single (mono-causal) remedy. The positions of Pateman and Shrage are consistent with a decriminalization of prostitution. Indeed although neither Pateman nor Shrage discuss questions of prostitution and the law in any detail, it is also consistent with a feminist legal view of prostitution to decriminalize prostitution itself, but to legally punish the prostitute's clients. Although this position has not been argued for before in any depth, it can be justified by the following argument used by Nancy Erbe in another context:

> "To accept the assumption that men are entitled to sexual service from women and girls is to accept incest offenders' and prostitute customers' assertions that sexual deprivation justifies their behavior - sex without responsibility for the consequences. In other words, sexual deprivation justifies sexual abuse. Men cannot, justify sexual abuse on the basis of their own sexual deprivation. Men cannot blame the victims of men's actions for the evil men perpetrate upon them. Men are responsible for their sexual behavior. No amount of wife neglect, daughter affection, or prostitute enticement erases the fact that a man determines his participation in exploitative sex with women and children". [32]

If police arrested and charged <u>male clients</u> as they left brothels, instead of arresting prostitutes, and if society made a concentrated and sincere attempt to enable these women to subsist without prostitution by gaining a better education and employment - all within the context of a serious attempt to deal with drug addiction (and this in turn means waging a war on organised crime, political and police corruption), then the spread of AIDS through the "second wave" would be diminished. Of course, no elected, so called "representative" government within a capitalist society would attempt such a bold programme - for there is no doubt that rich and powerful men consider women's bodies as just another commodity to be bought (Japanese politics in recent times supports this statement well). It is for this reason that I believe that an adequate response to the AIDS pandemic, that does not merely consist of putting a single bandaid upon a haemorrhage, must be linked up t a general programme of radical and far-reaching socio-economic and eco- political reform.

This is certainly the case for the problem of prostitution, and the time to begin <u>deep</u> social reforms in this area is <u>now</u>.

(3) <u>TESTING FOR AIDS</u> Public policies relating to AIDS testing have many complex legal ramifications, especially with respect to health insurance, disability, insurance and life insurance. [33] As I am not a legal theorist, I shall not discuss these issues here. More important though to the theorist of social ethics is the controversial issue of testing and the physicians fear of contagion. E.H. Loewy writing in the March 1986 issue of <u>Chest</u> points out that fear of contagion has led to some physicians refusing to care for AIDS patients. [34] Society has expected doctors to take reasonable risks in dealing with infectious disease; this is a tacit social contract and doctors have taken greater risks in infection, especially during the "Black Death" of the 14th century. [35] Lowey says:

> "Infectious disease not yet subject to cure elicits an unaccustomed fear and also challenges our God-like invincibility. It brings us face to face with two facts: we are finite, and we are mortal. And we - great men and women that we are - don't like it. [36]

AIDS raises a serious problem for psychiatrists counselling AIDS patients who are attempting to cope with the inevitable threats of a fatal disease. Dr. C. Thompson and other members of the Department of Psychiatry Charing Cross Hospital, London describe the problems in dealing with a 27 year old male AIDS patient with suicide tendencies. The patient attempted suicide during his stay in the psychiatric hospital, cutting his hands and smearing himself and his surroundings with blood. Clearly the patient needed help, but Thompson believes that few psychiatric hospitals are capable of supplying this without creating a health hazard for other patients and hospital staff. [37]

In the Australian context, the issue of AIDS testing in hospitals has become an explosive issue. Dr. Noel Kinny,

Federal Secretary, Australian Association of Surgeons writes:

> "It is clear that there are very real risks of the infection spreading to the uninfected group when contact with the infected group takes place under conditions which permit the possible transfer of the disease.
>
> One such set of conditions is supplied by the operating theatre, especially in regard to surgery, where surgeons and other health care workers may be exposed to a real risk of transmission of the disease, especially if unaware of the patient's potential infectivity.
>
> Surely surgeons have every right to seek to protect themselves and their fellow health care workers to the greatest extent possible, and to seek to limit the further spread of the disease in the community.
>
> It is a sad commentary on the present state of our laws, and an indictment of those who make and administer those laws, that surgeons seeking to apply rational approaches to the problem as they care for their patients should not only be exposed to public vilification by closet homosexuals in positions of power, but also should be exposed to the risk of being dragged before the quasi-judicial and pseudo-judicial tribunals which now purport to dispense justice in this country". [38]

The Australian Medical Association is seeking the compulsory testing of migrants, along with hospital patients and health workers. According to the Federal Vice-President Dr. Bruce Shepherd:

> "AIDS is one of the worse ways to die yet one of the greatest tragedies is that we are worrying more about the privacy and sensibility of the victims than we are about preventing innocent people from catching it". [39]

How is HIV blood a danger to doctors, nurses and hospital workers? Consider the most common possibility, the taking of blood by nurses, for various purposes. The wearing of gloves when taking blood, makes it difficult to find veins according to many nurses, because often they rely upon the sensitivity of the fingers to detect the vein - especially in overweight patients. Needle notches have eliminated the problem of removing bloody needles from syringes by hand, although taking the needle from the patient's arm to the needle notcher may lead to blood dripping onto the nurse's hand. Another way in which this may occur is when a swab is placed over the needle point entry after the needle is removed, where blood may seep onto the fingers through the swab. More obviously, during major surgery in operating theatres, surgeons will come into contact with quantities of blood, and operations on HIV infected patients will require careful cleaning of operating theatres and strict sterilization of instruments. Now there is no ethical problem if a patient consents to such a test prior to surgery. What if he/she refuses? Is mandatory testing justified in this situation, as it obviously is with respect to all donations of blood and blood products, ova semen and organs for transplantation?

The testing of all hospital patients with or without their consent in situations where doctors and hospital workers are likely to come into contact with blood products, seems at first glance to escape the decisive objections that have been made against proposals such as the mandatory testing of every person in Australia on a regular basis. [40] Nevertheless there is still a problem with <u>false positives</u> and false negatives as Adam Carr describes:

> "If we assume that 500,000 Australians belong to increased-risk categories, and that 10% of these are HIV infected, and that, of the remaining 15.6 million people, 0.03% are infected (as in the US), and if we assume that the antibody test is 99% accurate both for specificity and selectivity, then testing the 500,000 increased risk people would produce 445,500 true negatives, 49,5000 true positives, 4,500 false positives and 500 false negatives". [41]

As well as this, there are problems that may arise by patients who are in the so-called window period - HIV is present, but the antibodies have not developed - or in rare cases where HIV is present, but the antibodies have disappeared. To deal with the problem of false negatives and false positives raised by use of the ELISA test, the Western Blot test or particle agglutination assays or membrane assays could be used for confirmation or falsification of the test results. The detection of HIV nucleic acid by gene amplification techniques such as the polymerase chain reaction (PCR) which is capable of detecting a single HIV gene solves the problem of the "window in time", but this complex molecular biological technique is a laboratory test. It would be extremely expensive and time consuming to perform extensively. [42]

Even if testing was conducted on every hospital patient, and AIDS recommendations and guidelines followed for healthcare workers and laboratory personnel [43] there is still a finite risk of HIV infection among health care workers who come in contact with infected blood, blood products and other body fluids that may contain the HIV. [44] Ways in which infection can occur through accidents include needle-stick injuries, splashing of fluid in eye/membranes, open wound contamination and scalpel wound. Many of these accidents arise because the pressure of hospital work, in times of inadequate funds and staff cuts, means that to save time certain risks have to be taken. For example, a nurse doing the rounds of a ward, would be likely to dispense with gloves in taking blood from a vein of a patient under the stress of a heavy work load. The safety procedures required to prevent blood from getting on the fingers may be perceived to be too time consuming. But this is not an argument for dispensing with HIV safety precautions! On the contrary, if nurses and doctors are to adequately protect themselves from HIV infection from accidents, then time must be allowed for the necessary procedures to be carried out. This will mean that tasks from surgery to blood collection will become more time consuming. A moral and just society will recognise this and make a commitment to supply adequate funds to hospitals, so that situations such as doctors and nurses working double shifts do not occure - increased weariness is almost certain to produce accidents.

Thus the resolution of the AIDS health care workers debate is not in terms of testing, for that does not address the ultimate question of the safety of the health care worker, who is dealing with known HIV infected patients. My proposal, one which has surprisingly enough has not been discussed in the literature, is that hospitals and research laboratories have to become safer places through modifying work relations. Of course, even if all precautions are taken, accidents do happen, gloves may be cut but a faulty test tube full of HIV infected blood. But is it possible to design a pair of gloves which whilst being flexible, would resist a needle-stick? This proposal is not absurd in the light of the new materials revolution. For example, vests exist today, which are flexible, yet can resist a 44 magnum bullet at point blank range! The glove could use certain high tech cut resistant materials and could slide over normal surgical gloves, leaving only those minimum areas exposed necessary for sensitivity. Another possibility is for the development of a spray on chemical, along the lines of products like _Pentaid_, that dries to form a thick skin-like film, with the difference that the film contains a powerful anti-HIV chemical. The film however, would have to be able to be peeled off easily, which does not occur with conventional plastic skin products. Surgical gloves could perhaps be worn over the film.

4. PRISONS

"Prisons are not created to promote health. Nevertheless, the AIDS epidemic demonstrates forcibly how important prison health policy is for the community as a whole". [45]

In New York State, more than half of all deaths of prisoners are due to AIDS. [46] It is obvious that prisoners are a high risk group, the dangers being through consensual anal sex, homosexual rape and needle sharing. [47] With respect to Australian gaols, there is still the potential for gaols to become breeding grounds for AIDS infections, although there is by no means an explosion of AIDS cases in most Australian prisons. For example, 11 prisoners tested HIV antibody positive within South Australian gaols at December 31, 1988. [48] However, the Correctional Services Minister, Mr. Blevins, saw the drug problem in South Australian gaols as a serious one. This problem exists within the context of a major prison crisis within South Australia, as well as other states: the gaols are overflowing. By 1995 in South Australia, there will be a short fall of 269 beds/cells within the prison system, resulting in the prison system becoming unmanageable, according to the Correctional Services Minister, Mr. Blevins. [49] Whilst drug convictions rose frin 1569 in 1982 to 2165 in 1987, imprisonments fell from 81 down to 43. But driving offences more than doubled from 141 to 351, with a rise in driving convictions from 4914 to 7017. The problem of overcrowding in the gaols certainly makes it more difficult to control drug abuse, and thus must further contribute to the AIDS problem.

Screening and segregation has been strongly challenged in the literature as an over-inclusive policy, since only a small number of seropositives will engage in behaviour which transmits HIV. Gastin (et al) argue as follows:

> "Segregation of seropositive prisoners in an environment with the potential for repeated exposure to HIV could result in a significantly increased health hazard. It is conceivable that continued sexual relations or needle sharing with other infected prisoners could contribute to the development of the full blown disease.
>
> The decision to impose mandatory screening and segregation in prison facilities sends a harmful public health message to the public, as if the state were developing an "AIDS colony". It conveys an image that will affect public perception of the nature of the disease and ways to control it. If prison screening and segregation were adopted as policy in geographic areas at high risk for AIDS, substantial parts of the prison population would need to be housed in separate facilities.
>
> A less restrictive policy to control the spread of AIDS would seek to reduce unsafe sexual behavior and IV drug use in prison, activities already proscribed. Comprehensive and continuing education on HIV transmission and on specific risk-reducing behavior should be implemented. Further, stringent measures to prevent dangerous sexual and needle-sharing behavior should be established, including

better lighting, increased staffing, improved training and supervision, monitoring and enforcement. In sum, prison screening and segregation would not achieve a valid public health benefit, would adversely affect the health and privacy of positive testing prisoners, and would divert attention from less restrictive, more effective, policy alternatives. [50]

Macklin gives an independent, but equally powerful statement of this argument:

"Some defenders of prisoners' rights have voiced concern about the danger to inmates who are victims of homosexual rape while in prison. They stand to be doubly victimized if they are placed in jeopardy if becoming infected with AIDS. A possible solution would be to test all prison inmates and segregate those who are found seropositive. One reply to this proposal notes that the costs would be prohibitive, given the fact that most jails and prisons are already overcrowded, and to construct separate, duplicate facilities for inmates with AIDS, AIDS-related Complex, and those who are seropositive would be impossible, practically speaking. It has also been observed that in all likelihood such duplication of facilities would be "separate and unequal". Prison guards would shun inmates segregated for reasons relating to AIDS, educational and recreational programs for those inmates would be minimal or nonexistent, and even basic amenities might well be absent. What is needed, this reply concludes, is better protection for inmates against homosexual rape, rather than an effort to prevent victims of rape from also being victims of AIDS". [51]

Finally, these recommendations are consistent with the World Health Organization's recommendations at its Special Programme on AIDS, that occurred in Geneva on November 16-18, 1987. The conclusion reached was that prisons' AIDS control measures should not differ from AIDS control measures in the general community. The guidelines included measures such as:

"(1) Prison administrations in close collaboration with health administrators recognise their responsibility to minimise the chances of transmission of HIV in prison (and consequently in the general community when prisoners are released).
(2) Prisoners should be treated in the same way as other members of the community, including the same right of access to:
Up to-date information on AIDS and education programmes designed to minimise spread of the disease (particularly) high-risk sexual behaviour,

prostitution and intravenous drug abuse) and the prevention meausres outlined in those programmes;
Testing for HIV infection on request, confidentiality of results, and timely pre-test and post-test counselling and support from appropriately trained people acceptable to the prisoner;
Medical, nursing, inpatient, and outpatient service of the same quality as that for AIDS patients in the community at large;
Compassionate early release and the opportunity to die in dignity and freedom;
Information on treatment programmes and freedom to reguse such treatment.
(3) All prison staff should receive up-to-date information and education on AIDS prevention and control in prisons, as part of a broader occupational health and hygiene training, including recognition of possible AIDS-associated conditions, appropriate compassionate identification and release procedures, and the most humane management of prisoners so identified.
(4) Prisoners should not be subjected to any discriminatory practice relating to HIV infection or AIDS, such as involuntary testing, unnecessary segregation, or isolation, except where that is required for the prisoner's own well-being". [52]

Compulsory testing is performed on prison inmates in gaols in South Australia, Western Australia, Northern Territory and Queensland. These practices are over-inclusive and do not penetrate to the heart of the AIDS problem in gaols. Indeed there is an extensive body of literature which is explicitly concerned with the more basic problem: why are there so many people in goal and why do the numbers continue to grow? [53] Even for those of the Right, it must surely be a puzzle that requires an explanation. Why are more serious driving offences being committed? What does this say about the state of our transport system and our lifestyles? It would require a book in itself to follow through in detail the many causal pathways that would require investigation to supply answers to these questions. Nevertheless it is clear once more, that any adequate social understanding of the problem of AIDS in prisons must involve examining the wider question of the role of prisons in society, the philosophy of punishment and the social causes of crime. [54] With the prospects of Australian gaols, and <u>a fortiori</u> American and British gaols becoming unmanageable within five years, it is time to ask - what is causing this, and how is the problem solved. The cause of the problem is not dealt with by building, bigger and more expensive gaols.

(5) SCHOOLS AND THE WORKPLACE

"In August, 1985, the Los Angeles City Council

unanimously passed an ordinance banning discrimination against persons with AIDS in employment, as well as housing, medical and dental services, business establishments, city facilities, city services and other public accommodations. So far as employment is concerned, the law prohibits discrimination against people with AIDS or AIDS-related conditions in hiring, promotion, and termination practices. Also prohibited is segregating employees with AIDS or AIDS-related conditions". [55]

Discrimination against AIDS victims raises many difficult moral and legal problems. In many cases it involves groups such as homosexuals and IV drug users, who are already labelled as "deviant" by society, and who suffer further discrimination upon the basis of AIDS. As well, in the U.S. coloured people make up a disproportionate number of persons with AIDS - 38% of those with AIDS are minorities, 87% of women with AIDS are coloured, 91% of children with AIDS are non-white, nearly half of the AIDS cases in New York City involve heterosexuals and 80% of these are black or Hispanic. [56] In the following section I shall deal with the issue of discrimination against homosexuals. In this section I address the issues of discrimination against AIDS victims in school and in the workplace, beginning with the issue of AIDS and schools. [57]

Partida, writing in the <u>Pepperdine Law Review</u>, said this on the issue of whether children with AIDS have a right to attend school:

"Because so much about AIDS is still a mystery, society's right to be free from communicable disease must be factored in the balance between governmental objections and the rights of individuals with AIDS. Balancing these factors under a rationality test [all persons similarly circumstanced shall be treated alike] - the lowest level of judicial scrutiny - would most assuredly validate the policy excluding children with AIDS from school because this would be a reasonable method of protecting healthy school children. It is therefore necessary to determine whether a higher standard of review is mandated by the Constitution". [58]

This is done under U.S. Law by "strict scrutiny review". Partida points out that laws subjected to strict judicial scrutiny are upheld only if (1) the State demonstrates a compelling interest in the action taken and (2) the action taken was precisely devised to meet the desired governmental goal. Partida feels that U.S. case law raises doubts about whether the State has a compelling interest to exclude children with AIDS from school, yet feels in the light of Roe

v. Wade (1973) that if the State has a sufficiently compelling interest in the potentiality of life so as to proscribe abortion during the third trimester of pregnancy, then this same interest in protecting life would be sufficient to meet the first condition of the strict judicial scrutiny test. This judgement is essential and unargued.

The second condition requires that some alternative could not have been used to obtain the same end. Partida is also less than compelling here, concluding that the means-end test is met, without considering any number of options.

"... the constitutionality of excluding AIDS children from school can be determined under the equal protection clause of the fourteenth amendment. Under equal protection analysis, laws excluding children with AIDS from school will be upheld because each possible tier of judicial review can be satisfied. Even so, deprivation of a right so important as education, which includes social interaction, should not be taken lightly by the courts, and the compelling State interest in protecting its citizens must not be abused". [59]

Krusen writing in 1987 in Dickinson Law Review [60] notes that in

"the case of District 27 Community School v. Board of Education (1986), the court noted that automatic exclusion of all children with AIDS would violate their rights under section 504 of the Rehabilitation Act of 1973. The court noted that having AIDS was a physical impairment because HIV destroys lymphocytes and this in turn limits a person's life activities. Because the transmission of HIV by casual contact is only a very remote possibility, this was a case of discrimination".

Krusen notes that in School Board of Nassau County v. Arline (1987) an elementary school teacher who lost her job after episodes of tuberculosis maintained that her dismissal also violated section 504 of the Rehabilitation Act, as her susceptibility to TB constituted a handicap. The district court found for the defendant employer concluding that TB is a contagious disease that is not a handicap within the sense of the term of section 504 of the Rehabilitation Act. The court felt that it could not believe that Congress intended contagious diseases to be considered handicaps. The Eleventh Circuit Court of Appeals, in its examination of the appeal disagreed and believed that the language of the provisions did support the conclusion that infectious diseases are handicaps, requiring protection under section 504 of the Rehabilitation Act. This position was affirmed by the United States Supreme Court in March 1987. The Justice recognised that whilst individuals with contagious diseases may pose a health risk to others, universal exclusion of the contagions is a "discrimination based solely on fear". The contagious condition should be investigated by medical experts on a case-by-case basis to determine the specific risks of contagion:

> "The foundation of every legal evaluation of the issue of appropriate educational placement of the AIDS infected child lies in the medical community's declaration that the disease is not transmitted through casual contact....
>
> The most important issue ... is whether current scientific data is worthy of such high esteem. When making a choice that could unleash a killer among our nation's youngest citizens if the decision is incorrect, does society want to rely on the scientific knowledge of a disease that appeared only six years ago, and whose causative agent has been the subject of research for a mere three years? Unfortunately, a better alternative is not available at this time". [61]

Nevertheless, as Brockman points out, section 504 of the Rehabilitation Act fails to supply discrimination protection for AIDS victims.

> "The U.S. Justice Department in interpreting of Section 504 of The Rehabilitation Act of 1973, maintained that this section prohibits discrimination only when the discrimination is on account of the handicap. Section 504 does not apply to cases where disease may be spread, or because of fear, either rational or irrational. Thus to fire a worker merely for having AIDS is discriminatory, but to fire because of the fear, howerver irrational, of spreading the disease, is not discriminatory. [62]

It is clear, that in the United States, and Australia, a specifically written legal protection against discrimination for AIDS victims is required, rather than trying to deal with this new health challenge on the basis of laws written in the past. [63] "Irrational fear" is not a good basis for legal decision making. In the case of school age children with AIDS, exclusion of the child with AIDS is justifiable only if there is some demonstrated risk of transmission of the disease - such as the presence of open lesions, as recognised by the CDC guidelines. These arguments apply <u>a fortiori</u> to the issue of AIDS in the workplace. [64] In most occupations there is very little risk of contracting AIDS at all because contact is typically <u>casual</u>. (This observation excludes more controversial areas such as the "sex industry", the "medial industry" and for strategic reasons, the military). Therefore exclusion of people from the workplace who are AIDS sufferers or HIV antibody positive, is justifiable only if there is some demonstrated risk of transmission of the disease. This can only effectively be done on a case by case basis. Further, having rejected compulsory HIV testing even in gaols as being an effective public health strategy mean a fortiori that such a measure would be ineffective in the wider community context of the workplace. In rare situations, where employees deliberately attempted to infect someone it is more appropriate to treat this matter as a criminal rather than a civil issue. [65]

I turn now to discuss the most controversial issue in the AIDS debate: the issue of AIDS and homosexuality.

3. Homosexuality and AIDS

The central philosophical issue relating to AIDS and homosexuality - more basic than the already well discussed topic of discrimination and homophobia, and indeed standing as a foundation for these issues [66] - is that of the social legitimacy and morality of homosexuality itself, as Mendicino well puts it:

> "... the issue of the individual liberties of homosexuals is critical to all AIDS victims, who are likely to be subject to the same treatment as gays in a society that identifies the disease with a particular sexual practice. In the future, gays will not be able to rely on the safety of "the closet" to ensure the preservation of their rights. Self-preservation in the gay community depends not only on protections from the fatal virus but on the ability to persuade courts and legislatures to distinguish the reality of the disease from the metaphors that surround it". [67]

In the Australian context, it is not difficult to find writers from both the right and the left who regard AIDS as a gay plague". [68] Let us begin with the Australian Right. The National Party of Australia, at their Federal conference in July 1989, had a number of delegates who forcefully maintained that AIDS is a disease only of homosexuals and drug users. One delegate told the conference "Don't be nice about it. They are poofters", he said "So rule number one, no poofters". [69] Ironically this sort of narrow minded garbage is, as Professor Ron Penny has maintained in reply, counter to the joint AIDS policy agreed between the Nationals and Liberals, which recognised AIDS potential to spread to the wider community - which is now occurring with infections being passed on by HIV positive IV drug users and their partners through heterosexual transmission. [70]

In recent writings of the Australian Right, we find the same theme reoccurring: AIDS is a gay plague, homosexuals are to blame, they must be punished. A Lansdown, in a savage review of Altman says:

> "If homosexuality is a freely adopted identity rather than a fixed characteristic, and if homosexual behaviour is a chosen behaviour rather than an unsought end uncontrollable compulsion, then homosexuals can be justly held responsible for the consequences of their sexual behaviour". [71]

and he asks "Why didn't - why haven't governments acted to prevent people engaging in all homosexual practices, which are by nature unhygienic?' [72] Ignoring every question of morality and oppression, this author has no plan for how governments could do this without policing every bedroom in the country. But then - who polices the police?

Norman Podhoretz, editor for the U.S. *Commentary*, and writer for *The Australian*, sees AIDS as a gay plague arising from the practice of anal sex - even in Africa - and there is something of a conspiracy by gay organizations so as not to jeopardise public support of AIDS research. [73] Podhoretz forgets that many hundreds of gays in Australia have already died from the conditions associated with AIDS. The following is a sample of his rhetoric:

> "Well, there are many excellent, moral and practical reasons for urging chastity and monogamy on the young, but AIDS is not one of them.
>
> If we are to tell the truth to our young people on this matter, what we will have to say is that the best way to avoid getting AIDS through sex is for girls to refrain from affairs with drug addicts, and, most of all, for boys to refrain from allowing themselves (in the striking old Victorian phrase) to be "used as girls" by other men. [74]

B.A. Sanatamaria, another "extreme right-wing" writer for *The Australian* would agree:

> "In the interest of insisting on their central point, they have misused millions of public money in perpetuating the lie that heterosexual practices are just as likely to be the source of the AIDS infection as homosexual practices.
>
> This despite the fact that 91.6 per cent of AIDS-infected people in Australia are homosexual, bisexual or intravenous drug users, while only 15 cases, or 1.2 per cent of aids infections, have been attributed to heterosexual transmission. Why lie about it? [75]

as would Hiram Caton:

"For me the most interesting response was from the homosexuals. They betrayed no sign of shame or repentance for the wreckage they wrought. There were no appeals for counselling services to help them return to the straight life. Instead they persisted in the aggressive impertinence that has become their tradmark.

The homosexuals' response revealed extreme egotism and colossal impertinence. They not only refuse to accept any responsibility for the horrendous consequences of their depravity, they would shift the blame to the average bloke. They not only entertain no thought of relinquishing their high-risk self-indulgence, they demand the protection and perpetuation of it from the very community that they have so grieviously injured. Homosexuals sow the seeds of their own destruction in more than one sense. After apocalypse, Armageddon. [76]

There is also a strong element of condemnation of the gay life style in Australian Christian writing. Some publications such as <u>AIDS and Compassion</u> edited by J. McPherson [77] are exceptions, emphasizing compassion and understanding over simplistic condemnation, and thus I believe should be applauded. So should the remarks of John Woodley, University Church Chaplain, The University of Queensland, writing in <u>Social Alternatives</u>:

"... the package of sexual prohibitions put together by the New Right under such slogans as "pro-moral, pro-family, pro-life", owes more to authoritarian hierarchical and patriarchal attitudes than it does to any historical Christian view of society". [78]

Nevertheless, whilst most mainstream Christians have rejected the idea that AIDS is a judgement from God, they nevertheless believe that homosexuality, if not outrightly sinful is a moral inferior or problematic life style. This is seen for example in the judgemental statement on AIDS made by the Australian Catholic Bishops [79] and in the "Reformed" tradition by the attitude taken towards homosexuality by a leading magazine such as <u>On Being</u>. In an interview with Sy Rogers published in 1988, Rogers a former gay speaks of his "failed manhood". The interviewer says "You seem to be implying that homosexuality is really evidence of deeper things wrong in a person's life" to which Rogers replies "Absolutely. People are gay <u>because</u> ... and its the 'because' we have to get to". [80] He sums up his position as follows:

"Anyone who comes to Jesus Christ from a gay background needs to understand that in Christ they are now considered heterosexual. There's nothing in our genes that says we're born gay or straight. But it is God's intent for us to be heterosexual, just as it is His intent for us all to be virgins until marriage". [81]

Other Christian writers on AIDS, whilst rejecting the idea that AIDS is a punishment from God, nevertheless see AIDS as a natural outcome of an immoral lifestyle which is ultimately a rejection of God. [82] Perhaps the most dangerous view of all, as far as controlling the spread of AIDS, is the Catholic Church's dogmatic stand on the issue of condoms. Father Harman expresses this attitude clearly and concisely in the following dialogue with Hinch:

> HINCH .... If I am an AIDS antibody-positive husband, maybe got it from whatever manner .. blood transfusion or extramarital activity .. the Church would then say to me that I would be wrong to use a condom having sex with my wife?...
>
> FATHER HARMAN. The Church would say that, whether AIDS or not, you would be wrong to use a condom, insofar as the Church's stand is that every act of intercourse should be open to conception. [83]

It is the aim of the discussions in the sub-sections below to rationally undermine the positions of the authors cited above.

Before doing so however, it is worthwhile to consider another controversial writer, this time from the left, who has also been the most vocal Australian media critic of the Australian Health Department's treatment of AIDS as a national crisis. Adam's argument is that there is no evidence of unequivocal transmission of HIV through (strictly only) vaginal intercourse (with no sharing of dirty IV needles or anal sex.) [84] This argument, whilst a popular one in right wing circles [85] also finds a home amongst those of the artistic left, who fought for sexual awareness and expression in the 1960s and '70s. Let us examine Adams' arguments closely, for they fly in the face of the research of most AIDS experts e.g. Fourth International Conference on AIDS (Stockholm 1988). I will argue in turn that Adams' position is untenable.

Adams points out that the African case, where there are as many women as men affected is not unequivocal proof for the received AIDS theory. First, due to the scarcity of medical resources in much of Africa IV needles tend to be used repeatedly often without adequate sterilization, especially in mass vaccination programmes. Second, the controls and checks over blood banks that Australia has, are lacking in much of Africa, making HIV contamination of the blood supply a very serious problem. (No one to my knowledge doubts this). Adams however then argues that anal sex is frequently practiced by heterosexuals in Africa as a form of contraception. As well, a generally poor standard of publich health has led to populations where there are already pandemics of other sexually transmitted diseases, which may ulcerate the vagina and anus, leading to a greater probability of HIV transmission. Lorian in a paper in *The Lancet*, May 14 1988 [86] points out that HIV transmission is more to do with sexual practice than sexual orientation. What makes homosexual men a high risk group is the practice of anal sex. Heterosexuals who practice anal sex are likewise at risk. The reason is due to the physiological difference between the vagina and the anus: the vagina is constructed of tough platelike cells, whilst the rectum is constructed primarily of columnar cells which tear easily. The vagina is generally naturally lubricating, whilst the anus is not. Lorian points out that evidence of HIV transmission via artificial insemination with HIV contaminated semen is not a clear-cut example of vaginal HIV infection because A.I. is typically intrauterine, with some risk of bleeding.

In studies cited by Lorian as presentations at the International Conference on AIDS, Washington D.C. June 4, 1987 differentiated AIDS transmission among heterosexuals between anal and vaginal intercourse. Lorian noted that large numbers of infections may arise from (exclusive) vaginal intercourse, despite low HIV infectivity, because this sexual activity is the norm. There was a greater rate of infection among heterosexuals who practiced anal intercourse, the risk being 1.8 times more for anal than for vaginal intercourse - and the same for homosexual anal-receptive infectivity. Nonetheless, the male-to-female HIV infection ratio in Europe is 16:1, and in Africa is 1.7:1 which is approximately an equal sex distribution. This does not prove, but is suggestive of heterosexual transmission of HIV. Quinn says:

> "In addition to the equal sex distribution of cases, other evidence that suggested heterosexual transmission was the fact that women with AIDS were more likely than men to be unmarried (61% versus 36%), and nearly one third of the married AIDS patients had had at least one previous marriage or "union libre" (persistent cohabitation without formal marriage). One third of AIDS patients reported having had at least one sexually transmitted disease during the three years preceding their illness. In many areas of Africa, a large proportion of the AIDS cases comprise female prostitutes or men and women with a history of multiple sexual partners within the previous five years. However, additional factors that may influence transmission of HIV include frequent exposure to unsterilized needles (80% of AIDS cases), and a history of blood transfusion within

the previous three year period prior to the onset of illness (9%). More recent case-control studies have further demonstrated that AIDS is primarily transmitted in Africa by heterosexual activity, blood transfusions, exposure to blood-contaminated needles and syringe for medical or ritual purposes, and via perinatal transmission from mother to infant.

Seroprevalence data on HIV infection suggest that of these different modes of transmission, heterosexual transmission appears to be the predominant mode of infection in Africa. In a recent study of HIV infection among 6,000 healthy persons residing in Kinshasa, Zaire, a bimodal distribution of infection was evident with a peak prevalence under one year of age and among young adults aged 16-29 years. The first peak in seroprevalence among children under one year of age represented a combination of passive antibody transfer and transmission of virus from mother to infant. The low prevalence rate between ages 2 and 14 argues strongly against arthropod transmission, since arthropod transmission diseases usually have peak infection rates among these age groups. As sexual activity increased during adolescence, the rate of HIV infection increased dramatically, particularly among women aged 15-29 years. This increase was followed by a rise in HIV infection among men between the ages of 20 and 39 years. This patterns, in conjunction with the distribution of AIDS cases, is consistent with that of a sexually transmitted disease with higher prevalence rates among younger, sexually active women having sexual relations with older men. [87]

Along with the above, generally sound observations about AIDS in Africa, Adams quotes the paper by van der Ende (et al) in The British Medical Journal [88] which reported on a three year follow up study of 13 haemophiliacs positive for HIV antibody and their spouses. None of the patients' partners were positive for HIV antibody at any time during the follow up and both patients and partners denied being IV drug abusers or having homosexual contacts. All couples practiced vaginal intercourse, four partners had oro-genital sex, two couples had vaginal intercourse during menstruation and none practiced anal sex. They calculated that the rate of transmission of HIV by unprotected and protected intercourse was 0.04 - 0.06% and 0.08 - 0.1% respectively, concluding that in the absence of other risk factors, transmission of HIV from men to women by vaginal intercourse is infrequent - but not from their data non-zero. Adams when reading this data concludes that There was no transmission of HIV between couples. van der Ende (et al) noted that one partner had unexplained lymphadenopathy druing the three years of the study and although she was not HIV positive, it was thought that she might become HIV positive or antigenaemia in a longer follow up. It is therefore not possible to conclude, as Adams does, that exclusive heterosexual promiscuity between agents who do not practise anal sex and are not IV drug abusers, is safe. Even an infrequent transmission of an incurable, and possiblly lethal virus is an important public health issue.

In reply to the type of argument used by Adams, Dr. John Dwyer [89] points out that the

> "risks of being infected during vaginal intercourse are similar to the chances that a woman has of getting pregnant. One act, may in many cases be sufficient, especially if the woman has genital ulcers or vaginal tears and if the infected male partner is in the phase of his own HIV infection where his immune system is failing and the virus count in seminal fluid is high.
>
> For example two women with no other risk factors became infected with HIV after a single act of sexual intercourse; one woman had unprotected anal and vaginal sex with an IV drug user infected by HIV, the other had vaginal sex with a man who had heterosexual contacts in Central Africa. [90]

Vaginal infection with HIV has been documented by the National Health and Medical Research Council epidemiology research unit, that has documented to November 20, 1988 121 Australians who have contracted HIV through vaginal intercourse. Even though the homosexual/bisexual transmission category constitutes 88.5% of the cumulative national cases of AIDS and the heterosexual transmission category 1.3% (April 1989), this is hardly grounds for complacency, since with respect to known deaths in Australia, the homosexual/bisexual transmission category constitutes for up to April 1989 47.1% of the cases, and heterosexual transmission category 16.6% - figures which are obviously statistically significant. The recommendations of the Australian radical right are therefore flawed and must be rejected.

With respect to the issue of AIDS and homosexuality, perhaps the most important task which a progressive philosopher can perform is to attempt to undermine the ideological jusitfication for homophobia. My following contribution is with respect to two topics (1) the right's tendency to view homosexuality as sexual perversion and (2) the church's condemnation of homosexuality. One would hope that an enlightened society would pass a comprehensive set of anti-discrimination laws, similar to anti-discrimination laws with respect to sex and race - but for Australia, any such hope must lie in the distant future.

4. HOMOSEXUALITY, SEXUAL PERVERSION AND THE METAPHYSICS OF ANAL SEX

R.J. Stoller points out in his book <u>Perversion: The Erotic Form of Hatred</u>[91] that it is unjustifiable prejudice to regard homosexuality as a psychiatric disorder or disturbance, as for example the American Psychiatric Association's <u>Diagnostic and Statistical Manual of Mental Disorders (DSM-2)</u> [92] did until 1973. Homosexuality is a sexual <u>preference</u>, not a diagnosis. A proper diagnosis in medicine involves the following:

> "a syndrome - a constellation of signs and symptoms shared by a group of people, visible to the observer; (1) underlying dynamics (pathogenesis) - pathophysiology in the rest of medicine, neuropathophysiology or psychodynamics in psychiatry; (3) etiology - those factors from which the dynamics originate. [93]

Homosexuality is not a uniform constellation of signs and symptoms and different homosexuals have different psychodynamics underlying their sexual behaviour, as people with all sorts of personalities and of all shapes and sizes prefer homosexuality as their sexual practice. Further, there is no unitary cause for homosexual behaviour. [94] It is difficult then to regard homosexuality as a disease, disorder or disturbance.

Nevertheless homosexuality might be regarded as a <u>perversion</u> or <u>abnormality</u>, a view recently defended by the right wing sociologist Steven Goldberg [95] and the extreme right wing philosopher Michael Levin. [46] I shall attempt to undermine the arguments of these writers. I shall show that attempts to show that homosexuality is a perversion by any standard definition of the concept of perversion (or abnormality) fail. It is then concluded that there are no good reasons (taking the material examined here as constituting a representative survey) for regarding homosexuality as either perverse or abnormal.

A perversion or abnormality may be taken to be that which is <u>unnatural;</u> homosexuality is frequently taken to be an unnatural act along with coprophilia. But what is an unnatural act? Suppose that we explicated this problematic concept by the following: 'an unnatural act is an act contrary to or outside of nature'. If being 'outside of nature' means 'being contrary to natural physical law', then homosexuality along with all human activities, is natural. [97] Clearly advocates of the view that homosexuality is perverse because it is unnatural do not mean that homosexuality is unnatural in this sense, but rather that homosexuality violates the natural purpose of sex. According to orthodox Catholics (although not, perhaps according to the New Testament) God intended sex for the purposes of procreation ("God" may also be replaced here by the "selfish genes" of the sociobiologists). [98] Non-procreative sex frustrates the will of God (or the selfish gene's desire to increase its inclusive fitness - although most sociobiologists believe that homosexuality can be genetically explained), and is hence unnatural. The position could be modified slightly so that sexual intercourse that <u>could in normal circumstances</u> lead to reproduction, is natural. The main problem with this view is that if the God of the Catholics or the God of the sociobiologists really did regard only procreative sex as natural (or adaptive), then why is it that human beings have non-procreative sexual desires and engage in so much non-procreative sex? In any case if you wish to hold to this viewpoint, then you show that homosexuality is a perversion only to find that most heterosexual activities ar also perverse. This is a high theoretical price to pay.

This theoretical price must also be paid by anyone who wishes to use Thomas Nagel's model of sexual perversion to show that homosexuality is perverse. [99] Nagel takes perversions to be <u>unnatural</u> sexual inclinations rather than merely unnatural practices adopted for non-sexual reasons. Natural sex for Nagel follows a seduction model, one must be possessed by desire, not nly for one's partner's body, but for his/her desire and this state of embodiment must involve a complex series of feedback loops involving the awareness of each other's desire and increasing arousal. There is no good reason for accepting this idiosyncratic account of sexual perversion. Again it means that many standard heterosexual inclinations (e.g. for little foreplay and arousal coming from the early stages of sexual intercourse) are perverse. Further, there is no good reason to suppose that homosexuality is a perversion according to Nagel's account of 'perversion', as Nagel's peculiar form of reciprocity may be a preference or inclination of many homosexuals.

The same can be said about the model of sexual perversion given by Robert Solomon. [100] Like Nagel, Solomon believes that non-perverted sex is natural sex. Sexuality however is primarily a means of communicating feelings and emotions to other people through "body language". Here we note that nothing prevents homosexual sexual acts from expressing feelings and emotions of positive value.

Stoller defines the term 'aberration' as follows:

"By an <u>aberration</u> here I mean an erotic technique or constellation of techniques that one uses as his complete sexual act and that differs from his culture's traditional, avowed definition of normality". [101]

A perversion is a specific type of aberration:

> Perversion, the erotic form of hatred, is a fantasy, usually acted out but occasionally restricted to a daydream (either self-produced or packaged by others, that is, pornography). It is a habitual, preferred aberration necessary for one's full satisfaction, primarily motivated by hostility. By "hostility" I mean a state in which one wishes to harm an object; that differentiates it from "aggression", which often implies only forcefulness. The hostility in perversion takes form in a fantasy of revenge hidden in actions that make up the perversion and serves to convert childhood trauma to adult triumph. To create the greatest excitement, the perversion must also portray itself as an act of risk-taking." [102]

Homosexuality, if taken to be an "aberration" does not necessarily involve hostility. Hence homosexuality is not a perversion. By Stoller's account of an aberration we would establish that any sexual practice (excluding purely procreational sex) is an aberration, as most cultures have accepted definitions of 'normality', which have rendered a wide range of sexual practices abnormal, and hence on Stoller's account, aberrative. Thus an aberration in culture C(1) with a criterion of sexual normality N(1) need not be an aberration in culture C(2) with a criterion of sexual normality N(2), C(1) = C(2) and N(1) = N(2). The account is thus culturally relative. Further, even if N(1) was an anti-homosexuality norm, it is possible that attitudes in the culture may change for purely non-rational reasons, so that a non-discriminatory homosexual norm N(2) was accepted. Thus something can be an aberration at one time and not at another. Finally, a culture's norms may be unclear, contradictory or unjustified. This is hardly the stuff to incorporate into sound scientific theorizing.

It is concluded that the standard definitions of 'perversion' do not lead us to regard the proposition that homosexuality is a perversion, as being to any degree tenable. These standard definitions are also conceptually obese; if accepted they entail that many paradigm examples of non-perverse sexual behaviour is really perverse. So much the worse for the standard definitions.

Levin argues that homosexuality is abnormal because it is "purely mechanical ... misuse of bodily parts". [103] This argument he regards as a prolegomena to policy issues involving the rights of homosexual and the rights of those desiring not to associate with homosexuals. He does not systematically detail this relationship, but it is not unreasonable to suppose that a radical right winger such as Levin would like very much to see homosexuality outlawed. He sees homosexuality as a threat to children, because for some obscure reason he seems to think that homosexuality is something a homosexual elementary school teacher will teach students. How this is done, without any crime being committed, remains equally obscure. Levin's analogy about our need to protect children's teeth from the dangers of sugar-coated cereals, is only of amusement, not argumentative value. In any case these irrational dogmas depend upon Levin's conclusion that homosexuality is unnatural, and if his argument for this conclusion is defeated, so are his arguments given in justification of specific repressive policy issues.

The basic intuition which Levin appeals to in his argument for the conclusion that homosexuality is abnormal is this:

> "The erect penis fits the vagina, and fits it better than any other natural orifice; penis and vagina seem made for each other. This intuition ultimately derives from, or is another way of capturing the idea that the penis is not for inserting into the anus of another man - that so using the penis is not the way it is supposed, even intended, to be used. [104]

Levin then attempts to show how such intuitions may be justified by recent work in the logic of functional ascription. He concludes that homosexuality is unnatural and an unwise thing to use one's body for. The unnaturalness of homosexuality explains the fact that homosexuals as a group are "unhappier" than heterosexuals. I shall not discuss the matter of alleged homosexual unhappiness here: let us generously concede the point for the sake of the argument. Note that Levin's argument stands or falls on the justification of the claim that homosexuality is a misuse of body parts.

For Levin an adequate explication of 'S is for F in O' is:

> "(i) S conduces to F in O,
> (ii) O's being F is necessary for O to occur or be maintained, or for the maintenance of O's genetic cohort,
> (iii) (i) and (ii) are part of the causal explanation of the existence or persistence of S in O and members of O's genetic cohort. [105]

More simply: "an organ is for a given activity if the organ's performing that activity helps its host or organisms suitably related to its host, and if this contribution is how the organ got and stays where it is". [106] Now one of the functions of the penis is to introduce semen into the vagina, and in doing this it has been selected for. But proto-human males who found coitus unrewarding, and consequently did not engage in coitus, would have left no descendents. Levin goes on:

"In particular, proto-human males who enjoyed inserting their penises into each other's anuses have left no descendents. This is why homosexuality is abnormal, and why its abnormality counts predentially against it. Homosexuality is likely to cause unhappiness because it leaves unfulfilled an innate and innately rewarding desire". [107]

Recall that Levin was to show that homosexual behaviour involved a misuse of body parts. His criticism of homosexuality is that (non-bisexual) homosexuality is a form of sexual practice which it engaged in exclusively to heterosexual coitus, does not result in the production of any descendants. If this was so, then we would expect (exclusive) homosexual practices, if genetically wired, to be selected against by natural selection. Such practices would be self-extinguishing. Obviously (exclusive) homosexuality is not dying out in modern society, if anything it is increasing in its frequency of occurrence in modern populations and a variety of sociobiological explanations have been given for this. Let us concentrate our attention though on the issue of whether an activity such as homosexuality does involve a misuse of bodily parts.

It is an implication of Levin's position that heterosexual intercourse is merely a form of reproduction or has as its very point, propagation. He says "if heterosexual intercourse is not directly connected to propagation, what is?" [108] This is a question-begging claim. Given that the incidence of reproductive sex is low compared to the incidence of non-reproductive sex for pleasure and love in the set of all human heterosexual sex acts, reproductive sex may be viewed as a bi-product of general heterosexuality, not as its cause. This view fits well with all the general uncontroversial biological knowledge about human sexuality. Human beings can reproduce only when the female has ovulated, but they may copulate at any time of the month. Sexuality is, as I have argued in previous books, a cultural phenomenon. Hence heterosexual intercourse is not in general directly connected to propagation. It may during periods when the human female is fertile lead to conception, but this uncontroversial fact does not establish the "sexuality - reproduction function" or that the very point of sex is reproduction. Without this (unsubstantiated) assumption Levin's argument disintegrates.

To see this consider the functional analysis of the penis, which sees the penis as an organ which is not only capable of urine elmination, and the ejaculation of semen, but also as conducing to sexual pleasure in the male. Thus the penis conduces to sexual pleasure in the male, and it is necessary for such pleasure to occur, or at least occur intensely and swiftly. The intuition appealed to here is that the penis is not merely a reproductive and waste elimination organ, but is also an organ which functions as a sexual organ, an organ for sexual pleasure. To use one's penis for sexual pleasure then is not abnormal. To use it as a paint brush or coast hanger, is. But homosexuals use their penises for sexual purposes, rather than as garden tools. Hence homosexuality is not abnormal.

Levin may still argue that the anus is not "meant" to be subjected to the thrust of a fully erect penis, and the penis is not meant to come into contact with the contents of the bowel. This has some plausibility. Bowels can be easily damaged and diseases contracted as the case of AIDS shows. But all these considerations show is that anal sex without a condom has a health risk (recognising that condoms may break more frequently during anal sex than vaginal sex due to friction factors). Heterosexuals, as the letter pages of the pornography magazines show (and often their pictorials as well), may engage in anal sex and some heterosexuals prefer anal sex to coitus. In anal sex the penis gets considerable friction against the bowel lining, and the head of the penis is substantially stimulated by the usually tight anal sphincter. The clitoris can be manually stimulated. Anal sex, it is said, has its advantages over some coital positions if mutual pleasure is your goal. Homosexuals need not engage in anal sex to obtain mutual pleasure - they may mutually masturbate each other just as heterosexual couples may do in foreplay, with the difference that the former masturbation is to orgasm. This involves no misuse of body parts at all. Interestingly enough Levin has nothing to say about female homosexuality in his paper; perhaps he believes that it does not exist as did Queen Victoria.

It is doubtful whether even anal sex does involve a misuse of body parts. Whilst the bowel damage and the transmission of disease does not show that using one's bowel as a sexual organ involves a misuse of the bowel. The tight vagina of a virgin can be damaged by a large erect penis, thrust by an unsympathetic owner, and diseases such as AIDS may be transmitted during coitus. On the other hand, the contact between the penis and excreta on the sides of the bowel can be avoided by use of lubricated condoms - although of course there is a probability of breakage and misuse. However, the AIDS pandemic cannot be used to show that anal sex per se is "perverse", "abnormal" or "sick", without reference being made to promiscuity and "unsafe" sex. When this is done though, they cannot exclude heterosexual promiscuity from their catalogue of "perversions" as well, contrary to their intention.

I conclude that Levin fails to establish that homosexuality involves a misuse of body parts. Basic assumptions made by Levin without any thought of justification, turn out to be false. The critique of homosexuality will have to be conducted on independent grounds by theorists of the right.

Steven Goldberg offers the following definition of 'abnormal behaviour':

"Behavior is abnormal if it forces the individual manifesting it to suffer unnecessary pain. The pain of negative social sanction (such as social ostracism) is unnecessary if the behavior that elicits the negative sanction is caused by a factor that can reasonably be termed "abnormal". A causal factor can reasonly be termed abnormal if it unnecessarily limits one's autonomy and maturation. A causal factor unnecessarily limits one's autonomy and maturation if it is composed of irrational motivating factors or a displacement of emotions and generates behavior that elicits the pain of negative social sanction." [109]

Goldberg devotes some space towards arguing that this definition of 'abnormal behaviour' is non-tautological, claiming that if one does this, then one cannot consider any causal factor as being abnormal. This is however not what is wrong with Goldberg's definitions: its vice is that it is viciously circular. To understand what 'abnormal behaviour' means we must first understand what 'unnecessary pain (of negative social sanction)' means. To understand what 'unnecessary pain (of negative social sanction)' means we need to know what the 'abnormality of a causal factor' means. This phrase leads us to the meaning of an 'unnecessary limitation on one's autonomy and maturation', and back to the 'unnecessary pain (of negative social sanction)'. These definitions turn in a closed logical circle and are hence incoherent and totally unsatisfactory. Circularity though, does not particularly worry Goldberg.

Nevertheless one could define 'abnormality' as follows: abnormal behaviour forces the individual manifesting it to suffer the pains of negative social sanctions. It is not too difficult to see the errors involved in this account. First, the absence of a negative social sanction about behaviour B immediately means that B is not abnormal. Abnormality hinges then upon the inventiveness and viciousness of a culture's ability to negatively sanction behaviours and this is hardly a satisfactory basis to found any scientific psychiatric theory upon. The reason for this is that the majority of the members of a culture could be suffering from severe mental illnesses (as Fromm argues) and may be quite irrational about the behaviour which they negatively sanction. They may even be inconsistent and negatively sanction heterosexual behaviour, whilst hypocritically engaging in this negatively sanctioned delight themselves; Worse, this definition means that even paradigm cases of sexual perversions, such as coprophilia, if done in private without any real danger of negative social sanctions being mobilized, are not abnormal. Alternatively, if the pervert did not feel pain from the enforcement of negative social sanctions, then the behaviour in question is not abnormal. But this is absurd.

Goldberg's definition of 'abnormality' would be of considerable use to the theoreticians of the world's political psychiatric camps. Many post Soviet citizens pressed for social change and basic human freedoms and were openly critical of the Soviet political system only to wind up in such camps in pre-<u>perestroika</u> days. There must be, according to Goldberg, something <u>abnormal</u> and <u>perverse</u> about someone who persists in doing something when he/she knows he/she will be punished. So all protesters are <u>abnormal</u>, no matter how just and rational their protest is. It is only one further step to go to say that such abnormal people require psychiatric help. The implications of this are obvious.

It is concluded that there are no good reasons to regard homosexuality as a perversion or an abnormality in any of the senses of these terms considered above. The arguments of Levin and Goldberg for the thesis that homosexuality is abnormal, have been examined and shown to be untenable.

5. Homosexuality and Conservative Christianity

According to the sixth edition of the Concise Oxford Dictionary of Current English, the word 'prudery' means extrme propriety in conduct and/or attitudes, especially regarding sexual matters. 'Propriety' means, according to the same distinguished source, "correctness of behaviour or morals". Now surely one could oppose "prudery" on moral grounds without inconsistently criticizing correct moral behaviour in sexual matters, so that OED definition must be incorrect. A better term than 'propriety' is 'strictness' or 'severity' if common usage is any judge. Prudery then involves a rigorous strictness or severity in conduct and/or attitudes regarding sexual matters in particular. It is a certain type of prudery which I wish to refute here: the moral attitude taken by the Christian tradition to premarital and non-marital heterosexual intercourse and homosexual intercourse, and their continuing occurrence in non-marital sexual relationships.

The conservative Christian prudery which I wish to consider here involves this claim: <u>all</u> acts of premarital and non-marital heterosexual intercourse and homosexual intercourse are moral evils or sins. [110] Here I shall argue that the general arguments given in support of this position are seriously flawed from both a logical and scriptural point of view. Thus it is not inconsistent with <u>Christian literalism</u> to maintain that at <u>least some</u> acts of premarital sexual intercourse <u>and</u> homosexual sexual intercourse are not morally objectionable. By 'Christianity' I mean a rationally defensible interpretation of the Old and New Testaments of the Christian bible and by 'literalism' I mean that position which regards all or most cognitive propositions in the scriptures as being true, provided they are given a rationally justifiable interpretation. No scriptural passage which contains a conceptual incoherence can be true, and thus some alternative interpretation must be sought in the realm of poetry. Note as well that it takes only one counter-example to defeat the Christian prudism outlined here. This by no sound argument shows that "anything goes" by way of sexual conduct and attitudes. All I claim is that <u>some</u> acts of premarital sexual intercourse by hets, and some acts of sexual intercourse by gays, are not immoral. This has been denied by the Church as was mentioned in the main discussion.

Tannahill notes that the Christian tradition is unique in its condemnation of all forms of sexuality, [111] and few traditions can have the pleasure to boast that their leading early thinkers - Tortullian, Jerome, Augustine, Abelard, Chrysostom, Aquinas etc. - viewed all forms of human sexual intercourse as shameful and fundamentally disgusting. Yet the thoughts of the founding fathers, however mad and perverted and even whilst polluting the waters of thought for hundreds of years, need not have an unbreakable grip upon the minds of their intellectual offspring. Certainly the view of th early Church FAthers and other early Churchmen, that sex is inherently evil, has been challenged since the Reformation. There is virtually no scriptural support for this view (including the writings of St. Paul) and much evidence against it. Proverbs 5:15-19 and the Song of Solomon 2:6 and 8:3, heterosexual intercourse in a monogamous marriage is described as being both the normal way of satisfying human sexual desires, as well as being good in itself. Indeed the Song of Solomon is correctly described as a celebration of marital sexual love and no reference to procreation occurs in it. Even if the Pauline doctrine in 1 Corinthians 7:1-7 is interpreted to mean that celebacy is a more valuable state than marital sexuality, it hardly follows that marital sexuality is an evil or is in anyway shameful. What is shameful and fundamentally disgusting is the views of the Churchmen on this matter. But since their views do not square with the scriptures, their own criterion of ultimate truth, we may dismiss them from further consideration.

Popular Christian writing on sexual morality, such as Herbert Miles' <u>Sexual Understanding Before Marriage</u> [112] and John White's <u>Eros Defiled</u> [113] present a wholesome view of marital sexuality, indeed these books are not inaccurately described as the modern Christian equivalents of <u>The Joy of Sex</u>. Both texts have been strong sellers - <u>Sexual Understanding Before Marriage</u> had by September 1975 nearly 100,000 copies in print. Both text are very liberated about the moral legitimacy of erotic delights in marriage. White for example, whilst regarding orogenital and penile-rectal orgasms as "<u>sub</u>-normal sexual practices", [114] nevertheless manages to say this: "if God gives you as a married couple a delight in the sensations provided by orogenital or rectual stimulation, be thankful and receive such pleasures". [115] Such delights, of course, are strictly reserved for the marital bed and both Miles and White believe that sociopsychology and the scriptures support them. I shall aruge that scriptural sources do not.

The critique naturally enough falls into two parts. First is an examination and critique of Miles and White's case for the sinfulness of premarital heterosexual sexual activity, and second is an examination and critique of their moral and theological objections to homosexual activity. If it can be shown that there are no sound moral objections to homosexual intercourse from a Christian perspective, then we have immediately established that not _all_ acts of non-marital sexual intercourse (of which premarital sexual intercourse is a subset) are immoral. This is so because homosexual marriages do not legally exist in most of the western world and would not in anycase be recognised as legitimate by the non-Gay Christian Church. Thus the sexually active homosexual cannot help but to engage in non-marital sexual relationships. If it can be shown that at least some homosexual relationships (and consequently the sexual acts committed in these relationships, provided that these acts are not immoral for non-sexual or independent reasons) are not morally objectionable, then we establish that not all non-marital sexual relationships and their consequent sexual acts, are morally objectionable. However it is still logically possible that _premarital_ sexual relations are morally unjustified because in the case of such relations, they could have been consummated in marriage. Hence the need now for a consideration of Christian ethics and premarital sexuality.

The point of departure in our argument must be with the question 'What is marriage from the Christian perspective?' This is not, as it may seem at first glance, an easy question to answer. [116] Is marriage a certain legal relationship involving a contract? This contract we suppose, must be socially recognizable. But for the Christian, what must be said about the actual or merely hypothetical post-World War III Adam and Eve, living (or dying) without social institutions to recognise contracts and living without "total" divine protection after the Fall? Either our Adam and Eve are married, in which case the Christian cannot claim that marriage is essentially a legal relationship requiring social recognition, or they are not married. The hypothesis that our Adam and Eve are not married conflicts with the account of Genesis 4:1 which says that Eve is Adam's wife and there is no reason not to suppose that this holds in general. Hence marriage cannot be purely a legal relationship. Nothing depends upon the Adam and Eve story in Genesis being _literally_ true for this conclusion to follow just as the social contract theory does not require the state of nature, or the original veil of ignorance to be historical existents. [117]

There is an argument to be found in 1 Corinthians 6:12-20 by St. Paul, which seems to view an act of sexual intercourse between a man and a woman as the constituent factor establishing a marriage. This thesis has been recently discussed and criticized by B. Ward Powers, [118] and Powers interpretation of Paul's position has been criticized in turn by Vivian Bounds. [119] This issue, as we shall soon see, is of importance to the issue of the morality of premarital sexual intercourse. Now Paul wrote in 1 Corinthians 6:16-17 that one should not have sexual intercourse with a prostitute because "he who unites himself with a prostitute is one with her in body [?]. For it is said, "The two will become one flesh" [Genesis 2:24]". Paul takes the body to be the temple of the Holy Spirit, so sexual sins are particularly serious. Paul does not realise however that if we accept that marriage involves becoming one flesh, (Genesis 2:24; Matthew 19:5, Mark 10:7; Ephesians, 5:3) and that in becoming one body" on becomes "one flesh", then if two people can become one body through an act of heterosexual sexual intercourse, then the same two people can become married through this act. But if at least these two people are virgins prior to their sex act, then all of their sex acts after the initial marriage-making sex act are cases of marital sex rather than premarital sex. Hence their sexual relationship is morally justified from a Christian perspective. Yet our couple are "living together in sin"!

Powers objects to the equation of the meaning of 'one body' and 'one flesh' on the grounds that it does not explain why it is wrong to seek union with a prostitute. [120] But no identification of the meaning of 'one flesh' and 'one body' occurs in this passage. The claim that "the two will become one flesh" is voiced as an explanation as to why one should not become one body with a prostitute. Therefore Paul is claiming that sexual relationships are quite unlike physical relationships for they involve a metaphysical transformation of persons. This explains why Paul went on to say in verses 18-20 of 1 Corinthians that sexual sins are more serious than all other sins because they offend against the body, a "temple of the Holy Spirit". Thus it is reasonable to agree with Vivian Bounds that Paul did believe that an act of sexual intercourse leads to marriage. If this is so, then my criticism of Christian prudery given in the previous paragraph immediately holds.

There are strong objections which could be made to Paul's position. Counter-examples such as the rapist and his victim becoming one flesh and body, and hence married could possibly be dealt with by demanding rational choice made on the part of the sexual agents, a condition not satisfied in the example of the rape. [121] But an outstanding problem is this: the prostitute must be "one flesh" with all of her customers, but is any individual customer "one flesh" with any other individual customer? If so, then two males can be married even if they never met. If not then why is it that the relation of <u>being one flesh</u> fails to be transitive? And what about celibate "marriages" - is the concept of a celibate marriage to be taken to be logically contradictory? The Pauline position seems to be untenable and some more rational position should be sought by the reasonable Christian. But for the many fundamentalist groups who use arguments such as Pauls, they are honoured with justifying "living in sin" for two virgin heterosexuals who met and have continuous sexual intercourse.

It is not necessary to resolve the issue about the true nature of Christian marriage here, for this issue has served its critical purposes. It is established that it is by no means uncontroversial what the true nature of Christian marriage is, and further one interpretation of this nature would seem to undermine Christian prudery. Now I shall address the arguments for the immorality of premarital and non-marital sexual relations given by Miles and White, taking 'marriage' itself as an undefined term. But it is intuitively clear who is not married: our two young virgin heterosexuals who meet, fall in love, develop a relationship full of trust, care and a mixture of other virtues and have sex continually are <u>unmarried</u> and immoral according to Miles, White and most Christians. Why?

There are basically two types of arguments that are advanced to show the immorality of the premarital sex of our two "hot" but loving virgins. The first type of argument is scriptural based on alleged Biblical evidences. The second type of argument is based upon social and psychological evidences, showing the social and psychological harm which inevitably arises from premarital sexual relations. For the sake of argument I assume that the alleged logical gap between "is" and "ought: can be soundly bridged, so that one can argue from factual premises to evaluative conclusions. I shall try to show in what follows that both types of arguments fail, beginning with the scriptural argument. [122]

I Corinthians 6 and 7 contains what has been taken by most Christians to be the clearest statement of an objection to premarital sexual relations. But this is mere prejudice. 1 Corinthians 6, which White cites as conclusive evidence for his position, contains as I have shown, a logical problem. It is therefore highly likely that the Pauline view of sexuality is untenable and too uncertain to base any sound reasoning upon. Miles cites 1 Corinthians 7:2 and 1 Thessalonians 4:3-5 also as evidence. [123] He points out that the word 'fornication' (porneia) has three different meanings as used in the New Testament. The word may refer to <u>all</u> sexual immorality in general (as in John 8:41; Acts 15:20, 29; 21-25; Romans 1:29; 1 Corinthians 5:1; 6:13; 18; 11 Corinthians 12:21; Ephesians 5:3). Miles claims that such a use must also include premarital sexual intercourse, including the case we suppose of our two "hot" but loving young virgins. But this is little more than a thinly disguised question begging argument - only because Miles is so confident that all cases of premarital sexual intercourse are morally objectionable does he include it under the heading of general sexual immorality to begin with.

The word 'fornication' is used in Matthew 5:32 and 19:9 as a synonym for the word 'adultery', but in four other passages the words 'adultery' and 'fornication' are both used, which indicates in Miles' opinion that a definite distinction between the two words is being drawn. The passages are Matthew 15:19; Mark 7:21, 1 Corinthians 6:9 and Galatians 5:19. Miles concludes: "Since adultery only includes the behavior of married people, the word fornication would have to mean (among other things) sexual intercourse and other sexual abuses of single people. This is a direct reference to premarital relations. [124]

Miles' argument is invalid. If the word 'fornication' includes all forms of sexual immorality, then a distinction can be drawn between the words 'adultery' and 'fornication', without 'fornication' referring at all to "premarital relations". All the term need refer to is any case of sexual immorality, not involving adultery. There are any number of cases of this: fetishes, sadistic activities, human-animal contacts, and so on. Unless we were already convinced that all premarital sexual relationships were objectionable, then we would have no reason at all as Christians to draw Miles' conclusion.

This leaves us with 1 Corinthians 7:2 and 1 Thessalonians 4:3-5 to consider. The above remarks can be repeated for these passages, with one qualification. Paul says in 1 Corinthians 7:2 that "since there is so much immorality, each man should have his own wife, and each woman her own husband". This would seem to be an inescapable reference to premarital sex, for what other sexual immorality could Paul be referring to? The "other" sexual immorality is prostitution, a topic which must have been fresh on Paul's mind after writing 1 Corinthians 6:12-20. Further we know that in the maritime and commercial city of Corinth, prostitution flourished. According to Hans Licht in Sexual Life in Ancient Greece:

> "Of the wantonness and licentiousness of life in this metropolis of ancient trade, so wealthy and so favoured by nature, it would be difficult to give an account that would err by exaggeration. ... What human fancy elsewhere was content merely to imagine in the way of licentiousness, found in Corinth its home and visible exemplification... The priestesses of venal love crowded about the city in incalculable numbers. In the district of the two

harbours were swarms of brothels of every degree and prostitutes without number lounged about the streets. To a certain extent the focus of unmarried love and the high school of the hetairae was formed by the notorious temple of Venus, in which no fewer than a thousand hetairae or <u>hieroduli</u> (temple-servants), as they were euphemistically called, practised their profession and were always ready to gree their friends". [125]

It is therefore not unreasonable to take prostitution to be the form of immorality referred to by Paul in 1 Corinithians 7:2.

It is of interest to note that most of the kings of the Old Testament had their <u>concubines</u> (e.g. 2 Samuel 15;16; 16:21-22). Now a concubine is a woman who cohabits with a man, usually having sexual relations with him, whilst not being his wife. If the king was unmarried, then he engages in allegedly illicit premarital or non-marital sexual intercourse. If the king was married then he commits adultery. Strangely enough, whilst the Old Testament contains a description of King David's punishment for adultery with Bathsheba (and the murder of her husband Uriah the Hittite in 2 Samuel 11), there is no condemnation of King David keeping his supply of at least ten concubines (2 Samuel 15:16) who by definition were kept on hand for sexual gratification even if they were not actually used. Is there therefore two moral laws: one for the rich and one for the poor? If you feel that historical relativity solves this problem, (translation: that having concubines is ok for David but not for us) then how can you show that historical relativity does not also undermine the Christian's view of the general immorality of homosexuality?

I turn now to a consideration of the social and psychological objections to premarital sexual relations as stated by Miles. [126] The first objection is that premarital sexual intercourse may result in an unplanned or unwanted pregnancy. Whilst advances in contraceptive methods have occurred in recent decades, most teenagers do not have access to effective contraceptives. Hence premarital sexual relations are taken to constitute to a major social problem, and are judged to be morally wrong for that reason (granted we recall, that the is-ought gap can be bridged).

Now the force of this argument can be met in a number of ways, even accepting the severity of the problem of unwanted teenage pregnancies. First, one could take this argument to show that teenagers must have access to effective contraceptives if many social tragedies are to be avoided. Second, Miles' point counts for nothing in the case of our imaginery virgins (1) who may want a child and are prepared to support it, (2) who have effective contraception, even if this involves sterilization or (3) are past the child bearing age any way.

A second objection which also has much emotional force is that premarital sexual relations increase the likelihood of one contracting syphilis, gonorrhea, herpes and AIDS. The contraction of these diseases is a threat to those who practice sexual promiscuity, but is no more a problem to our example of the two virgins who decide to live together than it would be to the paradigm case of a Christian married couple.

Premarital sexual relations are also said by Miles to have a detrimental effect upon the attitude of youth's about the nature of sex. Unsuccessful sexual experiences may shatter the illusions of youth about "perfect sexual fulfilment in their future marriage". [127] Guilt feelings may also be produced which may tend to undermine the couples relationship, feelings that what has been done is wrong. These feelings arise from a conflict between the couple's sexual actions and their own internalized value system. Premarital sexual relations may also promote distrust and suspicion. In reply it may be said that none of these negative consequences may arise. Early sexual experiences if unsuccessful may be looked upon with amusement as a successful learning experience. If the couple did not believe that what they were doing was wrong, and if it was not, then guilt feelings would not be produced. If distrust and suspicion arises in premarital relationships, then perhaps this is more an indication of possessiveness and the desire for ownership of one's love object than an indication of any essential defect in premarital relations in general. In any case we can show that not all premarital sexual relations are morally objectionable on any of these grounds. In the case of our imaginery couple who meet as virgins, without guilt and suspicion, and who obtain sexual happiness, Miles cannot voice any objection, except perhaps to deny that there could be any such couple even approximately. Surely though it is a matter of commonsense knowledge that actual approximates to my imaginery couple exist.

It follows then from the argument of this section that the mainstream Christian moral position on premarital sexual relationship, is unjustified. That at least some premarital sexual relationships are morally wholesome, has not been excluded by either socio-psychological or Biblical arguments. Thus it is logically possible for one to be even a fundamentalist Christian and be involved in a premarital sexual relationship, without being in a state of sin.

According to Miles:

"Homosexuality is an abnormal practice that is a sin against God and His purpose for life. It is a sin against the other person involved. It destroys the normal functions of life and erodes and deforms personality development. Reason, intelligence, common sense, and Christian principles should lead any man (or woman) to reject homosexuality as an acceptable means of meeting sexual needs". [128]

As I have already rejected the view that homosexuality is abnormal, I shall address the question here as to whether reason and Christian principles do indeed lead one to reject homosexuality as an acceptable means of meeting sexual needs.

One of the first references to homosexual activity can be found in the Sodom and Gomorrah story in Genesis 19, where the cities of Sodom and Gomorrah were taken to be destroyed by God because of "offences against nature". That these offences against nature are homosexual acts is generally taken to be shown by Genesis 19:6-11. These verses describe the Sodomites surrounding Lot's house and calling for Lot to surrender his angelic visitors for the purpose of sex. The Hebrew word ya dha means both "to know" and "to have coitus". Indeed "to know" is often used as a metaphor for sexual relations. Some such as John McNeill feel that ya dha in Genesis 19:5 means "to know" without being a metaphor for sexual relations. [129] This interpretation does not square with Genesis 19:8 where Lot offers to the Sodomites his two virgin daughters and McNeill makes no satisfactory attempt to account for Lot's statement. [130] But even if the Sodomites did want to have sex with the angels, this hardly shows that homosexual practices are morally wrong. If the angels were female would one conclude that heterosexual practices are therefore morally wrong? Genesis 19:6-11 is a story about a group of would-be pack rapists who get to see the light the hard way. [131] Lot's behaviour, by the way is hardly God-like. If he was such a hero then he should have stood against the mob, not given in to them and allow his daughters to be offered up like so much meat.

More tougher stuff is found in Leviticus 18:22-23 and Leviticus 20:13. Homosexual relations are clearly and uncontroversially condemned as being "abominations", punishable by death. If one wishes to accept this as the word of God, then one must also accept the following propositions as being also voiced by God: (1) it is wrong to eat the fat of cattle, sheep and goats (Leviticus 7:23); (2) the rabbit is "unclean" (Leviticus 11:6); (3) emissions of semen involve defilement that requires purification (Leviticus 15:16-18); (4) one should not plant two different kinds of seeds in one's fields (Leviticus 19:19) and (5) one should not wear clothing woven of two different kinds of material (Leviticus 19:19). These commands seem to us today to be at worse silly, at best irrelevant. Further God's punishments for sin revolt against the contemporary moral conscience: not only are adultery and homosexuality to be punished by death (Leviticus 20:10; 20:13) but someone who curses his mother or father (Leviticus 20:9) or has sex with a woman during her period must be respectively put to death and cut off from their people. These considerations erode the credibility of Leviticus as anything more than a record of post-exilic Israelite criminal and legal codes.

Judges 19:22-29 contains a variation of the Lot story of Genesis 19. Only here the owner of the house allows a concubine to be raped and murdered. My previous remarks on Genesis 19 can be repeated here.

In the New Testament the three principle references to homosexuality are Romans 1:25-27, 1 Corinthians 6:9 and 1 Timothy 1:9-10. Let us take each of these verses and examine whether these verses lend support to the thesis that all homosexual acts are immoral.

In Romans 1:25-27, Paul describes the "shameful lusts" that all the godless men who have known God, but failed to recognise him and worship him, have been delivered over to. Among such "lusts" are "indecent acts with other men" and these godless men were "inflamed with lust for one another" (Romans 1:27). Now this passage is a condemnation of those who knew God and rejected Him. Their fates were grim and depressing as the spiritual vacuums in their lives were filled eith "shameful lusts". It just so happened that these lusts were predominately of a homosexual orientation. This however shows nothing whatsoever about any alleged moral wrongness of the God-loving homosexual Christian who lives without such lust. The theologians will still tell us that Paul has said that the Godless men abandoned "natural" relationships with women to practice homosexual acts, which must therefore be unnatural. But what is being contrasted here is natural relationships with women-marriage, with <u>lustful</u> relationships with men, relationships which must be adulterous since if natural relationships with women were abandoned then they must first have existed. Hence whatever type of sexual relationship these Godless men would have adopted after "abandoning" their marriages, Paul would have found these relationships morally objectionable (excluding celibacy and possibly masturbation). Hence Romans 1:25-27 lends no support to any Scriptural argument for the immorality of homosexual sexual love.

The key Greek words in 1 Corinthians 6:9 and 1 Timothy 1:9-10 are <u>malakoi</u> and <u>arsenokoitai</u>. The first edition of the Revised Standard version of the Bible translates both terms by use of one word 'homosexuals'. The New International version of the Bible uses the words 'homosexual offenders' in 1 Corinthians 6:9 and 1 Timothy 1:9-10 contains no explicit reference to homosexuality at all. The King James version of the Bible translates them as 'neither the effeminate nor the abusers of themselves with mankind'. It is obvious that the Christian prude must opt for the RSV as the "correct translation". It is doubtful whether any justification can be given for this. Coleman argues that

<u>malakos</u>, which really means 'soft', metaphorically was used by the Greeks to refer to males who played the passive role in homosexual intercourse. [132] McNeill on the other hand points out that <u>malakos</u> is usually employed in the Scriptures in a moral context signifying moral softness or weakness. It is therefore by no means clear that reference is being made to homosexuality at all in these passages. [133]

Finally there have been arguments given from time to time, for the view that Jesus was a homosexual or at least had some homosexual sexual experiences. [134] If a case could be made for this proposal then it destroys with one blow the Church's opposition to homosexual practices in general (and if Jesus did not marry, their opposition to all instances of non-marital sex). The present author shall not pursue this matter here.

Through an examination of the arguments found in Herbert Miles' <u>Sexual Understanding Before Marriage</u> and John White's <u>Eros Defiled</u>, an examination and critique of Christian prudery has been conducted. The conclusion reached is that even taking all <u>prima facie</u> cognitive parts of the Scriptures (translation: the non-poetic stuff that could be either true or false) at face value without any deep historical examination, there is no good reason to believe that the Scriptures condemn <u>all</u> acts of non-marital sexual intercourse. This is a surprising conclusion to reach from within the confines of the Christian scheme of things, and flies against the position of both the Catholic and Reformed traditions. But tradition may be wrong, and it in fact is.

If God has as part of His/Her characterizing essence goodness, then given that He/She can recommend no evil, God's recommendations for morally good sexual relationships cannot differ from the conclusions reached by a correct sexual ethics. Thus in reply to the anguished Christian who feels that the smoking ruins of the received view of sexual morality leaves one in a moral vacuum, we must point him/her in the direction of the theories of sexual ethics. [135] The above arguments undermine, I believe, the Christian Church's <u>rational</u> or argumentative, opposition to the homosexuality issue.

NOTES AND REFERENCES

1. M. Gronfors and O. Stalstrom, "Power, Prestige, Profit: AIDS and the Oppression of Homosexual People", <u>Acta Sociologica</u>, Vol. 30, 1987, pp. 53-66.

2. J.S. Mill, "On Liberty", in J.M. Robson (ed.), <u>John Stuart Mill: A Selection of His Works</u>, (Macmillan, London, 1966), pp. 1-147.

3. A sample of the literature of paternalism: R. Sartorius (ed.) <u>Paternalism</u>, (University of Minnesota Press, Minneapolis, 1983); J. Kleinig, <u>Paternalism</u>, (Rowman and Allanheld, New Jersey, 1983); J.C. Moskop, "Competence, Paternalism, and Public Policy for Mentally Retarded People", <u>Theoretical Medicine</u>, Vol. 4, 1983, pp. 291-302; J.R. Clarke (et al), "The Limits of Paternalism in Emergency Care", <u>Hastings Center Report</u>, Vol. 10, December 1980, pp. 20-22; C.E. Harris, "Paternalism and the Enforcement of Morality", <u>Southwestern Journal of Philosophy</u>, Vol. 8, 1977, pp. 85-93; J.C. Callahan, "Paternalism and Voluntariness", <u>Canadian Journal of Philosophy</u>, Vol. 16, 1986, pp. 199-220; B. Gert and C.M. Culver, "Paternalistic Behavior", <u>Philosophy and Public Affairs</u>, Vol. 6, 1976, pp. 45-57; A. Buchanan, "Medical Paternalism", <u>Philosophy and Public Affairs</u>, Vol. 7, 1978, pp. 370-390; D. VanDeVeer, "Autonomy Respecting Paternalism", <u>Social Theory and Practice</u>, Vol. 6, 1980, pp. 187-207; and "Paternalism and Subsequent Consent", <u>Canadian Journal of Philosophy</u>, Vol. 9, 1979, pp. 631-642; N. Fotion, "Paternalism", <u>Ethics</u>, Vol. 89, 1979, pp. 191-198; R.J. Arneson, "Mill versus Paternalism", <u>Ethics</u>, Vol. 90, 1980, pp. 470-489; E.P. Brandon, "Rationality and Paternalism", <u>Philosophy</u>, Vol. 57, 1982, pp. 533-536; A. Soble, "Paternalism, Liberal Theory and Suicide", <u>Canadian Journal of Philosophy</u>, Vol. 12, 1982, pp. 335-352; D.W. Brock, "Paternalism and Autonomy", <u>Ethics</u>, Vol. 98, 1988, pp. 550-565; J. Feinberg, <u>Harm to Self</u>, (Oxford University Press, Oxford, 1986); P. Hobson, "Another Look at Paternalism", <u>Journal of Applied Philosophy</u>, Vol. 1, 1984, pp. 293-304; R. Cater, "Justifying Paternalism", <u>Canadian Journal of Philosophy</u>, Vol. 7, 1977, pp. 133-145; J. Woodward, "Paternalism and Justification", <u>Canadian Journal of Philosophy</u>, Supp. Vol. 8, 1982, pp. 67-89; R. Young, "Autonomy and Paternalism", <u>Canadian Journal of Philosophy</u>, Vol. 8, 1982, pp. 47-66; F. D'Agostino, "Mill, Paternalism and Psychiatry", <u>Australasian Journal of Philosophy</u>, Vol. 60, December, 1982, pp. 319-330; B.J. Boughton, "Compulsory Health and Safety in a Free Society", <u>Journal of Medical Ethics</u>, Vol. 10, 1984, pp. 186-190; O. O'Neill, "Paternalism and Partial Autonomy", <u>Journal of Medical Ethics</u>, Vol. 10, 1984, pp. 173-178;

G. Dworkin, "Paternalism", *Monist*, Vol. 56, 1972, pp. 64-84; G.B. Weiss, "Paternalism Modernised", *Journal of Medical Ethics*, Vol. 11, 1985, pp. 184-187; R. Tur, "Paternalism and the Criminal Law", *Journal of Applied Philosophy*, Vol. 2, 1985, pp. 173-189; C.L. Ten, "Paternalism and Morality", *Ratio*, Vol. XIII, 1971, pp. 56-66, and "Paternalism and Levels of Knowledge: A Comment on Rainbolt", *Bioethics*, Vol. 3, 1989, pp. 135-139; G.W. Rainbolt, "Prescription Drug Laws: Justified Hard Paternalism", *Bioethics*, Vol. 3, 1989, pp. 45-58; M. Strasser, "Mill and the Utility of Liberty", *Philosophical Quarterly*, Vol. 34, 1984, pp. 63-68.

4. Mill, op.cit., note 2, pp. 13-14.

5. ibid p. 17.

6. E.D. Pellegrino, "Autonomy and Coercion in Disease Prevention and Health Promotion", *Theoretical Medicine*, Vol. 5, 1984, pp. 83-91. Citation p. 89.

7. E.D. Cohen, "Paternalism that does not Restrict Individuality: Criteria and Applications", *Social Theory and Practice*, Vol. 12, 1986, pp. 309-335.

8. J. Feinberg, "Legal Paternalism", *Canadian Journal of Philosophy*, Vol. 1, No. 1, 1971, pp. 105-124.

9. R. Routley and V. Routley, "The Irrefutability of Anarchism", *Social Alternatives*, Vol. 2, 1982, pp. 23-29.

10. D.A. Conway, "AIDS and Legal Paternalism", *Social Theory and Practice*, Vol. 13, 1987, pp. 287-302.

11. ibid, p. 300.

12. *Washington Post*, Nov. 9, 1985, at D3, col. 1, quoted from Anon. "The Constitutional Rights of AIDS Carriers", *Harvard Law Review*, Vol. 99, 1986, pp. 1274-1292. Citation p. 1282.

13. J. Grutsch and A.D. Robertson, "The Coming of AIDS: It Didn't Start with Homosexuals and it Won't End with Them", *American Spectator*, Vol. 19, 1986, pp. 12-15. Cited from L. Gostin and W.J. Curran, "The Limits of Compulsion in Controlling AIDS", *Hastings Center Report*, Vol. 16, December 1986, pp. 24-29, p. 26.

14. W.E. Parmet, "AIDS and Quarantine: The Revival of An Archaic Doctrine", *Hofstra Law Review*, Vol. 14, 1985-86, pp. 53-90.

15. Gostin and Curran, op.cit., note 13, p. 26.

16. Anon, op.cit., note 12, p. 1283.

17. ibid, pp. 1283-1284.

18. Gostin and Curran, op.cit., note 13.

19. D.F. Musto, "Quarantine and the Problem of AIDS", <u>Milbank Quarterly</u>, Vol. 64, 1986, pp. 97-117.

20. J.A. Gleason, "Quarantine: An Unreasonable Solution to the AIDS Dilemma", <u>Cincinnati Law Review</u>, Vol. 55, 1986-87, pp. 217-235.

21. N.L. Ford and M.D. Quam, "AIDS Quarantine", <u>Journal of Legal Medicine</u>, Vol. 8, 1987, pp. 353-396.

22. R. Elsberry, "AIDS Quarantine in England and the United States", <u>Hastings International and Comparative Law Review</u>, Vol. 10, 1986, pp. 113-157.

23. Quoted from D.J. Mayo, "AIDS, Quarantines, and Noncompliant Positives", in C. Pierce and D. VanDeVeer (eds.) <u>AIDS, Ethics and Public Policy</u>, (Wadsworth, Belmont, 1988), pp. 113-123. Citation p. 113.

24. R. Hicks, "AIDS: The Second Wave", <u>The Australian Magazine</u>, July 1-2, 1989, pp. 8-18. Citation pp. 10-11 "Marianne's Story". On AIDS and prostitution cf. W.H. Patterson, "Prostitution and Sexually Transmitted Disease", <u>Medical Journal of Australia</u>, Vol. 140, 1984, pp. 252-253; R. Taylor, "AIDS and Prostitution" in A. Carr (ed.) <u>Meeting the Challenge: Papers of the First National Conference on AIDS</u>, (Australian Government Publishing Service, Canberra, 1986), pp. 130-133; R. Taylor, "'He Who Pays the Piper': AIDS and Prostitution in Sydney", in Carr (ed.) ibid pp. 133-138; "Infected Prostitutes Continue to Work", <u>New Scientist</u>, 14 April, 1988, p. 26; M.J. Rosenberg and J.M. Weiner, "Prostitutes and AIDS: A Health Department Priority?" <u>American Journal of Public Health</u>, Vol. 78, 1988, pp. 418-423; D.A. Cooper and A.J. Dodds, "AIDS and Prostitutes", <u>Medical Journal of Australia</u>, Vol. 145, 1986, pp. 54-55; J.K. Kreiss (et al), "AIDS Virus Infection in Nairobi Prostitutes", <u>New England Journal of Medicine</u>, Vol. 314, 1986, pp. 414-418; J. Mann (et al) "Condom Use and HIV Infection Among Prostitutes in Zaire", <u>New England Journal of Medicine</u>, Vol. 316, 1987, p. 345; S.E. Barton (et al) "Female Prostitutes and Sexually Transmitted Diseases", <u>British Journal of Hospital Medicine</u>, Vol. 38, 1987, pp. 34-45. On the social and legal ramifications of prostitution cf. L. White, "Prostitution, Identity, and Class Consciousness in Nairobi During World War II", <u>Signs</u>, Vol. 11, 1986, pp. 255-273; D.K. Weisberg, <u>Children of the Night: A Study of Adolescent Prostitution</u>, (Lexington Books,

Lexington, 1985); M. Kanter, "Prohibit or Rgulate? The Fraser Report and New Approaches to Pornography and Prostitution", Osgoode Hall Law Journal, Vol. 23, 1985, pp. 171-194; M.H. Silbert and A.M. Pines, "Early Sexual Exploitation as an Influence in Prostitution", Social Work, Vol. 28, 1983, pp. 285-289; J.A. Scutt, "The Economic Regulation of the Brothel Industry in Victoria", Australian Law Journal, Vol. 60, 1986, pp. 399-406; M.S. Caughey, "The Principle of Harm and Its Applicaton to Laws Criminalizing Prostitution", Denver Law Journal, Vol. 51, 1974, pp. 235-262; E.M. Abramson, "A Note on Prostitution: Victims Without Crime - Or There's No Crime but the Victim is Ideology", Duquesne Law Review, Vol. 17, 1978 - 79, pp. 355-379; C. Rosenbleet and B.J. Pariente, "The Prostitution of the Criminal Law", American Criminal Law Review, Vol. 11, 1973, pp. 373-427; M.K. Lindsay, "Prostitution - Delinquency's Time Bomb", Crime and Delinquency, Vol. 16, 1970, pp. 151-157; D.E. Wade, "Prostitution and the Law: Emerging Attacks on the "Women's Crime"," UMKC Law Review, Vol. 43, 1975, pp. 413-428; J. Benjamin, "The Bonds of Love: Rational Violence and Erotic Domination", Feminist Studies, Vol. 6, 1980, pp. 144-174; K. Barry, Female Sexual Slavery, (Prentice-Hall Inc., New Jersey, 1979); J.R. Walkowitz, "Male Vice and Feminist Virtue: Feminism and the Politics of Prostitution in Nineteenth Century Britain", History Workshop Journal, Vol. 13, 1982, pp. 79-93; M. Neave, "The Failure of Prostitution Law Reform", Australian and New Zealand Journal of Criminology, Vol. 21, 1988, pp. 202-213; R.J. McMullen, "Youth Prostitution: A Balance of Power", Journal of Adolescence, Vol. 10, 1987, pp. 35-43; L. Dominelli, "The Power of the Powerless: Prostitution and the Reinforcement of Submissive Feminitiy", Sociological Review, Vol. 34, 1986, pp. 65-92; L. Savitz and L. Rosen, "The Sexuality of Prostitutes: Sexual Enjoyment Reported by "Streetwalkers", Journal of Sex Research, Vol. 24, 1988, pp. 200-208; M.E. Brown, "Teenage Prostitution", Adolescence, Vol. XIV, 1979, pp. 665-680; D.K. Weisberg, "Children of the Night: The Adequacy of Statutory Treatment of Juvenile Prostitution", American Journal of Criminal Law, Vol. 12, 1984, pp. 1-67; R.I. Parnas, "Legislative Reform of Prostitution Laws: Keeping Commercial Sex out of Sight and out of Mind", Santa Clara Law Review, Vol. 21, 1981, pp. 669-696; J. Cassels, "Prostitution and Public Nuisance: Desperate Measures and the Limits of Civil Adjudication", Canadian Bar Review, Vol. 63, 1985, pp. 764-804; C.D. Perry, "Right of Privacy Challenges to Prostitution Statutes", Washington University Law Quarterly, Vol. 58, 1980, pp. 439-480; R. Symanski, The Immoral Landscape: Female Prostitution in Western Societies, (Butterworths, Toronto, 1981); J. Kaplan, "Non-Victim Crime and the Regulation of Prostitution", West Virginia Law Review, Vol. 79, 1977, pp. 593-606; J.R. Walkowitz, "The

Politics of Prostitution", in C.R. Stimpson (et al) *Women: Sex and Sexuality*, (University of Chicago Press, Chicago, 1980), pp. 145-157; N. Erbe, "Prostitutes: Victims of Men's Exploitation and Abuse", *Law and Inequality*, Vol. 2, 1984, pp. 609-628.

25. B. Russell, "Prostitution", *Marriage and Morals*, (George Allen and Unwin, London, 1958), pp. 116-124.

26. C. Pateman, *The Sexual Contract*, (Polity Press, Oxford, 1988).

27. cf. J.R. Richards, *The Sceptical Feminist*, (Penguin Books, Harmondsworth, 1980; D.A.J. Richards, *Sex, Drugs, Death and the Law*, (Rowman and Littlefield, New Jersey, 1982) and "Commercial Sex and the Rights of the Person: A Moral Argument for the Decriminalization of Prostitution", *University of Pennsylvania Law Review*, Vol. 127, 1979, pp. 1195-1287.

28. Pateman, op.cit., note 26, p. 194.

29. ibid, p. 208.

30. L. Shrage, "Should Feminists Oppose Prostitution?", *Ethics*, Vol. 99, 1989, pp. 347-361.

31. ibid, p. 349.

32. Erbe, op.cit., note 24. Citation p. 621.

33. M. Scherzer, "Insurance", in H.L. Dalton (et al((eds.) *AIDS and the Law: A Guide for the Public*, (Yale University Press, New Haven, 1987), pp. 185-200; M. Neave, "AIDS and the Life Insurance Industry Code of Practice", in Department of Community Services and Health (ed.) *Report of the Third National Conference on AIDS* (Australian Government Publishing Service, Canberra, 1988), pp. 651-656. G.M. Oppenheimer and R.A. Padgug, "AIDS: The Risks to Insurers, the Threat to Equity", *Hastings Center Report*, Vol. 16, October 1986, pp. 18-22; R.R. Faden and N.E. Kass, "Health Insurance and AIDS: The Status of State Regulatory Activity", *American Journal of Public Health*, Vol. 78, 1988, pp. 437-438; J.D. Hammond and A.F. Shapiro, "AIDS and the Limits of Insurability", *Milbank Quarterly*, Vol. 64, 1986, pp. 143-167; B. Schatz, "The AIDS Insurance Crisis: Underwriting or Overreaching?" *Harvard Law Review*, Vol. 100, 1987, pp. 1782-1805; J.N. Hoffman and E.Z. Kincaid, "AIDS: The Challenge to Life and Health Insurers' Freedom of Contract", *Drake Law Review*, Vol. 35, 1986-87, pp. 709-771; Rationale for AIDS-Related Testing", *Harvard Law Review*, Vol. 100, 1987, pp. 1806-1825.

34. E.H. Loewy, "AIDS and the Physician's Fear of Contagion", Chest, Vol. 89, No. 3, March 1986, pp. 325-326 and E.J. Emanuel, "Do Physicians Have an Obligation to Treat Patients with AIDS?", New England Journal of Medicine, Vol. 318, 1988, pp. 1686-1690.

35. A.M. Campbell, The Black Death and Men of Learning, (AMS Press, New York, 1966).

36. E.H. Loewy, op.cit., note 34, p. 325.

37. C. Thompson (et al), "AIDS: Dilemmas for the Psychiatrist", Lancet, Vol. 1, No. 8475, February 1, 1986, pp. 269-270.

38. Dr. N. Kinny, "AIDS - Closet Gays Accused", The Australian, Monday July 10, 1989, p. 12.

39. Quoted from the Sunday Mail (Adelaide), July 23, 1989, p. 2. This debate is a strong confirmation of the following allegation by Daniel Fox:

    "Controversies about disease reporting in the present as in the past must be understood as political conflicts; that is, conflicts about power and about values. The critical issues have never been scientific or technological. Debates about reporting have always been about ideology, about the distribution of authority within the medical profession, about the relationship between medical and general politics, and about competing social values".

    D.M. Fox, "From TB to AIDS: Value Conflicts in Reporting Disease", Hasting Center Report, Vol. 16, December 1986, pp. 11-16. Citation pp. 15-16.

40. On the testing issue cf. T.L. Crenshaw, "HIV Testing: Voluntary, Mandatory, or Routine?" Humanist, Vol. 48, January-February 1988, pp. 29-34; M.L. Closen (et al) "AIDS: Testing Democracy-Irrational Responses to the Public Health Crisis and the Need for Privacy in Serologic Testing", John Marshall Law Review, Vol. 19, 1986, pp. 835-928; L.O. Gostin (et al), "The Case Against Compulsory Casefinding in Controlling AIDS-Testing, Screening and Reporting", American Journal of Law and Medicine, Vol. 12, 1987, pp. 7-53; T.L. Banks and R.R. McFadden, "Rush to Judgement: HIV Test Reliability and Screening", Tulsa Law Journal, Vol. 23, 1987, pp. 1-35.

41. A. Carr, "Uses and Abuses of the HIV Antibody Test", in Report of the Third National Conference on AIDS, op.cit Note 23, pp. 658-661. Citation pp. 660-661.

42. G.J. Murakawa (et al) "Direct Detection of HIV-1 RNA from AIDS and ARC Patient Samples", *D.N.A.* Vol. 7, 1988, pp. 287-295.

43. Anon. "Recommendations for Preventing Transmission of HIV in Health Care Settings", *Canadian Medical Association Journal*, Vol. 138, 1988, pp. 213-219.

44. P. Rigby, "Doctor with AIDS Sue for $175m", *The Advertiser* (Adelaide), Thursday September 22, 1988; D.M. Barnes, "AIDS Virus Creates Lab Risk", *Science*, Vol. 239, 1988, pp. 348-349; D.M. Barnes, "Health Workers and AIDS: Questions Persist", *Science*, Vol. 241, 1988, pp. 161-162.

45. T.W. Harding, "AIDS in Prison", *Lancet*, November 28, 1987, pp. 1260-1263.

46. R.V. Berkmoes, "AIDS Deaths Fuel Concern for Spread in Jails", *American Medical News*, Vol. 29, 1986, p. 7; G.E. Glass (et al) "Seroprevalence of HIV Antibody Among Individuals Entering the Iowa Prison System", *American Journal of Public Health*, Vol. 78, 1988, pp. 447-449.

47. H. Rowe, "Death Row: AIDS is Turning a Prison Term into a Potential Death Sentence", *California Lawyer*, Vol. 7, 1987, pp. 49-51.

48. P. Hackett, "AIDS Problem in Jails Understated Letter Reveals", *The Advertiser*, Wednesday June 21, 1989, p.10.

49. P. Hackett, "Prison Crisis Looms, Govt. Warned", *The Advertiser*, Tuesday July 4, 1989, p. 3.

50. L. Gostin (et al), "AIDS Screening, Confidentiality, and the Duty to Warn", *American Journal of Public Health*, Vol. 77, 1987, pp. 361-365. Citation p. 364; cf. also G.P. Wormser, "AIDS in Prisons", in G.P. Wormser (ed.) *AIDS and other Manifestations of HIV Infection*, (Noyes Publications, New Jersey, 1987), pp. 48-66; P.A. Wagner, "AIDS and the Criminal Justice System", in W.H.L. Dornette (ed), *AIDS and the Law*, (John Wiley, New York, 1987), pp. 177-193; L.J. Moriarty, "AIDS in Correctional Institutions: The Legal Aspects", *Criminal Law Bulletin*, Vol. 23, 1987, pp. 533-549.

51. R. Macklin, "Predicting Dangerousness and the Public Health Response to AIDS", *Hastings Center Report*, Vol. 16, December 1986, pp. 16-23. Citation p. 21.

52. Anon., "WHO Consultation on Prevention and Control of AIDS in Prisons", *Lancet*, November 28, 1987, pp. 1263-1264.

53. cf. I. Taylor, <u>Law and Order: Arguments for Socialism</u>, (Macmillan, London, 1981) for arguments and references.

54. On the philosophical issue of punishment cf. C.S. Niro, "A Consensual Theory of Punishment", <u>Philosophy and Public Affairs</u>, Vol. 12, 1983, pp. 289-306; A.H. Goldman, "The Paradox of Punishment", <u>Philosophy and Public Affairs</u>, Vol. 9, 1979, pp. 42-58; G. Sher, "An Unsolved Problem about Punishment", <u>Social Theory and Practice</u>, Vol. 4, No. 2, 1977, pp. 149-165; W. Quinn, "The Right to Threaten and the Right to Punish", <u>Philosophy and Public Affairs</u>, Vol. 14, 1985, pp. 327-373; K. McCormick, "Mentezin: On the Problem of the Rehabilitation of Criminals", <u>Ratio</u>, Vol. 18, 1976, pp. 156-162.

On the problems of prison management cf. W.C. Paterson, "Changing Philosophies and Prison Management", <u>Australian and New Zealand Journal of Criminology</u>, Vol. 21, 1988, pp. 214-226.

55. T.F. Silverstein, "AIDS and Employment: An Epidemic Strikes the Workplace and the Law", <u>Whittier Law Review</u>, Vol. 8, 1987, pp. 651-680. Citation p. 664; cf. also R. Roden, "Educating through the Law: The Los Angeles AIDS Discrimination Ordinance", <u>UCLA Law Review</u>, Vol. 33, 1986, pp. 1410-1441.

56. E. Harrington, "A Fatal Bias: AIDS and Minorities", <u>Human Rights</u>, Vol. 14, No. 3, 1987, pp. 34-37, 52. Citation p.34.

57. On AIDS in the schools cf. D. Nelkin and S. Hilgartner, "Disputed Dimensions of Risk: A Public School Controversy over AIDS", <u>Milbank Quarterly</u>, Vol. 64, 1986, pp. 118-142; L. Hammett, "Protecting Children with AIDS Against Arbitrary Exclusion from School", <u>California Law Review</u>, Vol. 74, 1986, pp. 1373-1407; R. Weiner, <u>AIDS: Impact on the Schools</u>, (Education Research Group, Arlington, 1986); F.A.O. Schwartz and F.P. Schaffer, "AIDS in the Classroom", <u>Hofstra Law Review</u>, Vol. 14, 1985, pp. 163-191; S.M. Price, "Fear and Loathing in the Classroom: AIDS and Public Education", <u>Journal of Legislation</u>, Vol. 14, 1987, pp. 87-105; G.J. Heaney, "The Constitutional Right of Informational Privacy: Does It Protect Children Suffering from AIDS?", <u>Fordham Urban Law Journal</u>, Vol. XIV, 1986, pp. 927-969.

58. G.A. Partida, "AIDS: Do Children with AIDS Have a Right to Attend School?" <u>Pepperdine Law Review</u>, Vol. 13, 1986, pp. 1041-1061. Citation p. 1052.

59. ibid, p. 1060.

60. B.A. Krusen, "AIDS in the Classroom: Room for Reason Amidst Paranoia", <u>Dickinson Law Review</u>, Vol. 91, 1987, pp. 1055-1083.

61. ibid, p. 1083.

62. L.N. Brockman, "Enforcing the Right to a Public Education for Children Afflicted with AIDS", <u>Emory Law Journal</u>, Vol. 36, 1987, pp. 603-648. Citation p. 634.

63. L. Taylor, "AIDS Sufferers 'Need Legal Protection'", <u>The Australian</u>, Monday May 8, 1989, pp. 1-2.

64. On AIDS and employment cf. R. Pargetter and E.W. Prior, "Discrimination and AIDS", <u>Social Theory and Practice</u>, Vol. 13, 1987, pp. 129-153; H.E. Cooperman, "AIDS and Pregnancy Discrimination", <u>Trial</u>, Vol. 24, 1988, pp. 14-17; M.J. Lazzo, "Recent Developments: Public Health and Employment Issues Generated by the AIDS Crisis", <u>Washburn Law Journal</u>, Vol. 25, 1985-86, pp. 505-535; J.P. Vladeck, "Is AIDS a Disability?", <u>The Practical Lawyer</u>, Vol. 32, 1986, pp. 13-21; M. Landolt, "Are AIDS Victims Handicapped?", <u>Saint Louis University Law Journal</u>, Vol. 31, 1987, pp. 729-747; R.A. Harder, "A Legal Guide for the Education of Legislators Facing the Inevitable Question: AIDS: The Problem is Real - What Do We Do?", <u>Journal of Contemporary Law</u>, Vol. 13, 1987, pp. 121-160; B.M. Dickens, "Legal Rights and Duties in the AIDS Epidemic", <u>Science</u>, Vol. 239, 1988, pp. 580-586; P.A. Curylo, "AIDS and Employment Discrimination: Should AIDS be Considered a Handicap?", <u>Wayne Law Review</u>, Vol. 33, 1987, pp. 1095-110; A.S. Leonard, "AIDS and Employment: Bibliographic Resources", <u>The Labor Lawyer</u>, Vol. 3, 1987, pp. 299-309; J.H. Leader, "Running from Fear Itself: Analyzing Employment Discrimination Against Persons with AIDS and Other Communicable Diseases Under Section 504 of the Rehabilitation Act of 1973", <u>Willamette Law Review</u>, Vol. 23, 1987, pp. 857-936; R.E. Stein, "Strategies for Dealing with AIDS Disputes in the Workplace", <u>The Arbitration Journal</u>, Vol. 42, 1987, pp. 21-29; T.E. Loscalzo, "AIDS in the Workplace: How Should Corporate America Cope?", <u>Delaware Journal of Corporate Law</u>, Vol. 12, 1987, pp. 527-561; M.A.E. Rousseau, "The AIDS Epidemic and the Issues in the Workplace", <u>Massachusetts Law Review</u>, Vol. 12, 1987, pp. 51-69; A.S. Leonard, "AIDS and Employment Law Revisited", <u>Hofstra Law Review</u>, Vol. 14, 1985, pp. 11-51; D. Brahams, "AIDS and the Law", <u>New Law Journal</u>, August 14, 1987, pp. 749-751; N. Fafan and D. Newell, "AIDS and Employment Law", ibid, pp. 752-754; W.F. Banta, <u>AIDS in the Workplace</u>, (Lexington Books, Massachusetts, 1988); M.D. Witt (ed.) <u>AIDS and Patient Management</u>, (National Health Publishing, Owing Mills, 1986); M.D. Kirby, "AIDS Legislation - Turning Up the Heat?", <u>Australian Law Journal</u>, Vol. 60, 1986, pp. 324-

332; D. Buchanan and J. Godwin, "AIDS - the Legal Epidemic", <u>Legal Service Bulletin</u>, Vol. 13, 1988, pp. 111-137; D.W. Myers and P.S. Myers, "Arguments Involving AIDS Testing in the Workplace", <u>Labor Law Journal</u>, Vol. 38, 1987, pp. 582-590; D.B. Ritter and R. Turner, "AIDS: Employer Concerns and Options", <u>Labor Law Journal</u>, Vol. 38, 1987, pp. 67-83.

65. J.H. Carey and M.M. Arthur, "The Developing Law on AIDS in the Workplace", <u>Maryland Law Review</u>, Vol. 46, 1987, pp. 284-319; D. Robinson, "AIDS and the Criminal Law: Traditional Approaches and a New Statutory Proposal", <u>Hofstra Law Review</u>, Vol. 14, 1985-86, pp. 91-105; D.P. Brigham, "You Never Told Me ... You Never Asked; Tort Liability for the Sexual Transmission of AIDS", <u>Dickinson Law Review</u>, Vol. 91, 1986-87, pp. 529-552; R. Smith Fredrickson, "Tort Liability for AIDS.', <u>Houston Law Review</u>, Vol. 24, 1987, pp. 957-990.

66. On the issue of blaming and discrimination with respect to homosexuality cf. S. Seidman, "Transfiguring Sexual Identity: AIDS and the Contemporary Construction of Homosexuality", <u>Social Text</u>, 19/20, Fall, 1988, pp. 187-205: "AIDS has provided a pretext to reinsert homosexuality within a symbolic drama of pollution and purity". (p.189); D. Nelkin and S.L. Gilman, "Placing Blame for Devastating Disease", <u>Social Research</u>, Vol. 55, 1988, pp. 361-378; R. Poirier, "AIDS and Traditions of Homophobia", <u>Social Research</u>, Vol. 55, 1988, pp. 461-475; D. Altman, <u>AIDS and the New Puritanism</u>, (Pluto Press, London, 1986); R. Shilts, <u>And the Band Played On: Politics, People and the AIDS Epidemic</u>, (Penguin Books, London, 1987), S.J. Palmer, "AIDS as Metaphor", <u>Transaction Social Science and Modern Society</u>, Vol. 26, 1989, pp. 44-50. More general but relevant material includes J.D. Baldwin and J.I. Baldwin, "Factors Affecting AIDS-Related Sexual Risk-Taking Behavior Among College Students", <u>Journal of Sex Research</u>, Vol. 25, 1988, pp. 181-196; S. Harding, "The Decline of Permissiveness", <u>New Statesman and Society</u>, Vol. 1, No. 22, 1988, pp. 25-26; D.R. Bolling, and B. Voeller, "AIDS and Heterosexual Anal Intercourse", <u>Journal of the American Medical Association</u>, Vol. 258, 1987, p. 474; G.J.P. van Griensven (et al), "Risk Factors and Prevalence of HIV Antibodies in Homosexual Men in the Netherlands", <u>American Journal of Epidemiology</u>, Vol. 125, 1987, pp. 1048-1057; A.R. Moss (et al), "Risk Factors for AIDS and HIV Seropositivity in Homosexual Men", <u>American Journal of Epidemiology</u>, Vol. 125, 1987, pp. 1035-1047; M. Ross and P. Herbert, "Responses of Homosexual Men to AIDS", <u>Medical Journal of Australia</u>, Vol. 146, 1987, p. 280; G.A. Richwald (et al), "Sexual Activities in Bathhouses in Los Angeles County: Implications for AIDS Prevention Education", <u>Journal of Sex Research</u>, Vol. 25, 1988, pp. 169-179; L.J. Bauman

and K. Siegel, "Misperception Among Gay Men of the Risk for AIDS Associated with their Sexual Behavior", **Journal of Applied Social Psychology**, Vol. 17, 1987, pp. 329-350; J. Chettle, "Post Coitum Tristrum", **Policy Review**, Spring, No. 32, 1985, pp. 66-68; M.F. Goldsmith, "Sex in the Age of AIDS calls for Common Sense and 'Condom Sense'," **Journal of the American Medical Association**, Vol. 257, 1987, pp. 2261-2263, 2266; M.W. Ross, "Problems Associated with Condom use in Homosexual Men", **American Journal of Public Health**, Vol. 77, 1987, p. 877.

67. T.R. Mendicino, "Characterization and Disease: Homosexuals and the Threat of AIDS", **North Carolina Law Review**, Vol. 66, 1987, pp. 226-250.

68. These writings should be viewed in the context that homosexuality is still illegal in a number of Australian states; the "crime" of sodomy carries a maximum penalty of 14 years imprisonment in Queensland. A gay couple appeared in court in Queensland in 1988 on the charge of sodomy, although in private, but fortunately received a fine and a twelve month good behaviour bond rather than a lengthy gaol term. For legal reasoning criticizing these type of laws cf. A. Khan, "The Invasion of Sexual Privacy", **San Diego Law Review**, Vol. 23, 1986, pp. 957-977; D.A.J. Richards, **Sex, Drugs, Death and the Law**, (Rowman and Littlefield, Totowa, 1982).

69. T. Aubin, "No Gaiety as AIDS Debate becomes a Battle", **The Australian**, Monday July 3, 1989, p. 5.

70. J. Allender, "Experts Attack Nats' View AIDS Just Gay Disease", **The Australian**, Tuesday July 4, 1989, p. 5.

71. A. Landsdown, "The Politics of AIDS", **Quadrant**, Vol. 31, March 1987, pp. 28-34. Citation p. 30.

72. ibid, p. 32.

73. N. Podhoretz, "It is Clear AIDS is No Threat to the Public at Large", **The Weekend Australian**, January 9-10, 1988, p. 18.

74. N. Podhoretz, "It's Time to Sheet Blame for AIDS Home to Homosexual Men", **The Weekend Australian**, October 31-November 1, 1987, p. 24.

75. B.A. Santamaria, "AIDS and the Fatal Price of Gay Abandon", **The Australian**, Tuesday March 14, 1989.

76. H. Caton, "The AIDS Apocalypse", **Quadrant**, Vol. 29, November 1985, pp. 27-29. Citation p. 28.

77. J. McPherson (ed.) <u>AIDS and Compassion</u>, (St. Mark's, Canberra, 1988).

78. J. Woodley, "Surf, Sex and Sin (or How the New Right has Side-Tracked the Church's Social Justice Agenda)", <u>Social Alternatives</u>, Vol. 7, No. 3, 1988, pp. 17-20. Citation p. 18. It is also pleasing, at least to progressives to see the article by J.B. Nelson, "Need: A Continuing Sexual Revolution", <u>The Christian Century</u>, June 1, 1988, pp. 538-542:

"We must also confront homophobia, which has effects beyond gays, lesbians and bisexuals. Rooted as it is in male sexism, homophobia undermines male friendships, bolsters the oppression of women and contributes fearsomely to our social violence. Though its varied dynamics are complex, the root cause of homophobia is always fear, and the gospel has resources for dealing with fear" (p.541).

79. J.S. Murray, "When Bishops Cast the First Stone", <u>The Australian</u>, Friday December 30, 1988, p. 7.

80. Interview with S. Rogers, "Can God Change Gays?", <u>On Being</u>, Vol. 15, No. 7, August 1988, pp. 10-12.

81. ibid, p. 12.

82. G. Reid, <u>Beyond AIDS</u>, (Kingsway Publications, Eastbourne, 1987).

83. D. Hinch, <u>AIDS: Most of the Questions, Some of the Answers</u>, (Bay Street Publishing, Melbourne, 1987), p. 97.

84. P. Adams, "AIDS Ads: Making War on Love", <u>The Weekend Australian</u>, December 24-25, 1988, Weekend 2 and "The AIDS War and the Gust Factor", <u>The Weekend Australian</u>, April 15-16, 1989, weekend 2.

85. cf. M. Ragg, "AIDS - Why the Full Truth hasn't been Told", <u>The Australian</u>, Monday October 3, 1988, p. 11; M.A. Fumento, "AIDS: Are Heterosexuals at Risk?", <u>Commentary</u>, Vol. 84, 1987, pp. 21-27.

86. V. Lorian, "AIDS, Anal Sex and Heterosexuals", <u>The Lancet</u>, May 14, 1988, p.1111.

87. T.C. Quinn, "AIDS in Africa: Evidence for Heterosexual Transmission of the Human Immunodeficiency Virus", <u>New York State Journal of Medicine</u>, May 1987, pp. 286-289 and (et al), "AIDS in Africa: An Epidemiological Paradigm", <u>Science</u>, Vol. 234, 1986, pp. 955-963.

88. M.E. van der Ende, (et al), "Heterosexual Transmission

of HIV by Haemophiliacs", *British Medical Journal*, Vol. 297, 1988, pp. 1102-1103.

89. J. Dwyer, "Tuckey Versus the Rest", *The Australian*, Thursday, August 18, 1988, p. 9.

90. S. Kingman and S. Cannor, "The Answer is Still a Condom", *New Scientist*, Vol. 118, 23 June 1988, pp. 33-37.

91. R.J. Stoller, *Perversion: The Erotic Form of Hatred*, (Pantheon Books, New York, 1975), pp. 197-201.

92. American Psychiatric Association, *Diagnostic and Statistical Manual of Mental Disorders*, 3rd edition, (American Psychiatric Assocation, Washington D.C., 1968). For a critique of the APA's pre-1973 view of homosexuality as a disorder cf. J. Margolis, "The Question of Homosexuality", in R. Baker and F. Elliston (eds.), *Philosophy and Sex*, (Prometheus Books, New York, 1975), pp. 288-302.

93. Stoller, op.cit., Note 91, pp. 197-198.

94. cf. I. Bieber, H.J. Dain, P.R. Dince, M.G. Drellich, H.G. Grand, R.H. Gundlach, M.W. Kremer, A.H. Rifkin, G.B. Wilbur and T.B. Bieber, *Homosexuality*, (Basic Books, New York, 1962); C.W. Socarides, *The Overt Homosexual*, (Grune and Stratton, New York, 1968).

95. S. Goldberg, "What is 'Normal'?, Logical Aspects of the Question of Homosexual Behavior", *Psychiatry*, Vol. 38, 1975, pp. 227-243.

96. M. Levin, "Why Homosexuality is Abnormal", *Monist*, Vol. 67, 1984, pp. 251-283; cf also T.F. Murphy, "Homosexuality and Nature: Happiness and the law at Stake", *Journal of Applied Philosophy*, Vol. 4, 1987, pp. 195-204, D. Levy, "Perversion and the Unnatural as Moral Categories", *Ethics*, Vol. 90, 1980, pp. 191-202 and M. Ruse, *Homosexuality: A Philosophical Inquiry*, (Basil Blackwell, Oxford, 1988). Ruse's claim that there is something ultimately unsatisfactory about the homosexual lifestyle under the image of the gay bath houses, involves as R. Porter, "Talking Man to Man", *Nature*, Vol. 334, 1988, p.660, a logical slide from the ethics of homosexuality to the problem of promiscuity.

97. cf. M. Slote, "Inapplicable Concepts and Sexual Perversion", in Baker and Elliston, op.cit., Note 2, pp. 261-267. Citation pp. 261-262.

98. For a critique of sociobiology cf. my *Reductionism and Cultural Being*, (Martinus Nijhoff, The Hague, 1984).

99. T. Nagel, "Sexual Perversion", Journal of Philosophy, Vol. LXVI, 1969, pp. 5-17.

100. R. Solomon, "Sex and Perversion", in Baker and Elliston, op.cit., Note 92, pp. 268-287.

101. Stoller, op.cit., Note 91, p. 3.

102. ibid, p. 4.

103. Levin, op.cit., Note 96, p. 251.

104. ibid, p. 251.

105. ibid, p. 256.

106. ibid, p. 256.

107. ibid, p. 261.

108. ibid, p. 263.

109. Goldberg, op.cit., Note 95, p. 228.

110. I follow L. Berkhof, Systematic Theology, (Banner of Truth Trust, Edinburgh, 1984), p. 231. There are theological problems involved with this view or alternatively, presented to Christianity because of this view. Consider the story of the fall of Man, told in Genesis 3:1-24. Whether this is taken to be reality or a myth with a moral (like the state of nature of the contract theorists) there is a major problem in taking Eve to have sinned by allegedly disobeying God and "eating" of the tree of the knowledge of good and evil. If Eve had to "eat" the fruits of this tree to first become a moral agent (knowledge of good and evil being a necessary condition for moral agency) then how could she have sinned in eating the fruit? At the time of eating she allegedly lacked knowledge of good and evil, and hence could by no means know that disobeying God was morally wrong. Hence, taking sin to be no more than moral evil, it follows that Eve did not sin. This renders problematic the explanation of the origin of sin given by Birkhof (ibid, p. 221) which sees sin beginning with the misadventures in Eden.

111. R. Tannahill, Sex in History, (Hamish Hamilton, London, 1980), pp. 136-161, esp. p. 155.

112. H.J. Miles, Sexual Understanding Before Marriage, (Zondervan Books, Michigan, 1975).

113. J. White, Eros Defiled: The Christian and Sexual Guilt, (Intervarsity Press, Leicester, 1983).

114. ibid, p. 25.

115. ibid, p. 25.

116. Nor in general is an ontology of marriage a non-trivial matter to sketch. cf. S.R.L. Clark, "Sexual Ontology and Group Marriage", Philosophy, Vol. 58, 1983, plp. 215-227.

117. cf. J. Rawls, A Theory of Justice, (Belknap Press of Harvard University Press, Cambridge, Massachusetts, 1971).

118. B.W. Power, "Paul's Teaching in 1 Corinthians on Sex and Marriage: Some Questions of Interpretation", Interchange, No. 31, 1983, pp. 19-32.

119. V. Bounds, "Does an Act of Sexual Intercourse make you Married?" Interchange, No. 34, 1983, pp. 61-63.

120. Powers, op.cit., Note 118, pp. 21-22.

121. cf. St. Augustine, City of God, translated by J.W.C. Wand, (Oxford University Press, Oxford, 1963), pp. 15-16 and pp. 17-18.

122. Miles, op.cit., Note 112, pp. 199-206; White, op.cit., Note 113, pp. 43-74.

123. Miles, ibid, p. 205.

124. ibid, p. 205.

125. H. Licht, Sexual Life in Ancient Greece, (The Abby Library, London, 1971), pp. 340-341, quoted from Powers, op.cit., Note 118, p. 20.

126. Miles, op.cit., Note 112, pp. 48-59.

127. ibid, p. 52.

128. ibid, p. 144. White, op.cit., Note 4, p. 113 compares the homosexual's desires with "Starving people in besieged cities of the past [who] found their mouths watering for such delicacies as boiled rats".

129. J.J. McNeil, The Church and the Homosexual, (Darton, Longman and Todd, London, 1977), pp. 43-44.

130. He does follow D.S. Bailey's Homosexuality and the Western Christian Tradition, (Longman, Green and Co., London, 1955) and claims that Lot's offer of his daughters was "simply the most tempting bribe Lot could offer at the spur of the moment to appease a hostile crowd" (emphasis added). The word "tempting" however

gives the game away: tempting for what? A sexual reference is not eliminated, it is restated.

131. For further arguments along these lines cf. L. Scanzoni and V.R. Mollenkott, <u>Is the Homosexual My Neighbour? Another Christian View</u>, (SCM Press, London, 1978), pp. 54-61.

132. P. Coleman, <u>Christian Attitudes to Homosexuality</u>, (SPCK, London, 1980), p. 95.

133. McNeill, op.cit., Note 129, pp. 50-53.

134. A <u>suggestions</u> of such an argument although one not explicitly embraced by its authors M. Baigent, R. Leich and H. Lincoln, can be found in the controversial, <u>The Holy Blood and the Holy Grail</u>, (Jonathan Cope, London, 1982), pp. 278-283.

135. A more rigorous critique of the mainstream Christian view of homosexuality is John Boswell, <u>Christianity, Social Tolerance and Homosexuality</u>, (University of Chicago Press, Chicago, 1980) and also of relevance, D. Thompson, <u>Flaws in the Social Fabric: Homosexuals and Society in Sydney</u>, (George Allen and Unwin, Sydney, 1985). Somewhat ironically after this chapter had been written and printed a report has come that the Anglican Church in Australia has recognised that certain sexual relationships before marriage are ethical cf. "Church paper Approves Sex Before Marriage", <u>The Advertiser</u>, Monday July 24, 1989, p. 5.

4 AIDS, heroin and IV drug abuse: philosophical issues

1   AIDS and IV Drug Use : The Second Wave

2   Deeper Problems : The Legalization of Heroin and other "Hard" Drugs

3   The Case Against Legalized Drugs

4   Deeper Solutions : Philosophical Foundations of the Drug Abuse Crisis

5   Conclusion : State of the Argument

> "To fight crime with complete success is not possible, but that is no justification for not trying. There is no doubt that the fight can be waged with more determination and success than is being currently perceived. This applies more particularly to organised, than to random, crime.
>
> Why is it that governments as a rule don't wish to clean up crime, but merely to give an appearance of doing so? The answer is simple. Not only do they fear to turn over stones without knowing what may be hidden underneath, but they realise that the cost involved (including a likely loss in revenue) will not benefit the government, particularly in view of the inability financially to adhere to the election promises already made, as they prepare to tough it out until next election". [1]
>
> "Drug financiers, like all businessmen, don't want to invest their money in a wasting asset. But their financial clout is so immense that if they decided to make substantial transfers of money from US banks to, say, Swiss banks or British banks or German banks, they have the power to bring the dollar to ruin. Such is the immensity of the sums involved". [2]

1. AIDS and IV Drug Use: The Second Wave

In New York 36 per cent of reported cases of AIDS related to intravenous drug use (IVDU); the majority of infected women in the U.S. obtained their HIV infection by IVDU and 70 per cent of HIV infection in newborns is a result of IDVU transmission of HIV. [3] The increase in HIV infection amongst IVDU in America is alarming and the slowness of society and Health Authorities to respond to this second wave crisis, is even more alarming. As Fineberg puts it:

> "In 1987 (IVDUs) represented 16 percent of new AIDS cases; in the first half of 1988 that number had grown to 21 percent. Serum surveys reveal that 50 percent or more of the intravenous drug users in New York City have antibodies to HIV. Of the more than 1.2 million intravenous drug users in the U.S., fewer than 250,000 are estimated to be in treatment at any one time. In some cities the waiting period for those who seek treatment is longer than six months". [4]

Some authorities believe that in New York over 80 per cent of IVDU are HIV positive.

Indeed, by the end of 1988 in the U.S. one-third of the 32,000 new cases of full-blown AIDS were IVDUs. [5] In Australia the second wave of AIDS has already washed onto our shores, despite the denials that we have already reviewed and refuted, by leading right-wing and left growthism figures. The Federal Health Minister, Dr. Neal Blewett by contrast, is alarmed at the explosive potential for HIV to spread to the general community: "New infections among needle-sharing drug users [estimated at about 170,000] are expected to increase rapidly and infected drug-users will pass the disease to their sexual partners and their children". [6] Many Australian AIDS experts now believe that the IVDU based spread of AIDS to the general community is a greater threat to society than the drug problem itself. [7] The Albion St. AIDS Clinic in Sydney has found that the rate of HIV infection in IVDU has risen from 1 per cent to 14 per cent in just over two years.

Since the thesis that IVDU based spread of HIV is a very serious public health problem, is not seriously debated, let us address the next question: what is to be done? Some strategies listed by Ms. Marion Watson, Co-ordinator of the Drug Referral and Information Centre in Canberra, include these measures:

"- To provide needle exchange programs with the capacity to provide information, resources and counselling on safe needle usage and safer sex to intravenous drug users;

- to train those working in the AIDS field to counsel intravenous drug users and to train those in the alcohol and drug field to counsel on AIDS;

-to encourage consumer groups to form and thereby provide peer education to intravenous drug users and their partners and families in an acceptable form while also providing lobbying and advocacy services for the support of those who require it whether it be because of a seropositive diagnosis or other needs;

- to review the existing legislation that may or does prevent the intravenous drug users from protecting themselves (their families, and sexual partners) from transmitting or contracting the virus;

-to encourage research into the area of intravenous drug use, especially where it has some impact on HIV transmission;

- that an integrated focus be used to coordinate both the abstinence oriented programmes and the AIDS transmission prevention programmes;

-that a variety of prioritized outcomes to AIDS/Drug/ Treatment programmes be adopted, these are:

abstinence from drug use
using drugs but not injecting
injecting but not sharing equipment
injecting drugs but de-contaminating shared equipment". [8]

Professor Ron Penny, Chief Commonwealth Education and Services Adviser on AIDS, has more recently given a complementary list of strategies which will form a basis for a new Australian National Council on AIDS (ANCA) task force. Measures include:

-A media campaign to educate the public about the "second wave" of AIDS, particularly recreational users who may not perceive themselves to be at risk.

-A campaign using IVDU peer groups and support organizations to educate IVDU about safe IV needle usage.

-Expansion of preventive programmes such as needle exchange programmes.

-Education of prison workers and police about IVDU HIV infection transmission.

-Changes to Australian drug laws that impede safe IVDU needle practices. [9]

Of the prevention programmes designed to reduce the spread of IVDU HIV infection transmission, none is more important than the introduction of one-use only needle-syringes. [10] The problem with many past designs is that they can be used again if the plunger is not pushed all the way down, although it appears that this problem can be now dealt with. [11] The use of one-use only needle-syringes overcomes a problem well summed up by Ms. Sonja Ristov of a Victorian AIDS Group working with IVDU: "People are just going to mix up their drugs and share them (needles and syringes) ... people don't want to nick off to the chemist and go buy a fit (needle and syringes)". [12] Unfortunately it may take several years to replace all syringes now on the market. [13] This in itself is an outrage, for a single technical innovation could have a substantial impact on reducing needle sharing. Indeed if all needle-syringes in Australia were one-use (including those used in hospitals which otherwise may be stolen), the transmission of HIV by needle sharing would virtually cease. It is worth considering that a single IV needle can be passed around and used by 30 to 40 people in prison in a day without disinfection. [14]

The society-wide use of one-use only needle-syringes would effectively solve this problem of 30 to 40 people in prison using the one dirty needle, *if* the only needles that were available in society were one-use needles, and the needles were freely available in prison. Now the objection made against the provision of standard multiple-use needle-syringes in prisons - that of security, does not apply to one-use needle-syringes. The idea behind this objection is that a multiple use needle-syringe could be filled with HIV contaminated blood and used as a weapon. This would indeed threaten prison security. However, a one-use needle-syringe cannot be refilled with blood - if the plunger is forced back by some prison strongman, the syringe must be designed to split open and be useless. The only objection that could then be made to this programme is that the spent needle-syringe could be used as a stabbing weapon. Indeed it could. However, a needle is a very poor stabbing weapon compared to the weapons already available in prisons. It would not substantially endanger prison security.

It may also be argued that needle-syringe supply programmes are morally objectionable because they amount to a social consent to IV drug abuse - it legitimizes IV drug abuse. Now the typical response to this object is to give a utilitarian argument along the lines that the social cost of allowing HIV infection to spread is greater than any free advertisement for IV drug taking. The problem with this reply is that it grants too much. Allowing the distribution of needle-syringes does not produce a single additional IV drug abuser. People do not become IV drug abusers because of the availability of needle-syringes, anymore than people become cocaine addicts because matches are freely available for supplying heat to vaporize cocaine. It is true that some people may die from heroin overdoses, delivered by government supplied needle-syringes. People however also die from road accidents on government supplied roads. Supplying needle-syringes is not like supplying people with empty guns, to which they supplu the (heroin) bullets. (An Australian T.V. advertisement which used this image of AIDS and guns was therefore very misguided). Needle-syringes are not explicitly designed for killing - guns are (target shooting being something of a civilized trade-off). Making needle-syringes available even in vending machines, is qualitatively differnt from making guns freely available in vending machines. The analogy between needle-syringes and guns that is often drawn cannot be sustained because in the case of the gun problem, it is the gun itself which is the problematic tool rather than the bullets. Of course bullets are needed to fire the gun, but with the amount of reloading equipment available and the tonnes of bullets that must be available in the community, controlling bullets is not the answer to the gun problem, in America for example. If analogies are needed, heroin itself is more like a loaded gun than a bullet (although this image is itself problematic). It is also possible to use, with some irony an argument used by the U.S.

gun lobby to defend needle exchange programmes. They say "guns don't kill people, people with guns do". Likewise, we may say that "needle-syringes of herion don't kill IVDU, dosage mistakes do". As we shall see, it is a fallacy of the heroin debate to regard heroin "addiction"/dependence as a death sentence - for many heroin IVDU who do not contract HIV live normal enough lives apart from the dependency (this is <u>not</u> to assert that heroin is a "safe" drug). Thus the analogy between heroin IVDU, and holding a revolver to one's head and pulling the trigger is badly flawed for a number of reasons. There are thus no substantial moral objections to comprehensive needle-syringe exchange/supply programmes.

2. Deeper Problems: The Legalization of Heroin and Other "Hard" Drugs

There has been increased support by public health and public policy authorities for either the decriminalization or outright legalization of heroin and other "hard" drugs, not only to deal with the AIDS pandemic, but also with the drug problem and organised crime. [15] Indeed, these problems are so severe as to rank as the social equivalents of the environmental crisis (the link between these respective domains of crisis will be detailed later). The U.S. economy consumes $US75-$90 billion on marijuana and cocaine; the profit on marijuana and cocaine is 20-25 per cent of the total after-tax profits of all US corporations. [16] In Los Angeles more than 600 "crack" gangs rule the streets, with 70,000 teenage members. Their escalating wealth enables them to purchase automatic weapons (a favourite is the Soviet AK-47) hand grenades, explosives and in a few instances, rocket launchers. This array of weapons resulted in 387 killings in 1987. [17] Heroin is also being mixed with crack to create a deadly cocktail known as <u>raid</u>. "Raid" is the name of a common insecticide that crack addicts often inhale to come down from "crack highs". In poor black areas of New York such as East Harlem, crack and AIDS are devastating the community. Estimates of AIDS infections vary from 1 child in 60 to 25 per cent of children born being infected by HIV. Dr. Louis Cooper, director of pediatrics at St. Luke's Roosevelt Hospital in East Harlem said: "This improverished society was the tinder, the AIDS virus was the spark and crack the gasoline". This occurs along with alcohol abuse, inadequate housing and other diseases. [18]

The American drug problem is not merely a problem of the poor, but also strikes at the heart of middle class America:

> "While abuse of legal substances like alcohol is a serious domestic problem, the use of illicit substances by Americans has created a drug trafficking enterprise that is the most serious international crime problem of this decade. The sale of illicit drugs accounts for almost 38 per cent of all organised criminal activity in the

United States and, according to various estimates, generates between $27 and $110 billion dollars in support of organized crime. Some estimates are even higher. Classified documents from the National Security Agency and the Central Intelligence Agency (CIA) reportedly indicate that the international narcotics industry's annual revenues exceed $500 billion.

At the individual level, drugs ruin lives. In a study of 598 eighth-, ninth-, tenth , and eleventh-grade students at two Philadelphia high schools, investigators from the Polydrug Research Center found that 33 percent of the students who dropped out of school before graduation had abstained from regular (at least weekly) drug use. In contrast, of the students who graduated, 65 percent had abstained. This study is one of the first to show a direct relation between drug use and dropping out of high school. Although drug use probably emerges along with other delinquent behaviors that characterize an entire negative worldview among students who are not doing well in school, it clearly interferes with academic progress and contributes to the nation's dropout problem." [19]

Australia as we have seen, has her own heroin problem [20], fed in 1989 by record opium crops in Asia's Golden Triangle, [21] and an emerging cocaine hunger, about to be fed by Latin American cocaine. [22] There are also thousands of amphetamine abusers in Newcastle and the neighbouring Hunter Valley centres, Cessnock, Muswellbrook and Singleton. Informers can allegedly name over 100 "speed" dealers in the relatively small city of Newcastle. [23] Needle sharing also occurs, which shows that the IVDU AIDS problem is not exclusively a heroin problem - it can arise with any drug that is consumed by use of an IV needle-syringe. Whilst the murder rate in Australia is relatively stable, rapes, burglaries and serious assaults have doubled in the past decade and robberies have increased from 29.74 per 100,000 people to 42.78. Whether or not this can be linked with the drug problem will be discussed later. Nevertheless a rising tide of violence is, correctly or incorrectly, linked in the public's mind to the drug problem. Assistant Police Commissioner Werner has this to say about the rising tide of violence in Australia:

"Ten years ago police weren't murdered in the streets; young girls did not have to fear predatory rapists breaking into their homes; armed gangs did not regularly invade homes and restaurants armed with knives and machetes; houses did not have to be fortified against burglars, selfish drug addicts did not regularly traumatise bank staff and customers in pursuit of easy money, bombings of consulates, houses and police buildings were almost unheard of and young men didn't go to discos with knives strapped to their bodies". [24]

Due to these problems, it has been proposed in both America and Australia, that heroin and perhaps other "hard" drugs be not merely decriminalized, but legalized. Programmes vary from the controlled provision of heroin in doctors surgeries or special clinics, to the more radical laissez-faire approach to drugs, where individual choice is all that matters. [25] The following argument for the legalization of drugs, by Rodney Allen, will be analysed and criticized in the next section. Its addition will give the reader an appreciation of the controversial nature of this area.

Rodney Allen - The Legalization of Drugs

My local federal Member of Parliament (Gordon Bilney) has recently declared himself in favour of the legalisation of all presently illegal drugs, including heroin. I don't think he is envisaging opium and marijuana industries freely promoting and selling their products to the general public. Rather, he mainly wants the government to be able legally to supply heroin to registered addicts free of charge. This would still amount to the prohibition of heroin. It would certainly not be freely available to the general public, nor would any private citizen or company be able to manufacture or market it. It would be prohibited in much the same way that liquor was prohibited in the Indian state of Maharastra up until the mid-1970s. There, one had to be a registered alcoholic in order to get a limited supply of liquor.

Gordon Bilney's proposal certainly has a lot of merit. It would cut back the amount of urban street crimes, for addicts would no longer need to maintain their habits by robbery and mugging. The spread of AIDS would be mitigated by the provision of hygenic resources for addicts. Fewer people would die immediately as a result of heroin usage, since the drug would be available without such lethal 'cutting' additives as strychnine.

Unfortunately, though, the provision of free heroin to registered addicts would not destroy or massively diminish the illegal market in hard drugs. Criminal entrepreneurs would still push drugs to actual and potential users unwilling or unable to limit themselves to a State regulated supply. The forces of law and order would still be engaged in a losing battle against armies of drug traffickers, smugglers and dealers. Only a wider legalisation of narcotics could drain the drug scene of its enormous profitability, and so allow the tidal wave of drug-related crime to recede.

Maybe, then, we should seriously consider fairly full legalisations - the wide though regulated freedom to produce and market, to buy and sell, all 'recreational' drugs. After all, virtually all societies allow the fairly free use of two harm causing and socially costly drugs - alcohol and tobacco. These are causing vastly more death and damage than that associated with the consumption of any other drug. According to Australian Department of Health statistics, 21,271 deaths were caused by drugs in 1986. Of these, 17,070 were caused by tobacco and 3,465 by alcohol. Only 736 deaths were caused by the use of other drugs, including 249 stemming from the use of opiates.

Moreover, the prohibition of other drugs - marijuana, cocaine, heroin - is simply not working. Anyone who wants these substances and has enough money can purchase them. Our society has created the crimes of drug use and drug dealing through legal proscription, but has failed to make this prohibition effective. Lives and treasure are expended in the war against drugs; but the drugs keep on coming. Short of the introduction of unthinkably draconian penalties - the public execution of drug users, for example - there is no way that Western societies can purge themselves of the presently illegal drugs by police action. We have probably reached the stage where ineffective prohibition is producing worse social consequences (violence and corruption, the wastage of social resources, and the actual encouragement of drug consumption through the glamour of illegal use and the profitability of illegal marketing) than would free availability.

In the United States the war against drugs is a feverishly intense battle which the established authorities are losing. Virtually every day there is some shootout between police and drug traffickers. Violent Colombian and Jamaican gangs kill each other and police in the streets in a struggle to establish supply lines to consumers. The US authorities have mobilized their Coastguard and Air Force in an effort to control the supply. Yet every drug known to mankind, including derivatives such as 'crack' and exotica such as 'ecstasy' are readily available to those with the money to buy. The drug scene has so impinged on suburban consciousness (syringes littering the streets; children buying drugs at school) that it was a major issue in the recent US Presidential election campaign. The candidates, however, offer no solution beyond more of the same - more resources for law enforcement. Perhaps they are envisaging the invasion of those Latin American countries such as Colombia whose economies are fuelled by the supplying of cocaine and other drugs to the US market. In fact, the foiling policy of prohibition has turned Colombia into a tripartite battleground. The long-standing violent struggle between a conservative landowning class and socialist revolutionaries has expanded to encompass a new protagonist - the 'narcos', the cocaine barons and their private armies. Meanwhile, back in U.S. White House, three secret service officers are currently under investigation for both drug use and drug dealing.

In Australia, the influx of 'hard' drugs is barely controlled. Police estimate that only about 10% of the 'hard' drugs entering the country are seized. Junkies do not need to worry about the availability of their drugs, only about the money to pay for them. The relatively 'soft' drug, marijuana, is fairly well entrenched throughout Australian society. Its production is both a cottage industry and a big business. Consumption is not confined to students and hippies, but is widespread throughout all sections of society. The term 'smoko' has taken on a new meaning in the Australian workplace, as young workers pass around their 'joints'. The most respectable families in the most respectable suburbs generate teenage 'dope' dealers.

Wouldn't legalisation merely make matters worse? Not necessarily. For one thing, it would limit the scope for criminal profit and corruption. Moreover, a public policy of permissive distaste might actually reduce drug usage by depriving the drug scene of its underground glamour and attractive rebelliousness.

We should also realise that the drug problem is not centrally about use, but rather abuse. Some of the substances now illegal - most notably marijuana - can be reasonably used, moderately, to add a little joy and conviviality to otherwise humdrum lives, or a little relaxation to otherwise stressed lives. Drug abuse - the element of actual badness in drug use - consists in people making themselves sick, poisoning or incapacitating themselves by excessive consumption, making themselves into parasitic dependents on their wider society, and endangering others by attempting such tasks as driving cars or buses while 'stoned'. These undesirable consequences are of course already realised by the legal consumption of alcohol. Prohibition by the criminal law is a blunt and ineffective instrument for containing drug abuse. It certainly proved to be a counterproductive measure against alcohol abuse in pre-war America. Ultimately, the abuse of drugs can only be contained by whole communities persuading their members through their educational and socialization processes, to eschew self-poisoning and social parasitism and irresponsibility. A public policy of permissive distaste - of legal tolerance combined with moral condemnation - may well be more effective than prohibition in achieving these ends.

There are two large obstacles on the path to liberalising reform of the drug laws in Australia. The most important of these is that the majority of people are implacably opposed to any degree of legalisation of the presently illegal drugs. Heavy opposition exists in the major political groupings of both left and right. Any government seriously contemplating reform would be courting electoral disaster. A recent opinion poll showed that only 29.7% of Australians supported the legalisation of marijuana (a large grouping, but still clearly a minority). Most of the majority are intensely agitated about the whole drugs issue. They perceive the illegal enjoyments of their fellow citizens as threats not only to the welfare of their children, but also to law and order and to social stability generally - threats that can only be overcome by an iron fist.

The other problem for liberalising reform is a puzzle - how can a capitalist market-oriented society tolerate a wider degree of drug availability whilst at the same time discouraging drug abuse? No-one has a clear conception of precisely how legalisation could be regulated so as to minimize abuse. In market societies, products are inevitably promoted or advertised; people are encouraged to consume them. Our society has not so far been very adept at discouraging cigarette smoking and excessive drinking in a context of market availability. How should a wider availability of other drugs be regulated? The more that availability is restricted, of course, the greater is the scope for criminal profiteering.

Should narcotics only be available under a medical prescription? Or should private citizens and companies be able to produce or import them, and to market them, to the general public? Under what conditions? Should our suburbs be able to sprout opium dens as well as bars and taverns? Perhaps narcotics could be made available in the same way that pornography has been made available. Perhaps one day we shall see a Drugs Censorship Board, classifying some drugs as 'X' rated (not really good for anyone) and others - e.g. light beer and mild marijuana - as 'G' rated family drugs.

The problem of how to reform the drug laws looms larger than whether to do it at all.

Community leaders, especially professionals dealing with drug usage and its effects, are increasingly voicing the opinion that some significant degree of legalisation is very desirable. The Director of the Australian Institute of Criminology, Paul Wilson, has publicly expressed two very pertinent points of view. Firstly, he has proposed that heroin be freely available to addicts - especially in view of the likely explosion of AIDS through the heterosexual population via syringe sharers. Secondly, he suggests that the production and distribution of marijuana be legalised - especially given the markedly less harmful effects of marijuana use compared with the consumption of alcohol. These two recommendations should, I think, serve as a starting point for enlightened reform of our drug laws.

One consideration that does not usually emerge in discussions of drug law reform is, surprisingly, liberal principle. The debate is conducted in utilitarian terms. Does prohibition produce better consequences for society, and for most people, than would legalisation? The missing consideration is whether people should have the right to consume whatever they choose, even if the social consequences of such permissiveness are less than optimal. One of the more important founding fathers of our present political culture, John Stuart Mill, proclaimed in his seminal essay, On Liberty, that individuals should be free to do whatever they choose, so long as their chosen activities do not seriously and directly cause harm to others. Mill himself was a utilitarian, and tried to justify his principle of individual liberty as a rule for producing the greatest happiness of the greatest number. He thought that individual liberty would be generally beneficial because each person is the best judge of his or her own interests. This is probably an implausibly optimistic assumption; and Mill himself might retract it if he could cruise the present day drug scene. Mill's principle is, however, the most articulate and influential formulation of the conception of freedom that is part of the longer tradition of liberalism, according to which freedom is a natural right. It implies that people have a right to damage themselves in pursuit of immediate pleasure if they so choose, provided that in so doing they do not seriously harm others.

Should our society tolerate people unnecessarily and self-indulgently making themselves sick or incapacitated? Mill in principle would answer affirmatively. Perhaps our society should, if it is seriously to respect individual freedom, allow everyone access to every offered product, even pleasurable poisons. Perhaps, if we wish to be properly liberal, we should resist all forms of social paternalism, and reject all legislation designed to protect people from themselves - everything from compulsory car seat belts to drug prohibition.

Unfortunately, the self-destructive conduct of individual drug abusers cannot be isolated from harmful consequences for the remainder of the community. Self-destructiveness is at the same time other-damaging. Notoriously, chronic drunkenness disrupts family and other social relationships, endangers lives, imposes costs (for example, health care costs) on society, and undermines productivity. It's possible that the economic shambles in the Soviet Union derives more from the fact that a lot of Russians are drunk for a lot of the time, than from centralized State direction of production. In general, it's not possible to define an area of human conduct where free individual action could not possibly damage other people; an area which should therefore be absolutely immune from social intervention.

Nevertheless, Mill's principle - even though it does not umproblematically define an area of absolute personal freedom - should be regarded as an important and independent constraints on public policy. Every society should allow some generous scope for self-abusive, reckless or corrupting conduct. Areas of personal freedom are essential if people are to be responsible and autonomous agents rather than dehumanized social automata. Societies with any pretensions to liberalism must establish and protect areas of individual liberty; even though the flip side of freedom is the possibility of its abuse. Certainly, the path of puritanical paternalism should not be blindly followed; for it leads beyond drug prohibition to such authoritarian nightmares as compulsory diets and enforced exercises. It leads in the end to the destruction of free people.

A clear implication of taking Mill's basic liberal principle seriously is this: if the freedom to consume alcohol is socially tolerable, then the freedom to use marijuana (a less harmful drug than alcohol) should equally be allowed.

It is also worth remarking that the most appropriate way for a freedom-respecting society to attempt to minimize drug abuse is through educational measures and socialization processes, rather than by legal prohibition. The emphasis should be on persuasion rather than force, because social objectives in general should be achieved in ways that respect everyone's capacity for reasoned decision making and free choice.

There is, therefore, a strong case for a wider degree of legalisation of drugs, on grounds both of liberal principle and utilitarian pragmatism. The wisest course for our society to follow in the present circumstances is that of liberalising reform of the drug laws. Unfortunately, we live in conservative times, so this case is unlikely to win easy and widespread acceptance. The conservatively inclined should realize, however, the it is conservative values - law and order, respect for individual freedom - that are being undermined by the present prohibitions.

Of course, drug dependence - the resort to chemical escapism, is not a good thing. It should be discouraged. Wider legalisation should occur in a context of publicly expressed disapproval and distaste, and of measures directed towards enhancing self respect and social responsibility. Most importantly, there must be a context of greater social justice. One horrifying future prospect is a complacently drug-free middle class exploiting a socio-economic underclass permanently pacified by easily available chemicals.

For the bottom line is simply this: people will only stop trying to escape social reality if social reality itself no longer makes even chemical escapism look like a sensible option. (End R.J. Allen).

3. The Case Against Legalized Drugs

As Rodney Allen has argued above, and as David Hawks argued in greater detail in his 1988 article in the <u>Medical Journal of Australia,</u> [26] the modest programme for the legalization of heroin is unlikely to deal satisfactorily with either the AIDS problem or the crime problem. Let us look then more closely at the arguments for the more comprehensive drug legalization programmes.

D.A.J. Richards significantly develops the "liberal" portion of Allen's above argument. [27] According to Richards, criminal sanctions are justified only insofar as they protect people from harm. However, he sees the prohibition of many drugs as not being based upon this, but upon unjustified dogmas:

> "Often, the distaste for forms of drug use reflects not neutral assessments of imminent risks to life or health, but ideological judgements about legitimate experience and even life style (the role of one drug as opposed to another drug or activity in different patterns of social life). The enforcement of such judgements through criminal prohibitions thus deprives people of the right to make reasonable judgements about the regulation of consciousness, mood, and experience (an aspect of the general good of control of one's mind) either where there is no risk to life or health, or where such risks might reasonably be taken in view of their role in the larger pattern of a well lived life. Not only do these prohibitions either fail to rest on any harm or on any harm sufficient to justify prohibition, but the harms they do combat are often incoherently pursued. What coherent theory of harms can explain the different ways our law treats alcohol and nicotine use in contrast to marijuana and cocaine use? A dominant cultural consensus of legitimate drug use (alcohol, nicotine) enjoys a kind of cultural hegemony at the expense of a genuine pluralism of alternative cultural patterns, ways of life, and spiritual perspectives. The true nature of the judgements underlying our prohibitory drug laws is reflected in both the substance and rhetoric of the "war on crime": The aim is not a reasonable concern with shifting patterns of drug use in ways that heighten the benefits and reduce the harms, but the ugly Manicheanism of the wars of religion." [28]

Richards offers the following alternative:

> "If our prohibitory drug policy is as wrong-heaed and as self-defeating as I believe it is, the answer is to discontinue forthwith the "War on

Drugs". We need rather a kind of negotiated settlement in which the current level of illegal drug sales and use might be a kind of working <u>modus vivendi</u> if sellers and buyers agreed to observe appropriate regulations of sale and use keyed to realistic assessment of harms. Both society and the drug trade would gain from this negotiated settlement, and that would be the key to its political realism and stable workability. Society would secure a regulatory interest in shifting patterns of drug use towards a balance of benefit over harm; the drug trade would secure markets unhampered by the substantial costs of the concealment of illegality (the crime tariff). It would suffice for the realism and workability of such a negotiated settlement that there is some equilibrium point or range of equilibrium points in which society would gain more control over both levels and kinds of drug use (than it currently has) and the drug trade would retain sufficient profitability even with lower prices because the exorbitant costs of illegality would evaporate (maintaining private armies, smuggling, etc.). Indeed, legality itself might be a status reward independently valuable to relevant businesspeople; people in the drug trade would be no less (and no more) reputable than Seagram. The measure of success of this program would not be ending drug use but shifting current patterns of drug use into less destructive forms through engaging (not degrading) the responsible judgement of people." [29]

There are a number of replies that can be made to Richards here. First, and most basic, the liberalism underlying Richards position can be rejected by the arguments given in chapter 2 of this book. The radically diverse cultural and religious traditions cherished by liberalism are hardly a basis for undermining paternalism - for these traditions (often highly paternalistic themselves) are rarely freely chosen by rational liberal men and women. If all that counts, according to the dominating cultural reductionism of our day, is the equal weighting of all "forms of life", then anything goes. Society however has the right to form laws not only to prevent harms, but for excellent utilitarian reasons to encourage and promote genuine social goods. It does this by so-called paternalistic laws such as minimal wage laws, maximum workday laws, social security laws, housing codes and so on, which are ideally decided upon by democratic consent, and given utilitarian justification. Even though they may limit the freedom of choice of particular individuals, these laws are usually seen to promote the general good. Richards is simply wrong about the foundations of law: laws do, and ideally should exist to promote general human welfare and social and individual good (and when they do not, such laws are bad and must be changed). This is more fundamental than Millian liberalism. For: why prevent harm? Surely because it reduces human welfare and diminishes human good. Neville recognises this as well, although his argument is different, but consistent with my own:

> "It seems to me that among the things highly valued in our society, though perhaps less to than in traditional societies, is a habit of taking care of people so that they live within a range of locally accepted human amenities. Harmful drugs might be justified in being controlled, therefore, because their uncontrolled availability would allow users to sink to socially shameful depths of abject filth, mindlessness, and disorder. This rationale for the desire to control harmful drugs is coordinated with our attempts at drug rehabilitation programs for people whose lives fit slum environments. Part of the rationale for those programs of course is the interest to control the social consequences of criminality in the drug life; but that could be satisfied by making the desired drugs freely available. The British experience seems to have shown that although availability reduces crime, it does not seem to make much of a difference to the level of social amenities drug users sustain for themselves. If we could eliminate the criminal costs to society, would we allow the abject victims of drug use to rot in their autonomy? I suspect not. We would hold the value of their enjoying the social amenities sufficiently important both to attempt to withhold the harmful drugs and to help them in their immediate situation. The reasons we cite for these attempts amount to saying that it is inhumane for society to let people victimize themselves to the extent common in the drug scene. This reflects not so much a principle of paternalism as a principle of social solidarity, of identification with the plight of the abject. [30]

Liberals such as Richards, offer another argument for the legalization of drugs, based upon personal freedom:

> "...drug use does not produce a drunken anarchy inconsistent with the aims of rational will as such. Humans use drugs for diverse purposes - for therapeutic care and cure, for relief of pain or anxiety, for stimulation or depression of moods, for exploration of imaginative experience (for creative, aesthetic, religious, therapeutic, or other reasons), for recreative pleasure, and the like. Humans consciously choose among these purposes depending on the context and their

individual aims. In so doing, they express self-respect by regulating the quality and versatility of their experiences in life to include greater control of mood and sometimes increased freedom and flexibility of imagination. For many, such drug use does not constitute fear-ridden anarchy, but promotes the rational self-control of those ingredients fundamental to the design of a fulfilled life. It is, of course, a banality of the literature of perceptive observers on drug experience that the quality of such experience varies according to the expectations, aims, and identity that the person brings to the experience. This should confirm that drug experience is neither satanic damnation nor divine redemption of the self, but merely one means by which the already existing interests of the person may be explored or realised." [31]

The argument from freedom for the legalization of heroin and other hard drugs is perhaps the weakest available argument for the liberal. Evidence exists, that even with tobacco smoking, the dangers of which have been advertised more than any other drug, misinformation among young people is widespread. [32] Drug taking is seldom a matter of informed choice. And even if it was, the use of drugs which lead to physical and/or psychological dependency, must involve an important diminishing of freedom or even enslavement. Someone who needs a drink or a sniff of cocaine or shot of heroin just to function as a social being is enslaved as surely as if they were in chains. [33] And perhaps even more so, because most such drugs supply us with temporary illusions and false escapes. [34] Drugs are indeed, the real opiates of the people, supplying us with false and irrational images of well being. A champion of reason such as J.S. Mill would no doubt view such an escape from rationality and truth, as living a life less than human, the life of moral cowardice.

Nadelmann [35] believes that most substances now banned, should be legally available to competent adults, with drug treatment and education programmes available to the public. His arguments for this, are in summary

1. Current drug policies fail - drug prohibition with minimal law enforcement resources has kept illicit drug prices at a higher level than if there were no laws.

2. Failure of international drug control.

3. Costs of prohibition.

Nadelmann describes the way he believes we should begin to think about drugs:

"The same false distinction is drawn with respect to those who provide the psychoactive substances to users and abusers alike. If degrees of immorality were measured by the levels of harm caused by one's products, the "traffickers: in tobacco and alcohol would be vilified as the most evil of all substance purveyors. That they are perceived instead as respected members of our community, while providers of the no more dangerous illicit substances are punished with long prison sentences, says much about the prejudices of most Americans with respect to psychoactive substances, but little about the morality or immorality of their activities.

Much the same is true of gun salesmen. Most of the consumers of their products use them safely; a minority, however, end up shooting either themselves or someone else. Can we hold the gun salesman morally culpable for the harm that probably would not have occurred but for his existence? Most people say no, except perhaps where the salesman clearly knew that his product would be used to commit a crime. Yet in the case of those who sell illicit substances to willing customers, the providers are deemed not only legally guilty, but also morally reprehensible. The law does not require any demonstration that the dealer knew of a specific harm to follow; indeed, it does not require any evidence at all of harm having resulted from the sale. Rather, the law is predicated on the assumption that harm will inevitably follow. Despite the patent falsity of that assumption, it persists as the underlying justification for the drug laws. [36]

I shall deal with the problem of international and local drug control later. First, however, I shall address the basic objection made by Nadelmann that prohibition serves only to keep illicit drug prices at a higher level than if there were no laws. The obvious but essentially correct reply to this, is that keeping drug prices high is the object of prohibition so as to deter people from becoming addicted. Further if it is known that some activity is bad, but is a severe social problem, legalization does not solve the social problem itself, it merely renames it. Why not solve the problem of child sexual abuse, murder and rape by legalizing them? Why not legalize robbery - it after all is a severe social problem, it cannot be eliminated, it is costly and so on. The reason, as Gee explains, is that legalization means, social approval:

"There is an ultimate argument against either partial or total legalisation of hard drugs, though it is rarely heard. To declare legal something which is known to be bad, has about it the ring of approval. The connection between unlawfulness and disapproval has been a phenomenon of all societies at all times. It is of little use to say that society can permit something yet disapprove of it. Of course it can. But we are not dealing with the minds of intellectuals or with logical concepts. The problem of drugs lies in the modern society, which combines affluence with discontent, hedonism with alienation, and includes a host of people seeking some mental prop. We are dealing with young people subconsciously choosing their lifestyle. In default of legal sanctions, warnings and exhortations mean little; to their minds, legality means approval. [37]

Nadelmann's comparison of drugs with guns is also an unfortunate example, using one controversial issue to support another. A parallel argument could be used to justify uranium sales. There is a strong body of arguments in environmental ethics, concluding that one would consider uranium salespeople/exporting countries guilty if countries that they sold it to made atomic weapons that were used for nuclear terrorism. Again the examples used by the liberals do not take us to where they hope to go.

Any debate about the legalization of heroin, crack, angel dust and so on, must address the issue of the legality and morality of alcohol and tobacco. There is no doubt that alcohol and tobacco are dangerous drugs and both are major causes of death in society. The Australian Medical Association believes that Australia's annual health bill for alcohol-related illness is at least $1 billion, with one in five to one in three people in hospital with alcohol-related problems, with 35-45 percent of road deaths involving alcohol. [38] In Australia the total alcohol-related deaths in 1984 was 3,174 compared to a massive 16,346 from tobacco, with total opiate deaths at 229 and total barbiturates at 105 deaths. [39] All of this shows that alcohol and tobacco are dangerous drugs - it does not show that heroin, crack, speed, raid, angel dust etc. are health foods! All that would follow is that Australia, and many other countries have a legal and illegal drug problem. Alcohol and tobacco kill so many people because they are not only socially accepted, but commercialized and more widely used. We do not know what the death statistics would be in a society in other respects like ours, but where speed and angel dust were the socially accepted drugs.

The issue of the American alcohol prohibition in the 1920s is always raised by liberals against prohibitions as an argument for the legalization of drugs today; it is they say a perfect parallel. Now this case is intuitively plausible, but not decisive. First the Prohibition did not in itself completely generate organised crime - the Mafia was carried to the U.S. by Italian immigrants in the late 19th century.

It had already penetrated well into the social fabric of cities such as Chicago before the Volstead Act. Corruption during the Prohibition then became as great as that of many Third World countries today. Despite this, alcohol use and alcohol-related diseases sharply <u>declined</u>. [40] Prohibition however failed because alcohol was ingrained in American culture, and the general public did not fully support a ban on alcohol. No law can function without public support. However no perfect parallel can be drawn between the Prohibition and today's heroin problem, because heroin users are a clear minority of the population. Alcohol users are the majority of the Australian population. Hence it is not satisfactory to use any alleged failure of alcohol prohibition as an argument for the legalization of "hard" drugs.

There is of course great controversy about the dangerousness of "hard" drugs such as heroin and cocaine, with some people arguing that heroin is less dangerous than alcohol, in careful use in a pure form. There is no doubt that given a chance of being operated on by a chronic alcoholic with shakey hands, and a "clean" heroin user, one would prefer the heroin user. There is also no doubt, as Robertson puts it in <u>Heroin, AIDS and Society</u>, that heroin is "a potentially very dangerous drug and the cause of much unhappiness and destruction to individuals and to society". [41] The most obvious problem is overdosing, which is not exclusively a problem of the "cutting" agent, but occurs when the dose exceeds the personal level of tolerance. However there can also be abrupt losses of tolerance and change of tolerances, which makes heroin use dangerous for the inexperienced. There is little doubt that cocaine, which is increasingly being mixed with heroin is a much more toxic compound. Although a lethal dose of cocaine is said to be 1.2 grains, some people have died with as low as 0.01 grains of cocaine. [42] Matters become worse when "hard" drugs are mixed, due to synergism.

Let us now consider the question as to whether legalizing heroin and other "hard" drugs would solve the problem of organised crime. I shall discuss this question in more detail very shortly, but for the time being let us give a general argument against the liberal. The sale of drugs is an extremely profitable enterprise for the gangsters in our society. No doubt legalizing a popular "soft" drug such as marijuana would destroy an extensive source of revenue for organized crime. This could also be done by the more conservative method of allowing users to grow their own marijuana for personal consumption, but prosecuting those in possession of large quantities used for commercial supply, the actual quantity being decided by public debate and rough consensus. This strategy could be defended on utilitarian grounds, if it was the case that marijuana was genuinely a "soft" drug and public opinion was so great that prohibition became merely nominal. Organized crime will then turn to the next illegal drug. If heroin and all other "hard" drugs are legal, then they will synthesize new drugs that are not regulated and supply them. Some uncommon opiates are on a per weight basis up to one thousand times as powerful as heroin, with a great ability to cross the blood-brain barrier. [43] Perhaps a new drug will erupt onto the drug scene, produced by underground chemists, which is addictive in one instance, thousands of times as powerful as heroin, totally chemically untreatable by substitute drugs and with zombie like effects? What then? Legalize it?

4. Deeper Solutions: Philosophical Foundations of the Drug Abuse Crisis

It is generally agreed that there are two distinct approaches to control of the drug problem: supply controls and demand controls. Liberals have argued, with great success that supply controls - such as the measures advocated the U.S. Bennett plan of tougher law enforcement and bigger gaols [44] - cannot succeed. However, they have typically assumed that legalization of "hard" drugs such as heroin, will constitute a way of dealing with the crime problem because they believe that heroin places a heavy financial burden on the user that leads to criminal activity. There is however evidence against even this liberal thesis: most heroin "addicts" are young socially disadvantaged males, 40 percent of which (in Australia) have convictions for non-drug crime preceding their first drug conviction. Further neither crime nor prostitution can account for the money spent on heroin: most users are also dealers in a complex drug market. [45]

The deeper supply response to the drug problem begins with the recognition that drug trading provides some developing countries with a significant fraction of their GNP - if Colombia had no cocaine exports, then there would be little difference between Colombia's economy and that of Argentina. Indeed the Colombian drug lords had offered to pay off the country's national debt in exchange for freedom from persecution. Drug money buys lots of goods and keeps people in work. [46] The problem here is expressed well in *The Gaia Peace Atlas*: "A global society marred by gross inequalities and dominated by consumerist ethics is a rich breeding ground for "alternative" routes to wealth". [47] Ultimately, to deal successfully with the drug problem, the problems of global inequalities, U.S. and Japanese superpower imperialism and domination, and the economic exploitation of the Third World must be addressed. This same conclusion can be reached by a consideration of the environmental crisis, an issue addressed in the final chapter of this book, where this type of argument is developed in detail.

The deep-supply response to the drug problem is also highly interested in the problem of organized crime within the national boundaries. Whilst some deny that organized crime exists in Australia [48] there is clear evidence that Australia is something of a paradise for organized crime and corruption. [49] A dramatic illustration of the operation of organized crime is the assassination of former Assistant Commissioner of the Australian Federal Police, Colin Winchester, who was gunned down outside his Canberra home on January 10 1989. The general theory as to the plausible culprits is, as Commissioner McAuley described them, the "caesars of the narcotics world", the Mafia. Winchester had apparently worked on a trap to catch drug growers on police-monitored marijuana plantations, codenamed "Operation Seville". It caught 11 people. [50] No such assassination of such a high ranking police figure has occurred anywhere else in the Western world within recent years. The situation is surely significant.

Justice Philip Woodward is quite correct in my opinion in our opening quote about the real reason supply-side drug control measures have not been successful: Repeating his important words for convenience:

> "To fight crime with complete success is not possible, but that is no justification for not trying. There is no doubt that the fight can be waged with more determination and success than is being currently perceived. This applies more particularly to organised, than random, crime.
>
> Why is it that governments as a rule don't wish to clean up crime, but merely to give an appearance of doing so? The answer is simple. Not only do they fear to turn over stones without knowing what may be hidden underneath, but they realise that the cost involved (including a likely loss in revenue) will not benefit the government, particularly in view of the inability financially to adhere to the election promises already made, as they prepare to tough it out until next election". [51]

It is easy enough in the Australian context to illustrate this. At the time of writing, former members of Chinese criminal triads would be allowed to migrate to Australia if they renounced their gang ties, providing other entry criteria are met. This was indicated in May 1989 by Ms. Janet Sekavs, the regional migration director for the Australian consulate. 1500 enquiries had been received and more than 1100 application forms sent out. The renunciation of triad identity is made before a Triad Renunciation Tribunal. It is fairly obvious that the Australian policy, part of our uncritical growth-manic immigration policy, is an effective way for many of the 16,000 triad members to get out of Hong Kong before it reverts back to China in 1997 (triad membership is illegal). Rumours of plans to rebuild Hong Kong in the Northern Territory, would of course save triad members a lot of fuss and bother. [52] After all, they have said that they would be good! However, it was reported in May 1989 that Australian Federal Police had smashed a $100 million plus drug racket, run by members of the Hong Kong based "Big Circle" triad group. The operation involved the arrest of 20 Asians and the seizure of 63.8 kgs. of heroin. [53] This speaks for itself.

The former chairman of the Hong Kong Independent Commission Against Corruption, Mr. Donald Stewart, has said that triad members move with comparative ease between Hong Kong, South-East Asia and Australia, and that their presence in Australia will increase as 1997 approaches. [54] The report published in The Australian had this to say:

> "Earlier this year the Chinese press in Australia reported the assault of an entertainer who had arrived from Hong Kong on a tour. Within hours of his arrival a number of men, one with an iron bar, had attacked the visitor, while screaming the name of a Hong Kong Triad leader.
>
> The Australian has been told the attack was in retaliation for an incident in Hong Kong and a warning that the tentacles of the organisation were long and powerful.
>
> And violence is increasing. Intelligence gathered so far has raised concern that Australia will face the same problems with heroin importations through Asia as the United States is facing with cocaine from Colombia. [55]

And the Sunday Mail (Adelaide) added these words:

> "At least 2000 Chinese have been identified as being involved in crime - mainly heroin trafficking - in Australia...
>
> Membership of triads is illegal in Hong Kong yet known members have travelled to Australia on tourist visas and simply stayed here, dealing in drugs and other illegal activities until caught....
>
> Despite the traditional focus on the Robert Trimboles of the Australian underworld, the reality is that this trade is dwarfed by the trafficking masterminded by Chinese syndicates...
>
> Crime writer Bob Bottom estimates the Chinese traffickers are responsible for $800 million worth of the annual $1000 million plus Australian heroin trade.

During its first four years, the NCA alone arrested 66 Chinese syndicate members and seized heroin worth $66 million. Federal and State police have added substantially to that score.

The NCA's biggest drug busts have collected heroin shipments worth $35 million and $20 million. [56]

The Australian newspaper had allegedly obtained evidence of a collusion between the Mafia, members of the Chinese triads and Vietnamese gangs, as well as evidence of two former government ministers with drug and Mafia connections: "The vast profits flowing from drugs are now able to finance a sophisticated protection network involving politicians, police, customs officials and others". [57]

The liberal hopes that legalization of drugs will prevent all of this woe, that the Mafia and triads will wither away or become respectable. There is no reason to believe that they will give up the taste of easy money. Even if prostitution and drugs were legalized they would still aim for easy money without toil, by extortion and thief-moving perhaps into computer based high tech crime and any new revenue area. Liberal writers on the drug problem and organised crime seldom consider the power of the Japanese Yakuza, which in many respects breaks the confines of their neat solutions Yakuza penetration into a country is usually undetected until it is firmly entrenched, as Japanese organized crime will appear first as seemingly legitimate businesses, involving construction, real estate investment and other speculations. The financial power of Japanese organised crime is immense - in excess of $US 5 billion a year. There is no doubt that with increased economic dependency of Australia upon Japan and the establishment of the networks of economic imperialism and control, penetration of the Yakuza into Australia will follow as a matter of course. This should make Australia cautious about large scale social engineering projects such as the multifunction polises, which to the minds of Australia's opportunistic businessmen and growthists, will totally reshape Australia's way of life. [58] The MFP project, advanced with no concrete information to the general public beyond the rhetoric of its academic supporters (who refuse to share information with critics in a scholarly fashion), and advanced with no democratic public debate (after all the public may reject the project) is perhaps an image of the sort of society that Australia is set to become. A society without effective scrutiny of its leaders, and without the encouragement of widespread public debate is a society that runs on organised crime and corruption. Queensland, with its gerrymander, which cannot by any stretch of the imagination be regarded as a representative democratic state, is a perfect illustration of this thesis.

My argument in short is that organized crime and corruption to the extent of becoming a massive social problem, are products of a particular social order. To analyse and detail this thesis at length would take another book. Certainly research in this area is an important task that needs to be conducted as soon as possible. From the evidence presented here, it can be concluded that the Australian government is <u>not</u> making an adequate effort to control the penetration of organised crime into Australia. Perhaps the most disturbing phenomenon of all is that arguments and evidence such as that given in this chapter, are increasingly being seen as no longer fit topics for discussion in our universities. Increasingly the role of intellectuals is being seen as one of serving business interests, to blindly support foreign investment projects and economic growth without penetrating and fundamental criticism and to become technicians, rather than Socratic visionaries. [59] One can only conclude, that this sort of heart-less and mind-less society, will reap what it sows. I believe, at this crisis point in human history as we struggle for survival into the third millennium, that intellectuals should be occupied with the fundamental questions about the purpose and justice of their societies, more than ever before. The profit and growth goals of business, are I will argue in the chapters to follow, a fit subject for social criticism.

Such then is the deep-supply approach to the drug problem. The <u>deep-demand</u> approach is not however radically different in structure from the deep-supply approach. Both approaches see the drug problem as a product of fundamental injustices, inequality and the alienation of modern society - its heart-lessness and mind-lessness if you like. The deep-demand approach, championed by Stanton Peel [60] and Fingarette [61] does not accept that there is a single biological or social cause of drug abuse; it sees the object of "addiction" as people, not mere bodies, and views drug taking as a culturally regulated activity. Fingarette illustrates the "moral/evaluative" approach to the drug problem with respect to alcoholism:

"In fact, alcoholics do have substantial control over their drinking, and they do respond to circumstances. Contrary to what the public has been led to believe, this is not disputed by experts. Many studies have described conditions under which diagnosed alcoholics will drink moderately or excessively, or will choose not to drink at all. Far from being driven by an overwhelming "craving", they turn out to be responsive to common incentives and disincentives, to appeals and arguments, to rules and regulations. Alcohol does not automatically trigger uncontrolled drinking. Resisting our usual appeals and ignoring reasons we consider forceful are not results of alcohol's chemical effect but of the fact that the heavy drinker has different values, fears, and strategies. Thus, in their usual settings alcoholics behave without concern for what others regard as rational considerations.

But when alcoholics in treatment in a hospital setting, for example, are told that they are not to drink, they typically follow the rule. In some studies they have been informed that alcoholic beverages are available, but that they should abstain. Having decided to cooperate, they voluntarily refrain from drinking. More significantly, it has been reported that the occasional few who cheated nevertheless did not drink to excess but voluntarily limited themselves to a drink or two in order to keep their rule violation from being detected. In short, when what they value is at stake, alcoholics control their drinking accordingly." [62]

Fingarette recommends this attitude towards the heavy drinker.

"What should our attitude be, then, to the long term heavy drinker? Alcoholics do not knowingly make the wicked choice to be drunkards. Righteous condemnation and punitive moralism are therefore inappropriate. Compassion, not abuse, should be shown toward any human being launched upon a destructive way of life. But compassion must be realistic: it is not compassionate to encourage drinkers to deny their power to change to assure them that they are helpless and dependent on others, to excuse them legally and give them special government benefits that foster a refusal to confront the need to change. Alcoholics are not helpless, they can take control of their lives. In the last analysis, alcoholics must want to change and choose to change. To do so they must make many difficult daily choices. We can help them by offering moral support and good advice, and by assisting them in dealing with their genuine physical ailments and social needs. But we must also make it clear that heavy drinkers must take responsibility for their own lives. Alcoholism is not a disease, the assumption of personal responsibility, however, is a sign of health, while needless submission to spurious medical authority is a pathology." [63]

This approach is theoretically fertile, especially in the light of conclusions reached by drug authorities such as Kaplan, that there is no satisfactory solution to the drug problem at all. [64] Many researchers have also felt however, that the drug problem is a function of deep social problems, alienation and despair. Robertson in *Heroin, AIDS and Society* says:

> "Availability of heroin is only comparative and obviously legal constraints and social convention make it inaccessible to the majority of the population. It is not therefore the only factor accounting for the increased popularity of heroin. Social conditions and unemployment give rise to many personal difficulties and the disproportionate distribution of heroin users in low socio-economic groups adds further weight to this. The hopelessness and despair associated with poor or non-existent prospects have been shown to be a powerful stimulus to criminality and alcohol abuse, and the associated use of psychoactive drugs by those with diminishing hope for the future is, on the face of it, rather obvious. [65]

ten Have and Sporken also agree

> "i. Heroin use can be intepreted as a socio-cultural problem. As such it represents a fundamental questioning of societal values and norms, a sign of some people's need for consciousness alteration and escape from the meaninglessness of social life.
>
> ii. In modern culture, there is a strong tendency to medicalise the use of heroin because medicine has become one of the most powerful mechanisms to reinforce the basic cultural norms and values.
>
> iii. Through calling heroin use a medical problem, society tries to reinforce those values which have become meaningless for some of its members. However, medicine cannot offer an adequate solution as long as it functions as a social supervision mechanism, articulating the prevailing cultural values.
>
> iv. Ethicists and philosophers ought not to restrict themselves to an analysis of the moral aspects of the medical management of heroin addiction (for example, personal freedom v paternalism). They should also analyse the role of medicine in defining and managing the drug problem. If medical practice results in diverting criticism away from cultural values by individualising social problems, a critical analysis of this process can help to throw more light on the philosophical basis of medical practice. [66]

As do Fraser and Kohlert:

> "A comprehensive attack on the use of illicit drugs cannot be successful without addressing the psychosocial and environmental conditions that produce substance abuse. Current policy makers have been particularly reluctant to address the environmental correlates of substance abuse, since that requires developing strategies to redress fundamental gender, racial, ethnic, and economic inequalities in our society". [67]

And Whitaker:

> "in reality, the rise in the use of drugs owes less to their intrinsic appeal than to many people's dislike of present day existence. Our starting point should be to ask ourselves what is so wrong with our society that more and more of our contemporaries should be driven to embrace and abuse drugs". [68]

A preliminary response to these challenges, will be given in the remainder of this book. [69]

5. Conclusion: State of the Argument

In conclusion, there are no fundamental differences between the position of the author (Smith) and the position paper of Rodney Allen with respect to the long-run social consequences of the drug problem. However, with respect to short term problems such as AIDS and heroin, the author believes that the use of one-use only needle-syringes and wider needle exchange programmes are more satisfactory responses to the AIDS crisis than legalization of heroin and other IV-used drugs. It is generally agreed that AIDS policy can only be successful if there is wide public support. Although the legalization-of-drugs-supporters are sincere and deep thinking even if they were correct, public fear of legalization guarantees that this method cannot succeed. My advocation of one-use-needle-syringes is a technical fix that is perhaps a little costly (for **all** multiple use IV needle-syringes in society must be recalled, destroyed and replaced _immediately_), but the cost of the further spread of HIV infections is infinitely greater. The social changes mentioned here and in the chapters to follow are also inescapable, I shall argue, if future human life is to have meaning and dignity, and the value and richness of what remains of nature is not to be completely destroyed.

NOTES AND REFERENCES

1. Justice P. Woodward, "Too Hot to Handle? Justice Woodward on the Continuing Rise of Organised Crime", *The Weekend Australian*, March 18-19, 1989, pp. 21-23. Citation p. 21.

2. M. Newton, "Dollar in Thrall to Drug Lords", *The Australian*, Tueaday February 28, 1989, p. 13.

3. H.V. Fineberg, "The Social Dimensions of AIDS", *Scientific American*, Vol. 259, October 1988, pp. 106-112. Citation p. 107.

4. ibid p. 108.

5. For background reading on the problem of AIDS and IVDU cf: W. Booth, "AIDS and Drug Abuse: No Quick Fix", *Science*, Vol. 239, 12 February 1988, pp. 717-718; H.M. Ginzburg, "Intravenous Drug Users and the Acquired Immune Deficiency Syndrome", *Public Health Reports*, Vol. 99, 1984, pp. 206-212; J.R. Robertson and C. Skidmore, "AIDS and Intravenous Drug Use", *British Medical Journal*, Vol. 294, 1987, p. 571; R.P. Brettle and B. Nelles, "Special Problems of Injecting Drug-Misusers", *British Medical Bulletin*, Vol. 44, 1988, pp. 149-159; J. O'Connor and S. Stafford-Johnson, "AIDS and Intravenous Drug Abuse", *British Journal of Addiction*, Vol. 82, 1987, p. 813; A. Wodak (et al) "Antibodies to the Human Immunodeficiency Virus in Needles and Syringes Used by Intravenous Drug Users", *Medical Journal of Australia*, Vol. 147, 1987, pp. 275-276; R. Ancelle-Park (et al), "AIDS and Drug Addicts in Europe", *The Lancet*, September 12, 1987, pp. 626-627; D.C.D. Jarlais and S.R. Friedman, "HIV Infection Among Intravenous Drug Users: Epidemiology and Risk Reduction", *AIDS*, Vol. 1, 1987, pp. 67-76; P.A. Selwyn (et al), "Knowledge About AIDS and High Risk Behavior Among Intravenous Drug Users in New York City", *AIDS*, Vol. 1, 1987, pp. 247-254; A.R. Moss, "AIDS and Intravenous Drug Use: The Real Heterosexual Epidemic", *British Medical Journal*, Vol. 294, 1987, pp. 389-390; M.P. Dolan (et al), "Characteristics of Drug Abusers that Discriminate Needle-Sharers", *Public Health Reports*, Vol. 102, 1987, pp. 395-398; G.M. Robertson (et al), "AIDS - Risk Behaviours and AIDS Knowledge in Intravenous Drug Users", *New Zealand Medical Journal*, 8 April 1987, pp. 209-211; G.A. Carlson and T.A. McClellan, "The Voluntary Acceptance of HIV - Antibody Screening by Intravenous Drug Users", *Public Health Reports*, Vol. 120, 1987, pp. 391-394; R.T. D'Aquila and A.B. Williams, "Epidemic Human Immunodeficiency Virus (HIV) Infection Among Intravenous Drug Users (IVDU)", *Yale Journal of Biology and Medicine*, Vol. 60, 1987, pp. 545-567; A. Johns (et

al) "Drug Users, AIDS, and the Government Response", <u>The Lancet</u>, July 2, 1988, p. 41; R.L. Hubbard (et al), "Role of Drug-Abuse Treatment in Limiting the Spread of AIDS", <u>Reviews of Infectious Diseases</u>, Vol. 10, 1988, pp. 377-384; D.C.D. Jarlais and S.R. Friedman, "Target Groups for Preventing AIDS Among Intravenous Drug Users", <u>Journal of Applied Social Psychology</u>, Vol. 17, 1987, pp. 251-268; W.R. Lange (et al), "Geographic Distribution of Human Immunodeficiency Virus Markers in Parenteral Drug Abusers", <u>American Journal of Public Health</u>, Vol. 78, 1988, pp. 443-446.

6. Dr. N. Blewett, quoted from R. Hicks, "AIDS: The Second Wave", <u>The Australian Magazine</u>, July 1-2, 1989, pp. 8-14. Citation p. 10.

7. A. Wodak and R. Penny, "A Report on the National Advisory Committee on the Acquired Immunodeficiency Syndrome's Workshop on Human Immunodeficiency Virus Infection and Intravenous Drug Abuse", <u>Medical Journal of Australia</u>, Vol. 149, 1988, pp. 373-375; C. Sweeny, "AIDS and the Needle", <u>Time</u> (Australia), January 23 1989, pp. 10-15.

8. M. Watson, "Australian Strategies for Dealing with AIDS and IVDU's", in Department of Community Services and Health, <u>Living with AIDS Toward the Year 2000: Report of the Third National Conference on AIDS</u>, (Australian Government Publishing Service, Canberra, 1988, pp. 372-373.

9. R. Hicks, "AIDS 'The Main Danger' From Drugs", <u>The Australian</u>, Monday July 3, 1989, p. 3.

10. P.D. Welsby, "One-Use Needle Syringes for Drug Abusers", <u>The Lancet</u>, August 1, 1987, p. 285.

11. J. Allender, "Single-Shot Shoot Out in the War on AIDS", <u>The Australian</u>, Friday February 24, 1989.

12. cf. also L. Edgoose and J. Baillie, "AIDS and Intravenous Drug Abuse: Risk Behavior", <u>Medical Journal of Australia</u>, Vol. 146, 1987, pp. 279-280; S. Connor, "Advisers are Bitter at AIDS Ruling", <u>New Scientist</u>, 7 April 1988, p. 17; S.K. Chaturvedi, "Does AIDS Fear Disuade Intravenous Drug Abuse?" <u>British Journal of Addiction</u>, Vol. 82, 1987, p. 101.

13. J. Allender, "'Safe Syringe' Project Stalled", <u>The Australian</u>, Tuesday July 25, 1989, p. 7.

14. S. Kingman, "AIDS and the Social Outcast", <u>New Scientist</u>, 10 March 1988, pp. 30-31.

15. On decriminalization and legalization cf. E.T. Miller (et al) "Decriminalizing Drugs: Variations in Endorsement Within Professional Roles", <u>Contemporary Drug Problems</u>, Vol. 7, 1978, pp. 181-193; H.M. Greenstein and P.E. DiBianco, "Marijuana Laws - A Crime Against Humanity", <u>Notre Dame Lawyer</u>, Vol. 48, 1972, pp. 314-339; M.G. Kurzman and H. Magell, "Deciminalizing Possession of All Controlled Substances: An Alternative Whose Time has Come", <u>Contemporary Drug Problems</u>, Vol. 6, 1977, pp. 245-259; J. Richman, "Sociological Perspectives on Illegal Drug Use: Definitional, Reactional, and Etiologic Insights", <u>Behavioral Sciences and the Law</u>, Vol. 3, 1985, pp. 249-258; H.B. Kaplan, "Conceptual Issues in Marijuana Decriminalization Rersearch", <u>Contemporary Drug Problems</u>, Vol. 10, 1981, pp. 365-382; R.C. Petersen, "Decriminalization of Marijuana - A Brief Overview of Research-Relevant Policy Issues", <u>Contemporary Drug Problems</u>, Vol. 10, 1981, pp. 265-275.

16. M. Newton, "Dollar in Thrall to Drug Lords", <u>The Australian</u>, Tuesday February 28, 1989, p. 13.

17. A stark portrayal of this crisis was given in the film <u>Colors</u>. cf. Also S. Macmillan, "Guns, Drugs 'at Root' of Soaring Murders", <u>The Advertiser</u>, Monday March 20, 1989, p. 6; C. Reid, "Week Like No Other in Rotten Big Apple", <u>Sunday Mail</u>, (Adelaide) August 13 1989, p. 22.

18. C. Reid, "Born to Die", <u>The Advertiser</u>, Saturday August 12, 1989, magazine p. 2.

19. M. Fraser and N. Kohlert, "Substance Abuse and Public Policy", <u>Social Science Review</u>, March 1988, pp. 103-126. Citation p. 104.

20. J. Krivanek, <u>Heroin: Myths and Reality</u>, (Allen and Unwin, Sydney, 1988); S. Davies, <u>Shooting Up: Heroin - Australia</u>, (Hale and Iremonger, Sydney, 1986).

21. M. Baker, "Heroin Flood Feared", <u>The Advertiser</u>, Saturday April 22, 1989, p. 6; "Losing the Poppy War", <u>Asiaweek</u>, July 28, 1989, p. 31.

22. E. Hannan, "Heroin Addicts 'Turn to Cocaine'", <u>The Australian</u>, Tuesday February 28, 1989, p. 4.

23. C. Egan, "How Middle Australia is Hooked on Speed", <u>The Weekend Australian</u>, March 25-26, 1989, p. 4.

24. Assistant Police Commissioner V. Werner, "Whitewash on Crime", <u>The Australian</u>, Tuesday January 17, 1989.

25. K.D. Berhard, "The Best Solution to Our Heroin Problem", <u>Religious Humanism</u>, Vol. 8, 1974, pp. 8-13; T. Szasz,

Ceremonial Chemistry: The Ritual Perception of Drugs, Addicts and Pushers, (Anchor Press, New York, 1975); A.S. Trebach, The Heroin Solution, (Yale University Press, New Haven, 1982); P. Adams, "Wowsers, Scumbags and Mates", The Bulletin, December 13, 1988, p. 99; G.J. Church, "Thinking the Unthinkable", Time (Australia), May 30, 1988, pp. 34-38; E. Marshall, "Drug Wars: Legalization Gets a Hearing", Science, Vo.. 241, 2 September, 1988, pp. 1157-1159; O. Brown, "Legalise Heroin or Wipe Out Youth: Adviser", The Advertiser, Monday June 19, 1989, p. 3; J. Allender and K. Harbutt, "AIDS Expert Calls for Clinics to Distribute Legalised Heroin", The Australian, Tuesday January 31, 1989, p. 2; S.M. Stoll, "Why Not Heroin? The Controversy Surrounding the Legalization of Heroin for Therapeutic Purposes", Journal of Contemporary Health Law and Policy, Vol. 1, 1985, pp. 173-194; P.P. McGuiness, "To Reduce the Problems of Crime and Corruption, Legalise Heroin", The Weekend Australian, March 18-19, 1989, p. 2.

26. D. Hawks, "The Proposal to Make Heroin Available Legally to Intravenous Drug Abusers", Medical Journal of Australia, Vol. 149, 1988, pp. 455-456.

27. D.A.J. Richards, "Towards New Perspectives on Drug Control: A Negotiated Settlement to the War on Drugs", Nova Law Review, Vol. 11, 1987, pp. 909-913.

28. ibid p. 910.

29. ibid p. 912.

30. R. Neville, "The State's Intervention in Individuals' Drug Use: A Normative Account", in T.H. Murray (et al), Feeling Good and Doing Better: Ethics and Non-Therapeutic Drug Use, (Humana Press, New Jersey, 1984), pp. 65-80. Citation pp. 71-72.

31. D.A.J. Richards, Sex, Drugs, Death and the Law, (Rowman and Littlefield, Totowa, 1982), p. 170.

32. H. Leventhal (et al), "Is the Smoking Decision on 'Informed Choice'? Effect of Smoking Risk Factors on Smoking Beliefs", Journal of the American Medical Association, Vo. 257, June 26, 1987, pp. 3373-3376.

33. E. Fromm, Escape from Freedom, (Holt, Rinehart and Winston, New York, 1963).

34. J. Adelson, "Drugs and Youth", Commentary, Vol. 87, 1989, pp. 24-28.

35. E.A. Nadelmann, "The Case for Legalization", The Public Interest, No. 92, 1988, pp. 3-31.

36. ibid.

37. K. Gee, "Heroin: To Be Legal or Not?", *Quadrant*, Vol. XXXIV, No. 257, July 1989, pp. 38-39. Citation p. 39.

38. K. Pakula and R. Girling, "Dying for a Drink", *The Australian Magazine*, May 13-14, 1989, pp. 20-33; Editorial, "Alcohol and Disease", *Acta Medica Scandinavica*, Vol. 223, 1988, pp. 97-99.

39. National Campaign Against Drug Abuse, National Drug Education Program, *An Australian Guide to Drug Issues*, (Australian Government Publishing Service, Canberra, 1986), p. 29.

40. J.C. Burnham, "New Perspectives on the Prohibition 'Experiment' of the 1920s", *Journal of Social History*, Vol. 2, 1968-69, pp. 51-68.

41. R. Robertson, *Heroin, AIDS and Society*, (Hodder and Stoughton, London, 1987), p. 38.

42. G.T. McLaughlin, "Cocaine: The History and Regulation of a Dangerous Drug", *Cornell Law Review*, Vol. 58, 1973, pp. 537-573; Committee on Drug Abuse of the Council on Psychiatric Services, "Position Statement on Psychoactive Substance Use and Dependence: Update on Marijuana and Cocaine", *American Journal of Psychiatry*, Vol. 144, 1987, pp. 698-702; J.B. Murray, "An Overview of Cocaine Use and Abuse", *Psychological Reports*, Vol. 59, 1986, pp. 243-264; S. Cohen, "Cocaine: Acute Medical and Psychiatric Complications", *Psychiatric Annals*, Vol. 14, 1984, pp. 747-749; and "Recent Developments in the Abuse of Cocaine", *Bulletin on Narcotics*, Vol. 36, 1984, pp. 3-14; A.M. Washton and A. Tatarsky, "Adverse Effects of Cocaine Abuse", in L.S. Harris (ed.) *Problems of Drug Dependence, 1983*, (NIDA Research Monographs, Series No. 49, 1984), pp. 247-254.

43. D.R. Jasinski (et al) "Etorphine in Man, I. Subjective Effects and Suppression of Morphine Abstinence", *Clinical Pharmacology Therapeutics*, Vol. 17, 1975, pp. 267-272.

44. T. Morganthau (et al), "Bennett's Drug War", *The Bulletin with Newsweek*, August 22, 1989, pp. 72-74.

45. C.E. Faupel and C.B. Klockars, "Drugs-Crime Connections: Elaborations from the Life Histories of Hard-Core Heroin Addicts", *Social Problems*, Vol. 34, 1987, pp. 54-68; I.D. Elliott, "Heroin: Mythologies for Law Enforcers", *Criminal Law Journal*, Vol. 6, 1982, pp. 6-43 and "Heroin Myths Revisited: The Stewart Report", *Criminal Law Journal*, Vol. 7, 1983, pp. 333-345.

46. R. Maddock, "Cocaine, Politics and the Economy", Flindersweek, June 13-25, No. 305, 1989.

47. F. Barnaby (ed.) The Gaia Peace Atlas: Survival Into the Third Millenium, (Pan Books, London, 1988), p. 122.

48. R. Hall, Disorganized Crime, (University of Queensland Press, St. Lucia, 1986).

49. cf. P. Dickie, The Road to Fitzgerald, (University of Queensland Press, St. Lucia, 1988); K. Moor, Crims in Grass Castles (Pascoe Publishing, Apollo Bay, 1989); B. Bottom (ed.) Big Shots, (Macmillan, Melbourne, 1985); B. Bottom, Connections, (Sun Books, Melbourne, 1985), Shadow of Shame, (Sun Books, Melbourne, 1988), The Godfather in Australia, (Shepp Books, Hornsby, 1988), Bugged! (Macmillan Melbourne, 1989); B. Bottom, "Faceless Big Shot", The Independent Monthly, Vol. 1, No. 1, July 1989, p. 12; B. Bottom, "Fitzgerald's Big Mistake", The Independent Monthly, Vol. 1, No. 2, August 1989, pp. 25-26; P. Charlton, "Queensland: The Joke Backfires", The Advertiser Magazine, Saturday July 1 1989, pp. 1, 5.

50. B. Woodley, "AFP on Trial in Winchester Inquiry", The Weekend Australian, May 13-14, 1989, pp. 14-15; J. Silvester (et al), "Slain Police Chief Led War on Mafia", The Advertiser, Thursday January 12, 1989, p. 1.

51. op.cit., note 1.

52. Agence France - Presse, "Former Triad Members May be Allowed in Australia", The Advertiser, Monday May 8, 1989, p. 3.

53. M. King, "Triad Links Snared in Australia's Biggest Drug Bust", The Advertiser, Saturday May 13, 1989, p. 3.

54. K. Harbutt, "AFP After Triad Death Peddlers", The Weekend Australian, July 22-23, 1989, p. 13.

55. ibid.

56. "Secret Triads Top NCA Hit List", Sunday Mail, June 25, 1989, p. 153.

57. K. Harbutt, "Mafia Joins Triads to Rule the Drug World", The Weekend Australian, October 29-30, 1988, pp. 1, 17.

58. D. Burstein, Yen: The Threat of Japan's Financial Empire, (Schwartz, Melbourne, 1989).

59. C. Boag, "Hire Education: Have We Got a Degree for You", The Bulletin with Newsweek, August 22, 1989, pp. 46-54.

60. S. Peele, "A Moral Vision of Addiction: How People's Values Determine Whether They Become and Remain Addicts", *Journal of Drug Issues*, Vol. 17, 1987, pp. 187-215 and *The Meaning of Addiction: Compulsive Experience and its Interpretation*, (Lexington Books, Massachusetts, 1985).

61. H. Fingarette, *Heavy Drinking: The Myth of Alcoholism as a Disease*, (University of California Press, Berkeley, 1988).

62. H. Fingarette, "Alcoholism: The Mythical Disease", *The Public Interest*, No. 91, 1988, pp. 3-22. Citation p.15.

63. ibid, p. 22. For controversy cf. W. Madsen, "Thin Thinking About Heavy Drinking", *The Public Interest*, No. 95, 1989, pp. 112-118 and H. Fingarette, "A Rejoinder to Madsen", ibid, pp. 118-121.

64. J. Kaplan, *The Hardest Drug: Heroin and Public Policy*, (University of Chicago Press, Chicago, 1983) and "Taking Drugs Seriously", *The Public Interest*, No. 92, 1988, pp. 32-50.

65. Robertson, op.cit. Note 41, p.42.

66. H. ten Have and P. Sporken, "Heroin Addiction, Ethics and Philosophy of Medicine", *Journal of Medical Ethics*, Vol. 11, 1985, pp. 173-177. Citation p. 177.

67. Fraser and Kohlert, op.cit. note 19, pp. 119-120.

68. B. Whitaker, *The Global Fix: The Crisis of Drug Addiction*, (Methuen, London, 1987), pp. 376-377.

69. Further supporting material includes: G. Harding, "Constructing Addiction as a Moral Failing", *Sociology of Health and Illness*, Vol. 8, 1986, pp. 75-85; L. Ray, "Problems of Substance Abuse: Exploitation and Control", *Social Science and Medicine*, Vol. 20, 1985, pp. 1225-1233; B.K. Alexander and P.F. Hadaway, "Opiate Addiction: The Case for an Adaptive Orientation", *Psychological Bulletin*, Vol. 92, 1982, pp. 367-381; A.P. Jurich and C.J. Polson, "Reasons for Drug Use: Comparison of Drug Users and Abusers", *Psychological Reports*, Vol. 55, 1984, pp. 371-378; P.C. Thauberger (et al), "Use of Chemical Agents and Avoidance of Ontological Confrontation of Loneliness", *Perceptual and Motor Skills*, Vol. 52, 1981, pp. 91-96; R. Eckersley, "Casualities of Change: The Predicament of Youth in Australia", (CSIRO, ACT, July 1988).

5 Privacy, medical confidentiality and AIDS

WITH RODNEY ALLEN

1   Introduction

2   Private Property and Private Ownership

3   The Problem of the Criteria of Possession of Private Property

4   A Critique of the Principle of Privacy in Ownership

5   Criteria of Acquisition

6   Individual Privacy and Medical Confidentiality

7   Conclusion

1. Introduction

The concept of privacy is confused. Yet both defenders and critics of this concept assume that it is a unified and coherent idea. But a little thought reveals a plethora of vague ideas and principles lurking behind the "privacy" label, the relations between which are problematic, if not outrightly incoherent. Yet many protracted political, social and philosophical disputes make essential reference to either the justification or unsoundness of this ideal, in both cases presupposing that the concept is clear and coherent. Some examples of this are (1) the "private-property-ization" of the nature of many moral offences, seen particularly in the definitions of such matters as theft, fraud, exploitation and corruption, in terms of proprietory interests; (2) in moral philosophy the assumption that egoism is the predominant natural moral characteristic of human kind, embodied in questions such as "Why should I be moral?" and "How is altruism possible, when we are all at heart egoists?"; (3) Within moral philosophy a pre-occupation with utilitarianism and with its associated problems of contractual morality, rights and obligations under promise and contracts; (4) Within social and political theory, a pre-occupation with the Hobbesian problem[1], the problem of achieving and maintaining social control and order. For socialists, consider also the very important conflict between defenders of the private ownership of the means of production and the criticisms of this ideal. Also consider problems which would (prima facie) exist in societies where there was no private ownership of the means of production, such as the limits (if any) of collectivist interference in the lives of individual people, such as in matter of religious beliefs, drugs, abortion, censorship and HIV infected individuals.

All these issues involving the concept of privacy raise the question of how it relates to the other social values such as freedom and equality, democracy, social justice and social welfare. For example, is privacy merely some form of freedom, or is it something sui generis that goes beyond freedom? If so, how should a concern for it, if indeed it is a value at all, be balanced against other social values, when they conflict? Are privacy claims justified at all?

There is no coherent ideology, which might be called "Privatism". It is true that the "petite bourgeoisie" have both a personal and social need for privacy, in a society where they may be threatened by both the "big state", "big business" and the "forces of revolution". But neither the

State, nor big business are very keen on being spied upon. They jealously guard their own secrets whilst invoking security, law-and-order, efficiency and national interest, as justifications for spying on everyone else. The by-product industries of security, espionage and counter-espionage continually expand, as secrecy breeds spies. This expansion is perceived as a threat to liberty and privacy by ordinary people, yet at the same time, it is demanded by many for their own protection. A similarly ambivalent attitude is held towards the rise of welfare - bureaucracies and their associated recording, surveillance and investigative mechanisms. Rightist political forces seek to protect the <u>privacy</u> of property and the <u>privacy</u> of the family, but are also keen on law-and-order, security and defence, and hence spies. Liberals look forward to the day when an individual's morals and life style, sexual and ingestive habits are private, but also to when governments and other authorities have no secrets, to open government, and an informed public. Socialists seek the liberation of people from ruling class domination, manipulation and exploitation, and the flourishing of autonomy and self-determination for people in general, but also the collectivization and communalization of the individual and the socialization of resources.

Generally speaking, a privacy is an immunity, a protective or defence perimeter against an external force, which may spoil or change something, or just add to it, or integrate it with something else. So the fundamental question in social philosophy that is raised by privacy claims is this: "What in societies should be immuned, or protected, from what?" We shall not attempt here to answer in full generality this question, but shall restrict our discussion to a critical examination, from a socialist perspective, of some of the most important privacy claims. We shall argue that most privacy claims are both confused and unjustified and incompatible with genuine socialist concerns; that many concerns for privacy are concerns for profit or privilege, irresponsible individualism or self-indulgence for self or chauvinistic interest, and that where a claim for privacy or immunity is justified, it may less misleadingly be understood as a soundly based claim for a specific form of freedom or justice.

Most writing on the concept of privacy has been within the context of American legal theory. [2] The U.S. Constitution itself does not explicitly state that privacy is a right, although the Third, Fourth, Fourteenth and Ninth Amendments, have been taken to provide a constitutional right to privacy. In <u>Roe v. Wade</u> (1973), Justice Blackmun concluded that an individual's right to privacy was broad enough, "to encompass a woman's decision whether or not to terminate her pregnancy". This right was never defined. T. Gerety, although believing that a woman's decision to have an abortion is an expression of her autonomy, points out that the Court cites no reasons only "uncertain precedents". [3]

Another (early) legal theorist R. Lisle, adopts the same attitude to an alleged legal right to privacy, which we adopt towards the philosophical right to privacy:

> "The right to privacy is for the most part an unnecessary right. With the modern definitions of property, thoughts and emotions which have been recorded in permanent form will be protected from exposition to the public. Under the laws of slander and libel, recovery can be had if the plaintiff is in fact unjustly exposed to hatred, ridicule, obloquy, or contempt before the public. Under breach of contract or trust, recovery can be had in many other cases". [4]

It is the aim of this chapter to provide philosophical support for the above point of view.

The literature on the topic of AIDS, privacy and confidentiality is also typically shallow and confused. William Dornette, for example says that "Everyone who learns of any indiviudal's HIV-infectious status must maintain confidentiality over a rather broad area". Nevertheless Dornette then goes on to say "Any disclosure should be limited to that needed to prevent further spread of the infection ... the devastating impact of the infection and the absolute importance of limiting further spread of this virus demand whatever meaningful controls that are necessary". [5] Dornette does not realise that this condition diminishes the impact and importance of privacy claims to virtually zero. Although the issue of privacy has been discussed in many other context, [6] these discussions have typically never attempted to explicate or justify the concept of privacy itself. It is also the aim of this chapter to provide a critical analysis of the concept of privacy, which is very much lacking in the ethical literature on the problem of AIDS.

We shall discuss the question of individual privacy and medical confidentiality, especially in the context of biobehavioural control with respect to AIDS. There we shall argue that individual privacy is not a distinct right and that whilst the physician has a _prima facie_ obligation to preserve the medical confidentiality of patients, this is not an absolute obligation and can be overridden by other weighty considerations. In our opinion it is well worthwhile to consider these traditional questions about the nature and justification of privacy, because no discussion of the right of privacy would be complete without a discussion of the socio-political institution needed to secure this right. Consequently we begin this chapter with a critique of the general theory of private property and conclude with a critical discussion of the many complex issues of individual privacy. In addition, in a world where an increasing value is placed upon the merits of private property and free enterprise (the New Right Philosophy) and governments sing the praises of privatization even with respect to fundamental social goods such as health care, it is well worthwhile in the interests of free thought to present a systematic critique of the ideology of private property and "privatism".

2. Private Property and Private Ownership

Private property is of course much more than a vague idea or principle, for it comprises most of the objects, things and ideas that people at least in capitalist societies want and use, and stands as a basic part of the relational fabric of such societies. Private property here has a value in an "economic" sense, an exchange - value, a money-measure. It comprises commodities that can be bought and sold, and in many cases, used "productively" as capital, yielding further returns as "private property".

Our concern here is with the ideology of private property; with why its defenders hold that it is a good thing. That is, we are concerned with the <u>normative principles</u> that constitute the social ideal of privacy in property, rather than with the <u>legal definitions</u> of private property, constituting various legal forms of private ownership. We follow the Marxian tradition in believing that legal forms are expressions of real social relations of control, the patterns of action constituting socio-economic structure. Indeed, we believe that the Marxian tradition has adequately documented the nature and role of private property in the capitalist mode of production and its effects in terms of the exploitation of labour, so we do not intend to deal further with these particular questions: we assume this material as part of our background assumptions. (Various problems facing the "Marxist" tradition will be discussed in the final chapter).

Since from a Marxian position, the concepts of "production", "mode of production" and "relations of production" are crucial to the analysis of social structure, it would seem necessary for this purpose to distinguish systematically between "private ownership of the means of production" and "private-consumption-wealth". This has produced a tendency in Marxist writings for an explicit concern with the socialisation of the means of production and thereby in many cases implicitly staking out the domain of consumption, at least in part as the appropriate realm of privacy. It is such a question, which we believe stands in need of justification. We will address our criticisms of privacy quite generally, making use of the distinction between "private - production - wealth" and "private - consumption - wealth", only when it appears relevant to the criticism of ideological pre-occupations.

We can divide our problems with privacy in property into two different, but related questions:

(1) The problem of the criteria of <u>possession</u> of private property.

(2) The problem of the criteria of legitimate <u>acquisition</u> of private property.

3. The Problem of the Criteria of Possession of Private Property

It would be a mistake to regard private property as that which one had <u>total and absolute control</u> over, either as an individual or as a collective. This is a mistaken explication because the idea of a socially maintained absolute freedom is incoherent: for if a society guarantees to some extent an individual's possession of private property, then it must restrict the use of such property to attack criminally or otherwise illegitimate uses of others' private property.

It is also a mistake to regard private property as that which is exclusively used or controlled by individual or group owners, since it is obviously unrealistic to pretend that such private owners universally and totally control access to their property, given the bureaucratic state, the expansion of legal regulation and other forms of state and non-state social intervention.

It is also a mistake in our opinion to assume that the only possible <u>subjects</u> of private property are individuals and that private property can be an attribute of individuals independently of social structure. Not only today is much more private property overtly and collectively owned by multinational corporations, but we believe that all social phenomena including the institution of private property are ultimately collective in nature, and are to be understood in terms of the structure of collectives: we reject the theses of both methodological individualism and social atomism. [7] Private property is constituted from, and sustained by, internal relations within and between social collectives. Consequently private property is a property of a subject, but the particular subject need not be in any sense an individual, and even if it were, this ownership would be derivative from and backed up by, social forces sustaining the general institution itself.

Yet another mistake would be to regard "free markets" and the processes of buying and selling as peculiar and essential to private property. Even "public" and "communal" property can be bought and sold, and hardly any private property can be "freely" sold in "free markets" in these days of monopolies, cartels, government intervention and legal regulation. Nevertheless the idea of market distribution is an important one for any comprehensive understanding of the capitalist economy. But it is not a central idea; we follow the Marxist tradition in giving theoretical primacy to the sphere of production rather than the sphere of distribution.

So far we have eliminated some inadequate explications of the concept of private property. It seems intuitively clear that private property is a power or entitlement of some type for its particular subject over its object. Perhaps we should try an alternative strategy and clarify the notion of private property by contrast with that of public property or the socialisation of property.

If public property were regarded as State owned property, then private property is property not owned by the State and socialism would be equivalent to state ownership. But is the property of the capitalist state, the "public" or "communalistic" property? The Marxist tradition, despite much internal disagreement, has given a resounding and communal "No!" to this question. The idea of the State as portrayed in neo-classical economics - as a neutral judge serving the interests of all, is a myth - the State in general serves the interests of the dominant economic classes in such societies. It is not necessary for this point to be made to equate the State primarily as the ruling class "servomechanism", for there is no contradiction involved in admitting that the capitalist state may well in some situations have interests which conflict with those of the ruling class itself, and the previous allegation. Rather the allegation is a statement of a propensity or tendency. We maintain that the distinction between the State and the rest of capitalist society, is irrelevant for the purpose of drawing a distinction in principle between public and private property, since the capitalist state is too closely attached to private capital to provide any meaningful contrast to private property, or a distinctive sense of public ownership.

The basic reason why not even a State that has largely absorbed the independent private economy of its society must be regarded as having socialised or communalised property, is that such States remain a coercive or hierarchic-bureaucratic social order. These characteristics are fundamental to States as we now know them, and the Marxist and elitist theory tradition at least agree on this point. As such they are centres of power over people, rather than means of returning power to the people. They contain within themselves the seeds of transformed class division, and indeed a transformed capitalist social structure. No matter how all-embracing, they continue to function basically in the interests of their upper echelons, and by way of typically bourgeois forms of exploitation, accumulation and expansion and imperialism. These remarks are quite consistent with mainstream socialist theory, which never did envisage progress towards socialism as consisting of the abandonment of capitalism and the retainment of the State. At best, the State has been regarded as a transitional mechanism, usually to guard against counter-revolution. Anarchists, nobody needs reminding, did not pin any hopes on the State.

Further, we reject the proposal that property becomes non-private (if not public or socialised) when control of its use is centralised under the guiding hand of the State, that is, that fragmented economic decision-making is the essence of privacy in property. The reasons are that economic decision-making in a private economy dominated by giant corporations, monopolies and oligopolies, is certainly not uncoordinated, or fragmented and a large bureucratic state may well fail to coordinate the fragmented decision-making of its various parts. The concentration of economic power in giant corporations has shown us that concentration <u>per se</u> does not diminish privacy of ownership, for this corporation may still be (in an intuitive sense) privately owned. If this concentration should take place within the State, we may come to regard the economy as non-private, although definitely non-socialist. But we would not have a meaningful contrast with private property.

It seems, on the basis of these arguments, that the attempts to explicate the idea of both private property and social or public property with reference to the State all fail. Still we believe it will be fruitful to approach the further elucidation of privacy in property by way of contrasting it with social or public property, and this in turn, by articulating the principles of genuine social ownership. It is sometimes necessary to find out where we are going, or could or should go, in order to know where we are.

We have already argued that social ownership cannot be equivalent to mere collective ownership. On the other hand, social ownership cannot quite literally be ownership by a whole society in all respects. To try to understand social ownership in this way would be to mystify it out of the realm of real possibilities. Just as it would be vacuous to maintain that every decision in a complex society can be equally made by each of the people, so it would be vacuous to maintain that every material resource of such a society can in some significant way be owned equally and uniformly by all its people. Real democracy and social ownership both require, not the impossibility of everyone equally controlling everything <u>in all respects</u>, but a structure which enables everyone to justly and with <u>social responsibility</u>, control those different things which affect their interests. Social ownership of a resource consists primarily in control of it by <u>users</u> - that is, those with a <u>direct</u> interest in it. Taking production, following Marx, to be the basic human interest and the developing force behind further interests, the basic form of social ownership of a resource would be ownership by those who use it productively, to provide goods and services to other members of society. Such ownership would be collective, since the production of anything is usually a co-operative enterprise. And it would be classless, consisting of ownership by all and only all the producer/workers concerned. Yet at the same time it would be cooperative and socially responsible production, geared towards the interests and well-being of other members of society, as indeed their production must be so geared. We will elaborate upon this. But we should note before passing on that the sort of initial interest which justifies admission to a social owning collective cannot itself be what is sometimes called a "proprietary interest", i.e. an interest in virtue of some prior private ownership of something involved in the enterprise. The effect of this would be to reduce social ownership to our contrasting starting point, private ownership.

A more immediate problem facing us here is the question of the social responsibility of the active - collector producers. Providing the dimension of general social responsibility is a major problem in describing the institutional nature of a socialist order. Reformist social democrats have long thought that social responsibility can be structurally guaranteed by the State, by increasing State control within the context of democratically guaranteed responsible leadership. Yet if we are correct in our claim that the State - even the so-called "Democratic State", is essentially a coercive order, then this hope is illusory, since coercive power is more likely to be used in the class interests of the coercers. It is utterly naive to believe that the class background of the holders of the State power will ensure a benign "rule". Even if they could, we would still be subject to coercive State Power, rather than subjects of the cooperative power of the People. If social revolutions could only amount to the transfer of State Power from one exploiting group to another, be this even a "new class" of intellectuals as Gouldner proposes, [8] then conceptions of socialism such as ours would be untenable.

Our response to this challenge is to point out that it is the structure of social relationships which determines, defines, constitutes and limits various forms of social power, including State Power and the power of Gouldner's emerging "flawed universal class" of intellectuals. Consequently we maintain that the object of socialist strategy is not simply the take over of existing sources of power and the use of these sources, but rather the transformation of existing social relationships and the transcendence of our reliance on the State and other so-called "flawed universal classes". Gouldner's position in particular offers no challenge to our own. His argument is, in an ultimate sense <u>circular</u> since it assumes basically a continuation of non-socialist social relationships. In his society to come, the "Intellectual Class" will control the important resource of "cultural capital", by contrast to the "moneyed capital" now owned by the Bourgeoisie and which for some reason will come to diminish in relative importance to "cultural capital". We puzzle at what precisely Gouldner's "generative mechanism" [9] is here; how in fact such a "vast" social transformation occurs. But we are as lay logicians, most puzzled at how a distinction between "cultural capital" and "moneyed capital" (or at least ultimately reducible to this in capitalist societies) can be sustained, given Gouldner's equation of "capital" with "income earning capacity". Ideas (at least some ideas) as any multinational book seller will tell you, are "moneyed capital", as are more concrete manifestations of capital such as art works, scientific instruments and so on. Nor is "moneyed capital" outside the sphere of culture: it is after all a human social product. Whilst we would need to develop these remarks in much more detail if we intended to produce a critique of Gouldner, our general strategy of defence should be clear, we hope, to both friends and foes.

Is it possible to describe a structure of social responsibility for ownership which is both non-anarchic and non-static? We have suggested that no form of ownership has <u>absolute</u> power as such. Both private and social owners alike would be under some form of constraint as far as their ownership is concerned. Private owners in a straight forwardly capitalist society are constrained by both the State and its laws, and the alienated operation of market relations. Social owners too, would be constrained and since one of our intuitive starting points for a conception of socialised wealth was that it must be somehow "commonwealth", it seems that social owners must be constrained <u>by</u> and <u>for</u> the interests of other community members affected by their operation. This is a basic principle of social ownership, but stated this vaguely, it seems to say no more than what defenders of the bourgeois State say, albeit misleadingly, falsely and ideologically, about their own laws.

We can, fortunately, go further. Social owners are generally collectives, and usually producers. These owning collectives exist within a community of people more or less indirectly affected by their operations as consumers, sharers of the environment and so on. With respect to any one resource, we can divide interested persons into: (a) day-to-day users of a resource and (b) members of the community who are or might be, more or less indirectly affected by use of the resource (e.g. consumers, clients, suppliers, neighbours, etc.) The day-to-day users would be social owners, and their basic proprietary right would be the right to day-to-day access and managerial rights. Their proprietorship would carry with it a general positive obligation of service to their wider community consumers, clients, guests, neighbours and so on; a community sanction enforced by <u>all</u> members of the community, and a loss of proprietorship could be attached to failure to reasonably achieve this. Thus the rights of social proprietorship would be (a) day-to-day access and management, and (b) an initiating share in general legislative role in this policy-making to ensure that the decisions of the day-to-day users are in fact in the best interests of society, the environment and the world if need this be(in the case of uranium mining for example). Therefore social ownership would render proprietorship into collective worker-management plus an initiating share in relevant policy-making, with wider communities of concerned persons also sharing in policy-making and inter-collective co-ordination.

One further important point. If property and wealth are to be genuinely social and if their structure is to be conducive to co-operation then the distribution of wealth must be just. Social justice is not a natural occurrence; it must be achieved by conscious social action. Therefore one entitlement that should not characterise social ownership is an unqualified right to the accumulation of further wealth based on the productive use of the owned resource. Social ownership should be subject to net transfers of wealth in response to wider social needs, as determined by co-ordinating "wider community" decisions. The distribution principle of socialism, is we maintain, need and subjecting social ownership to structurally regulated transfers of wealth would be necessary to accord with this principle and to ensure the "common-ness" of common-wealth.

An important corollary of this argument is that socialisation of ownership cannot be achieved singly and in isolation from the socialisation of all the basic relational structures of a society. A single commune - no matter how democratic, non-individualistic and non-hierarchic - cannot socialise what it owns, for it must necessarily lack a structural avenue of responsibility and related interests, including the possibility of organised transfers of wealth to and from it, in response to needs. Its wealth cannot be rendered common-wealth, the object of common conscious determination.

Social ownership, as we've described it, has two basic features; (a) the worker-collectivity of the owning subject; (b) the dimension of social responsibility, this being the constraint on owners by and for the interests of all concerned collectives and individuals, and people-in-general. Either principle is a sufficient condition to distinguish private and social property. However (a) is not a sufficient condition to distinguish between private and social ownership, although it is a necessary condition. For collective/worker ownership by itself (given differentiation, i.e. that each worker does not own equally everything in the society) is compatible with and would tend towards, the private appropriation of produced wealth in the sense of group/sectional accumulation, exclusive of the needs and interests of related collectives and society-in-general. So the essence of social ownership and control lies in the structuring of the use of resources to ensure the equitable satisfaction of all concerned and legitimate interests. It is a society-wide structuring of resource use to ensure responsiveness to all affected needs and interests.

4. A Critique of the Principle of Privacy in Ownership

We will now attempt to distinguish some basic principles of private ownership by way of contrast with the foregoing principles of socialized ownership and subject these principles to a philosophical critique.

Taking the "ownership-by-user-collectives" principle of socialised ownership first, it can easily be seen by contrast, that private ownership as we know it is not limited in this way. Private ownership of a piece of property does not necessarily include all the users of that property nor exclude non-users of the property. Moreover, a society with a class structure rooted in a specific mode of production will necessarily exhibit a general division between owners and users/producers, such that not all users are owners and not all owners are users. This would be the basic line of social fracture into classes, and in capitalist societies would represent the dividing line between the two most important and structurally antagonistic social classes. The structural necessity of such a division would derive from a mode of production dependent upon exploitative forms of control, as capitalism is dependent on both its two sides, capital and wage-labour.

Historically, privacy in property has developed in close interdependence with class-structured societies. Hence private ownership, especially of the means of production, has involved of structural necessity, a general division between owners and users. Yet these divisions seem characteristic of class structure rather than private ownership <u>as such</u> insofar as they are theoretically separable. This of course, is not to deny the causal primacy of the social relations of production and associated class structures in the development and maintenance of forms of privacy in ownership, nor the enormously important practical point that the division between owners and users cannot be overcome without transforming exploitative modes of production: we cannot make everyone into a worker-owner within a capitalist framework.

It seems to us that relations of <u>counter-responsibility</u> are the basic intrinsic features of the institution of private ownership. For the institution of private property is not an institution in the sense in which your local library might be, but rather it is an institution in the sense of a definite set of <u>society-wide</u> structural relations, as is the legal system, the political system, the family system and so on. And a moment's reflection on what we seem to have when we own some private property, in the light of our contrast with socialized property, should indicate that what we have in fact, in a society which allows us to use the owner resource for our own purposes and interests, is in a manner (within limits) indifferent to or contrary to, other socially legitimate interests. More than this, the social relations of private property in general structurally necessitate the pursuit of self and sectional interests, without which would occur the loss of a living, the non-satisfaction of one's needs. This structurally required selfishness is clearly evident in the straight forward operation of a capitalist market economy. So we conclude that the basic principle of private ownership is that the owned resource be available to the self-interested use and/or control of the owner; that owners be able to pursue their own interests exclusive of a concern for others, with the owned resource. Private property is in essence the "sectionalisation" or "egotisticalisation" of social resources.

A private property society is necessarily a mix of conflicts and competitions in accumulation and aggrandizement, a struggle generating winners and losers. This general struggle is a factor in, and has been refined through concrete historical development into class struggle; the monopolisation of productive resources by "winners" emerging on the basis of developing modes of production, and the struggle between social classes for the control of resources, a struggle which is unequal in favour of the one dominant class until (as Marx would have it) a new revolutionary moment arises, the historical uniting of a distintegrating economic order, new productive and social opportunities and a transformed political consciousness. Hence the privatization of property helps re-produce class structure. Private property itself is simply a structure of resource-egoism, a structure for the control of resources for production and consumption governed by the principle of universal <u>self-interest</u>, that each must fully and exclusively pursue his own interests.

Are we inconsistent in asserting that private ownership involves essentially self-interest given our anti-methodological individualist position? According to orthodox moral philosophy, self-interest literally means "individual interest", so that genuine concern for people makes one an altruist. Short of insanity and beyond childhood it is impossible for an individual person <u>not</u> to have some serious and genuine concern for some other individuals. For individuals always gain at least some of their self-identity and potential for selfishness from their status and role in social collectives and social structure. Their selves and their self-interests are in large part made possible by, and absorbed into a collective. Egoism, in the sense of self-creating and consequently self-serving sectarian concern for family, clan, gang and class is common and even when moderated by their interests and principles, to <u>some</u> extent necessary and valuable; this form of egoism that we are using here is our explication of privacy in property, we will call "sectarianism". In saying that private property is a structure of ownership governed by the principle of universal self-interest, we mean a structure which allows and/or requires the exclusive pursuit of <u>sectional-collective</u> interests, the interests of explicitly or implicitly collective owners. The egoism of private-property-ownership is exclusivist in the sense of being exclusive of the needs and interests of other parties directly or indirectly affected by the activity of particular owners. It displays itself as unfulfilled social potential for co-operation and assistance, as competitiveness and as the exploitation or neglect of "loser" interests and of general non-proprietary social interests such as the preservation of a human environment, health and education. Ideological criticism or justification of private property is contingent upon the "ego-ism-in-resource use" thesis.

There seems to be only two general courses open to the defender of egoism in resource use. One is the unpopular and clearly implausible course of bluntly maintaining that egoism in at least the economic sphere, is <u>intrinsically</u> good, regardless of its general consequences. The alternative with much more public relations potential, is to maintain that egoism, whilst morally wrong outside its proper economic sphere, nevertheless does produce generally good consequences for social well-being. It is something like this latter course which is usually adopted by apologists for capitalism and private property.

From this point, the main lines of justifying such ideologies are:

1. The delineation of the economic sphere - the sphere of commodity production, distribution and exchange - as the proper area for the unfettered play of basically self-interested behaviour.

2. The endorsement of the free market as the basic regulator of the economic process, and the judge of winners and losers in economic competition.

3. The endorsement of the State as the monopoly of the means to violence, the guarantor and defender of private property and the basic economic framework, and the minimal regulator of economic activity with consequent support for the myth of the State as <u>public</u> servant, allied with the warning from Private Property, that the State should not overstep its proper boundaries and interfere with legitimate private business activity.

4. The tying-in of the free market and free enterprise with the bourgeois values of <u>individual</u> self-realisation and <u>individual</u> freedom.

5. Support for mass political democracy as congenial to the free-enterprise system; but the confining of democracy to the State in its proper role as defender of property and assistant to private enterprise. The protection of private economic interests from democratic interference by the State, or worse still, the aroused masses.

6. <u>The basic point</u> that self-interested and acquisitive economic activity regulated basically by a free market, and within the "law and order" framework of a minimal State <u>will produce a greater aggregate amount of wanted goods and services</u> (i.e. the material conditions of "the greatest happiness of the greatest number") than would productive activity under any other governing principle.

7. The insistence that the utilitarian connection between egoistic economic behaviour and overall social well-being is guaranteed by <u>human nature</u> particularly the need of people for <u>individualised material incentives</u>. Emphasis that production will not occur to the greatest possible extent unless the socio-economic system provides such incentives, that the provision of avenues for acquisitiveness and inequality of wealth are necessary conditions of the greatest, most effective and most responsive amount of production.

8. There is, one further important sideline justificatory point concerning private property, which lies outside the basic "utilitarian-justification-of-economic-egoism" framework. This is to treat private property as a natural right to the fruits of one's labour. However, since this "just/right" line (dating from John Locke) is most clearly associated with ideological justifications of the <u>distribution</u> of private property, that is with ideology concerning the legitimate or proper ways for one to acquire private property or wealth, rather than with general justifications of the institution of private property, we shall deal with this argument under the heading "Criteria of Acquisition" below.

The salient lines of criticism of the utilitarian justification of economic egoism are these:

1. **It is wrong in its own terms**, in that (a) it is false that economic egoism as displayed concretely in capitalist economies results in the largest <u>most</u> effective possible productive response to the interests and wants of such people within such economies; (b) it is false that efficient, non-coerced productive work depends timelessly on the provision of individualised, relativised, material incentives and that human nature is essentially acquisitive, individually possessive and accumulative; (c) it is false that basic economic structures appealing to and sustaining economic egoism cannot be changed without destroying the possibility

of efficient productivity by doing violence to the essential human need for a relativised incentive.

2. **Its own Terms are Wrong** in that (a) it is mistaken in viewing the context of economic egoism abstractly as the free market in which everyone equally participates instead of historically as the developing capitalist mode of production with its antagonistic and unequal division between capital and labour, increasing monopolization of resources, and so on; (b) it is mistaken in emphasising individualist values (individual freedom, individual self-realisation) at the expense of human needs and interests which can only be realised collectively or co-operatively.

The lynchpin of the utilitarian justification is its concept of human nature - essentialist egoism, the idea that all people are essentially selfish, acquisitive, greedy, and will only work to the degree they are forced or offered a relativised and individualised material incentive. This is given as a reason justifying an economic system which admittedly sustains and encourages economic egoism. The evidence for this "reason" is presumably human behaviour as we know it - i.e. as conditioned by our socio-historical circumstances. People have after all, only lived in capitalist societies for a few hundred years. So at this point the argument becomes circular and question begging: it appeals for justification to the very same facts it is supposed to justify.

In fact, any attempt to uncover an unchanging and unchangeable human essence is foredoomed. It is difficult to discover any substantial unchanging elements of human beings, which are common throughout history, let alone lie outside the socio-historical process. The most recent attempt to do this has been human sociobiology, and this enterprise is in our opinion utterly bankrupt. [10] But in any case, genetic manipulation is not now just a possibility, but a threat, so even this old hard liner is not as hard as it used to be.

For us, human nature is most plausibly viewed, not merely in terms of attributes inherent for all human beings as tokens of a type, but in addition, in terms of tendencies and potentialities, which vary in the degree to which, and in the form in which they are concretely realised, largely because of socio-historical structuring. As Marx maintained, the real "human essence" is history, the continuous self-transformation of human nature. This does not mean that human nature is infinitely malleable, still less that any change can be achieved at any time; and still less that any change would be equally as valuable as any other. Marx's view consistently incorporated the ideas that there are quite general conditions of human life (the need to produce cooperatively) and that in consequence there are certain generally necessary developments in human history; that certain developments would be frustrating and destructive of human potential while others would be liberating and fulfilling, in the light of both the general conditions of human life and concrete historical conditions. He did not deny that there is a human nature in the sense of an abstract and generally necessary _form_ for human needs and interests, _and_ a potential for both self-destructive and self-fulfilling developments. This is in the sense of human standards generated from the general nature of human life, which can be usefully applied to concrete social conditions in the further light of concrete socio-historical analysis. Marx did deny however, that there is a "human essence" in the sense of a changeless, concrete, fully actualised nature. What is clear and relevant, even without Marx, is that it is fallacious to argue that some particularly predominant characteristic of human beings in a certain socio-historical context is unchangeable to any significant degree, and unmediated by socio-historical structure; that in its present concrete form it is none-the-less an absolute and timeless essence.

It seems that private property as "structure-for-economic-egoism" is bereft of a _general_ utilitarian justification. There seems to be no satisfactory way of showing in _principle_ that the principles of private property are morally valid. Egoism in resource use and control essentially and generally tends towards exploitation and inequality and critical lack of co-operation and planning: it should not be mystified into something which, when objectified and universalised as "the market economy" magically generates the greatest possible amount of material well-being for all, because it does not. We do not allege that the private enterprise system is _absolutely_ unworkable, for if it were, it wouldn't be even a proper object of discussion. The main critical points are that private property, its principles and inherent tendencies, are subject to serious ethico-political criticism; that the presupposed view of human nature is unjustified and that there is a preferable alternative to it. The previous discussion of socialized property displayed principles of organisation that are more in accordance with (rather than being, as with private property, largely contradictory to) the values of co-operation, equality and freedom as control over our lives.

Nevertheless, the ideology of private property has had a very strong hold over us. It is even the practice of many whose "higher" theoretical ideals are at variance with it. This means that private property cannot be changed merely by the ideological criticism of it, for what is at stake is not merely change in ideas, but change in social structure. Ideological criticism is not an end in itself. Its proper conclusion is revolutionary practice, the informed attempt to change those conditions which structure our practices, sometimes at variance with our "higher" theoretical ideals.

5. Criteria of Acquisition

In order to understand what something is, it is often necessary to understand how it comes about, the conditions which bring it into being. For example, it would be an inadequate understanding of childbirth that fails to place it in the context of the process of human reproduction. With normative matters too, it is necessary not only to understand abstract principles in isolation, but also the circumstances and processes which bring these principles into play, which "activate" them. For example, in order to understand what a promise is, we would need to know not only what rights and obligations are constitutive of a promise, but also how a promise comes about, the conditions under which a promise is properly made - that is, the overall process of promising.

With private property too, a full understanding would include knowing not only what it is or means to possess private property, but also how such possession properly comes about, the process of acquisition. Private property, just like many phenomena, is a process, a process with a certain structure and governed by certain principles. It is not simply and only a social structure, but a continuous "coming to being" of various concrete activities under that structure. The nature of private property includes the nature of its continuous coming to being, the process of acquisition and the principles governing its acquisition. How then do we suppose that people come to be, legitimately owners of private property?

The principles which we shall uncover in seeking to answer this question will also be from an overall social view, principles of distribution. They will raise the question of social justice, for they will articulate how, according to the conception of private property, wealth ought to be distributed. The principles governing the acquisition of private property are the very same principles which would, in a private property society govern the distribution of socially produced wealth. Looked at in this way, they appear as principles of social justice essentially involved in the conception of private property. So: in discussing "criteria of acquisition", we shall also be discussing alleged criteria of social justice; ideology concerning the nature of a just distribution of social wealth. This is also an element in the ideological justification of the institution of private property. Private property involves a conception of social justice, which in turn is used, circularly, to portray private property as a necessary element in a socially just order.

How does one come to acquire, legitimately, private property? The common answer is, by working for it: private property is held to be the appropriate and just reward for labour. This was John Locke's answer, long ago at the dawn of the rising of the bourgeoisie.

Although this answer appears to be - and is - seriously naive and misleading, it is still commonly embraced. And there is a reason why people cling to it. Everyone needs and wants access to material resources, under continuing conditions of scarcity. Thus any code of distributing them would need an attempt at justification in <u>moral</u> terms. Further, our present modes of appropriating private property are clearly associated with massive inequalities and inequities, whereby some people do not get enough even to survive. Hence the need to find an <u>ethical</u> rationale for this inhumane state of affairs. And hence the <u>work ethic</u> according to which everyone should earn what they get by working, and everyone should receive all and only what they deserve in virtue of the value of their work. This is an appeal to a recognisably ethical principle - that people should be treated according to their deserts, or merits. It is an attempt to find a principle which ethically grounds the basic nature of capitalism, whilst at the same time providing a congenial guideline for ironing out the obvious inequities and injustice in the system.

Moreover, leaving aggregate utility aside, no other ethical grounding for the distributional features of private appropriation appears readily available. Certainly, the appeal cannot be to equality or need, given the self-interested aggrandizing tendencies inherent in private appropriation. The mainstream justification of private appropriation really has two legs. They rest on these two foundations:-

1. **Aggressive utilitarianism:** "the-goose-that-lays-the-most-possible-golden-eggs" theory.

2. **Productive desert-ism:** the idea that private appropriation under free market conditions rewards each person proportionately to the value of their productive contribution - hence (allegedly) fairly and justly.

It is this latter ideological proposition which underlies the "work ethic" rationale for particular private appropriations, and which is supposed to outline and justify the basic nature of the distributions within a Capitalist economy. The path to private property is supposed to be a way of productive labour, or more generally, by way of contributing to the satisfaction of other people's wants. The right to private property is held to be conditional upon and proportional to the value of one's productive contribution. It is held to be intrinsically right that people should gain control over material resources only in proportion to the value of their productive contribution. Certainly the work ethic as understood here is deeply rooted in our consciousness. One of the spectres which rises from the grave yards of unemployment to haunt bourgeois citizenry is the Dole Bludger and other welfare recipients who have healthy bodies (or at least two legs and two hands) but laze about all day appropriating resources, and all those untold billions who are so lazy that if the threat of starvation was taken from their shoulders by giving them a "living" independently of the market-determined value of their productive contribution, would do nothing as well.

Productive desert-ism is false. It is not true that the "private property-market-capitalism" complex tends, because of its basic structure, to reward everyone proportionately to the value of their labour. Any simple supposition that it does would fail to take into account the egregious distinction between capital and wage labour. A capitalist economy essentially involves returns on capital (private ownership of the means of production) in the form of profit, interest, rent etc. as well as returns for labour in the form of wages. Even John Locke took this into account, pointing out that people could "alienate" their labour to another, thus surrendering their right to property in their product. C.B. MacPherson has very fully traced how Locke and others, integrated their views on labour and property with the reality of developing bourgeois production. [11]

Orthodox economics postulates that both capital and labour are "factors of production", that capital as such contributes to the productive process and thus has its own market-determined value. Should we then widen our horizons beyond labour, and view the market-capitalist system as rewarding proportionately to their productive contribution, whether as capitalist or wage-labour?

Marxian economics on the other hand, proposes a labour theory of value, according to which the value of a commodity is determined only by the labour embodied in its production, so that returns to the owners of capital as such come down to parasitic exploitations of labour, the appropriation of the "surplus value" produced by labour. Capitalism, Marx maintained, is structurally exploitative of labour. It generates only the appearance of "fair wages", an appearance reflected in bourgeois ideology. The bitter reality is, however, the exploitation of labour.

The "reswitching controversy" has shaken the assumptions that the neo-Classical critique is dependent upon. Joan Robinson [12] investigated a production function for output obtaining the various possible equilibrium points corresponding to various values of the profit rate for a given state of technical knowledge. She pointed out that there is a problem of measurement of capital as a factor of production, since a quantity of capital is a sum of values and not reducible to a single quantity. There is a long literature of attempts to salvage workable parts of capital theory from the onslaughts of the Cambridge school: we do not have the space nor the need to survey the literature here. Our point is that the assumption which the neo-classical critique is dependent upon is a matter of debate: neo-classical capital theory has become a very conceptually shakey topic indeed.

Whichever general approach to economic theory is correct, a sufficient number of points are sufficiently clear even to bewildered members of the economic laity, to constitute a successful critique of the idea that private enterprise capitalism basically distributes wealth in proportion to the value of people's work, or productive contribution. First, it is clear that capitalism essentially involves returns for the ownership of productive resources as such. Ownership as such yields dividends, i.e. more ownership, and this expanded ownership cannot be viewed as the deserved product of the owners' labour, even if the original could. In any case, wage labour is not rewarded by ownership of what it produces, but by wages which are most often sufficient only to sustain its consumption (in Marxian terms, maintain its labour power). So capitalist economies do not reward people on the basis of their labour. Certainly, there are no unitary "labour-measures" for the distribution of wealth. Some people "alienate" their labour to others, who then appropriate the product. In fact, the achievement of an economy which distributes wealth solely on the basis of labour, is regarded by Marxists as a central hallmark of "Socialism" as a transitional mode of economy in the movement towards "communism", the classless society.

Second: even if the ownership-of-resources-as-such (capital) is viewed as a productive contribution which should receive its own proper reward in its own right, it is clear that this reward will be chronically at the expense of returns to labour, if only because of the commanding economic position of capital, its nature as the mode of control of the productive resources needed by labour.

Third: it is clear that pure and free market forces cannot be available as determinants of the proper returns for capital and labour. Capitalist economies display inherent tendencies towards domination by large corporations, monopolies and cartels; there is irreversible State intervention and regulation; and there is increasing collectivisation of labour, through unions, all of which seriously interfere with the operations of free market forces.

Fourth: even if free market forces are available, it is clear that they would not regulate distributions solely on the basis of productive merits, but also on the basis of initial advantageous and disadvantageous positions within the market economy (who has money and who doesn't). Unless we assume - unrealistically and unhistorically - an equality between market participants, market-regulated distributions must be weighted towards the more effective demands of those in economically advantageous positions and relatively advantageous positions must arise in the <u>historical</u> operation of a market economy.

"Productive value" itself is of course a problematic term. If it means "market determined value", then the market would be supposed to measure nothing other than its own determinations. If on the other hand, "productive value" is used qualitatively to refer to a value in terms of satisfying human interests in general, then the market in a concrete historical setting cannot measure it, for it would discriminate in favour of effective interests. So, the ideology of "productive desert-ism" not only rationalises private appropriations in the interests of the dominant class: it is also false in that it distorts the concrete nature of private property and private appropriation in their historical setting. Our systems of private appropriation as historically developed do not and cannot distribute wealth to each of us according to what we deserve on the basis of our labour (given any intuitively plausible idea of "desert").

If "productive desert-ism" is largely false as a description of how private property is acquired, what is true? How <u>is</u> private property in fact acquired, if not by labour? If a labour theory of acquisition is not descriptively valid for private property, what sort of theory would be? The answer has been implicit in the foregoing. Private property is by and large acquired by the aggressive and self-interested usage of previously acquired property. Private property of itself breeds further property, or wealth. Acquisition is cumulative. Under private capitalism of course, both labour and capital generate income, but the appropriation of wage-labour's product and its surplus value by owners and their economically dominant position means the increasing concentration of wealth in a few hands. The road to property is basically via property ownership - hence the class structure, the difficulty of achieving social mobility, and the overall inherent tendency under capitalism for the rich to get richer and the poor to get relatively poorer.

There are as we have already seen three basic approaches to the problem of social justice in wealth distribution: the <u>utilitarian</u>, <u>desert</u> or <u>merit</u> approach, and the <u>egalitarian</u> "need" approach. We will argue later in support of the "egalitarian need" approach. It is important to realise in the ensuring discussion, that what we call the "egalitarian-need" approach is not one that requires uniformity, such that everyone gets the same amount of everything, irrespective of their particular needs, rather it is an approach according to which everyone should have their particular needs and interests satisfied to an equal degree, i.e. that they should receive as far as possible, equal shares in the conditions of human happiness. Equality as a social ideal does not mean the achievement of uniformity in everything, rather it means the achievement of equal degrees of interest satisfaction, the equal value of each person's life for themselves.

It is fairly widely acknowledged that a straightforward utilitarian approach to the problem of social justice would be seriously defective. [13] The basic reason for this is that a <u>pure</u> utilitarian approach would ethically license extreme forms of exploitation, if only thereby the general welfare, the aggregate good can be maximised. The happiness of many can be built on the extreme misery of a few, and the great happiness of a few can be built upon the relative and often extreme misery of many. Both these general types of situation seem compatible with simple ("act) utilitarianism, though not with our intuitive conceptions of justice. This incompatibility is implicitly acknowledged by mainstream philosophy's emphasis on "desert" as well as utility.

So the important question we must face here is whether or not "treating people according to their deserts", is (in vague terms) <u>the</u> fundamental distribution principle constitutive of social justice. This question is important for the critique of the ideology of private appropriation - for even if it is recognised that the ideology does not match the facts, even cannot match the facts, it nonetheles provides an ideal for reformists which does not question the massive inequalities of "privatised" economic systems, and which may be both reactionary and wrong. The criticism of ideology does not end in displaying how it mismatches the facts: it must proceed to question the ideological principles themselves.

Here, we will only be able to discuss the general principles of "desert" briefly and sketchily: anything else would require a lengthy excursion into complex theories of social justice. We shall also need to make some unargued, but <u>prima facie</u> plausible assumptions. We shall assume that valid principles of justice articulate manners or modes of treating people as <u>ends in their own right</u>, rather than as means to others' ends, or as means to some abstract and alien end. We shall also take it that valid principles of justice must have a <u>point</u>, that their realization must be the realization of something valuable and worthwhile; and further, that value-in-general should be understood as the conditions of the satisfaction of human interests, so that principles of justice must themselves be conditions of the satisfaction of human interests.

Now "desert" or "merit" is a complex concept. We can speak of a person's deserts in many different senses. Desert may take many different forms. We can speak of an individual's merits in the sense of their <u>potential</u> capacity for contributing to social well-being of themselves and/or others. These individual capacities can be treated as <u>forward-looking merits</u>. Alternatively, we can speak of <u>backward-looking merits</u>, such as an individual's past achievements in moral, intellectual or creative dimensions. We can also speak separably of an individual's moral merit, his intellectual merit, and his merits of all sorts of creative and semi-creative activities and roles. All this indicates that "treating people according to their merits or deserts" is not a simple matter. What sort of merit should be taken into account? What dimensions of achievement or capacity merit what sorts of treatment? And what level of "reward" is appropriate to what level of merit?

These sorts of questions arise in particular areas of philosophy where "desert" is a central concept, e.g. the philosophy of punishment. About punishment we need to ask: under what conditions do people <u>deserve</u> punishment? And what forms of punishment are appropriate to what forms of behaviour? It is not even clear that the concept of "desert" can provide by itself a valid ethical rationale for punishment at all - a completely utilitarian approach would deny this. If the relevance of "deserts" is granted, this still leaves unclarified the problem of matching forms of demerit with forms of punishment, and even that of determining what precisely should be punished. These matters still puzzle people whose thinking about punishment goes anyway beyond the confines of the legal system they happen to live under. And similar puzzles would arise for any attempt to apply a <u>general</u> "desert" criterion to anything connected with the distribution of "goods" and "evils" among people. Consider, for example, attempting to use the "desert" criterion to determine appropriate wage relativities. What characteristics of wage workers merit what degrees of wage relativity? Given that no easy answer springs to mind, how can we possibly know whether the market mechanism distributes income according to deserts?

Treating people on their merits, whatever form of merit is involved, is necessarily to treat them differentially, comparatively, proportionately to their relative merits. It is to treat people according to how well or badly they measure up to some standard(s), and thus at least implicitly according to how they compare with each other in respect of some standard.

It can be plausibly objected that to treat people on their merits is not necessarily to treat them differentially, since it is not logically impossible for any and every person to reach the same standard, whatever sort of standard is at issue. It might be said that there are two ways of comparing any two people in respect to any dimension of merit: (a) competitively, in such a way as to select the better from the worse, the winner from the loser, and (b) non-competitively against some standard of excellence which they may both approximate to the same degree. But whilst this distinction is important in many areas (educational practice for one) it is not one which can be used to show that treating people on their merits could be a non-relative, egalitarian procedure, if only everyone was good enough. <u>In the end</u>, it is impossible to distinguish a non-relative mode of grading, assessment or evaluation, and consequently, of rewarding people proportionally to their merits. As any teacher knows, relevant differences can always be found between any two students' performances, no matter how close they are. Human beings can only asymptotically approach perfection in any dimension: merit like length is infinitely divisible. Therefore to treat people strictly on their merits is necessarily to treat them differentially, to grade their rewards or punishments in proportion to discoverable differences between them (even though, for practical reasons, relevant differences between some people are sometimes overlooked in grading situations).

Treating people according to their needs and interests, however, is in one important sense, to treat them uniformly. While individual people do have different needs and interests, they all have the same second-order need, the need to have their needs and interests satisfied. So to treat people according to their needs and interests is to attempt to ensure that everyone, equally, has their genuinely human interests satisfied, that everyone is an equally well-developed and flourishing person. Whereas to treat people on their merits is to grade their interest-satisfactions relatively to their differing deserts.

The argument for the ethical priority of the "need principle" over the "merit principle" is this: the point of principles of justice in particular, and of morality in general, is to achieve the ordered <u>satisfaction</u> of human interests, taking each person as an end in their own right. Underlying the moral enterprise, and all practical evaluation, is this proposition: the satisfaction of human interests as such is good, and the frustration of human interests as such is bad. Without this starting point, we could not make sense of any human practice, or the whole, overridingly important, practical dimension of our lives. So the very point of justice is the satisfaction of interests. Yet acting on the merit-principle would necessarily ensure the <u>relative</u> frustration of some people compared to their "betters", by grading interest-satisfactions proportionately to the differing deserts of people. In this sense the merit principle contradicts the point of justice, the satisfaction rather than the frustration of human interests in general and therefore it cannot be seen as the most perfect, or the highest form of justice.

A further indication of the ethical priority of needs over deserts is that people's needs must be very nearly equally satisfied <u>before</u> they can be treated on their merits in a way which makes any moral sense. People cannot be treated <u>fairly</u> on their merits unless they are allowed a roughly <u>equal opportunity</u> to reach whatever standard or win whatever competition is at stake. Roughly equal opportunity is one of the criteria of fair competition and fair comparative evaluation, and it is surely only the outcome of fair competitions and fair comparisons that have any claim to the mantle of justice. Now, people's opportunities, their natural and social advantages and disadvantages vary hugely. To achieve a rough equality of opportunity across society would require a massive and ordered development of people's needs and interests. This in turn would be a necessary precondition of any fair, morally viable way of treating people generally on their merits.

However, whilst maintaining all this, we do recognise that the merit or desert principle is a principle of justice and it does articulate a way of treating people on the basis of themselves, rather as means to the satisfaction of other persons' interests. We can all no doubt think of cases in which it would be clearly right to treat individuals on their individual merits rather than equally according to their interests. In the case of punishment, if it is assumed that punishment is justified at all, it is morally counter-intuitive to institute some form of mass social punishment of everyone for the wrongs of an individual - if not outrightly incoherent. The supporter of egalitarianism has no need to be committed to such absurd conclusions at all. In general, it seems that it is right to treat individuals on their merits once their important needs and interests have been equally served and in the context of worthwhile, necessary, or otherwise justified activities, the point of which would be lost unless the participants were so treated. We cannot evade the point, that justice sometimes is a matter of responding to individual (and collective) deserts without ridding ourselves of blaming, praising, criticising and affixing responsibility. This is a large part of what it is to be treated, and to treat others as persons. More on this in the next chapter.

Nevertheless it is important - and consistent - to recognise the ethical priority of catering equally to everyone's needs and interests, in two related senses. (1) People must be roughly equally well-developed as human beings before they may be justly subjected to straightforward "merit criteria" in respect of their interest-satisfactions; (2) those activities in which people must in justice be treated on their merits must themselves be directed towards, or compatible with a larger social process of attempting to realise the highest possible equal level of development of all human beings, before they can be regarded as part of an overall framework of social justice. Thus, for example an academic examination conducted for the purpose of streaming candidates into a pre-established hierarchy of wealth and prestige, and between candidates some of whom are seriously disadvantaged would violate these conditions on the justice of treating people according to their merits.

Our conclusion then, is that the principle of treating people equally according to their needs and interests is prior to the "merit" principle as a principle of social justice, in the senses specified. This mean, that any ideology that appeals to "deserts" or "merits" as ultimate justifications for a preferred pattern of distribution of social resources is ethically mistaken. This in turn means that the form of ideology most clearly associated with the institution of private property is similarly mistaken.

6. Individual Privacy and Medical Confidentiality

We now turn to a consideration of the issue of individual privacy and philosophical problems of privacy in bioethics. We have already argued that privacy claims, as they relate to macrosociological issues are frequently confused and unjustified and incompatible with socialist concerns and we now argue that claims for privacy at the microsociological or individual level are best understood, if they are justified at all, as a soundly based claim for a specific form of freedom or justice. Privacy at the individual level, has often been taken as a major problem for socialists; socialism is thought to be a social system that erodes individual freedom and liberty. We argue here that this is not so and that this commonplace objection is mistaken.

There have been various definitions of 'privacy' offered in the literature. [14] Privacy has been regarded as a right to determine <u>what</u> information about oneself may be communicated to others; [15] or as the degree of control which an individual has over information about oneself [16] and as a condition of limited access to a person. [17] Here we follow Schoeman in distinguishing the issue of <u>how much</u> privacy one has from the issue of whether alleged privacy rights have been violated as well as the <u>condition</u> of privacy from the actual right to privacy itself. [18] Following Grcic we shall define privacy as "the right of a person not to have personal information about himself known by others". [19] This definition seems in our opinion to capture the commonsense meaning of the word 'privacy' and definitions such as this one frequently occur in the bioethics literature of privacy and confidentiality. [20]

It is our claim that there is nothing morally distinct about privacy claims. When we examine the justifications given of privacy claims, these justifications make use of moral concepts such as freedom and justice that can be adequately characterised and defended without any consideration of the concept of privacy at all. In other words discussions of privacy are really nothing more than disguised discussions of other moral values such as freedom, justice and utility. If there is nothing morally distinct about privacy claims, then the use of Occam's razor is justified in eliminating a moral concept which is nothing more than a conceptual "free-loader". This position can be justified by seeing whether there are any general philosophical arguments which establish that the moral interests involved in privacy cases are <u>best analysed</u> on an independent basis by reference to other moral values, without interference to a so called right to privacy.

Judith Jarvis Thomson has argued that there is no unique right to privacy, but rather the cases allegedly covered by this so-called right are subsumable under other rights. [21] That is to say, alleged privacy rights can be adequately explicated by concepts such as property rights and rights over one's own person. She uses a number of examples to defend her position. One such example involves the case of a man who owns a pornographic picture who wishes to keep the picture locked away in a safe so that no-one else can see it. If we use a special X-ray device to see the picture in the safe, then we seem to have violated his right to privacy. In Thomson's opinion however, what has been violated is a right to private property, or more accurately the negative right that others shall not look at the picture, this being one of the rights of private property. [22]

Grcic has argued that Thomson's argument is unsuccessful because her notion of the right over one's person is vague and her approach is too <u>ad hoc</u> because it is unclear <u>why</u> a property right means the right among other rights, not to have the property seen. Now it is certainly true that there is a considerable vagueness about why seeing this man's pornographic photograph violates his property rights, but perhaps this is a function of the somewhat silly example used where there is no really detailed reason why somebody seeing this photograph should violate the man's property rights. However, whilst we don't believe that the institution of private property is unjustified, within this framework, it is easy to give an example of where looking at an item violates property rights. If the photograph was an exclusive picture for a future <u>Penthouse</u> centre-fold, then looking at the photograph would violate an alleged right to private property, because successful advertising depends to a large extent upon secrecy. Why buy the magazine if you have already seen the pictures by spying?

Schoeman has argued that there is something distinctive about the right to privacy which is irreducible to either property rights or rights over the person. The example used to support this involves two types of sound wave interceptors. The first type records the speech carried by the soundwaves. The other type converts the soundwaves into usable energy without recording the speech itself. Consider the case of the neighbour with the soundwave interceptor that records speech:

> "My neighbour with the sound wave interceptor that records conversations does violate my rights; and Thomson agrees with this. The reason such usage of my sound waves violates my rights is that it interferes with my right to privacy, and not, as Thomson supposes, because it violates my right to

determine what happens to my sound waves. Reference to ownership of sound waves will not suffice, since, as we just observed, that ownership does not preclude certain usages, even without consent. Indeed, any ownership rights we acknowledge in such situations depend on establishing that a privacy right has been violated. The suggestion here is that without reference to privacy rights specifically we shall not be able to account for the wrongness of certain acts consistent with the innocence of certain others. Without reference to privacy, we will not be able to draw moral distinctions which are important to describe it". [23]

Thomson however is not committed to the absurd position that what is wrong with the voice recording sound wave interceptor is that it violates a property right over sound waves! Surely what is of importance here is the <u>information content</u> of the sound waves, not the sound waves themselves. In this sense, within the moral framework which accepts the legitimacy of private property, Thomson is free to argue that a person's speech content is his/her own, just as a radio station has ownership of the <u>contents</u> of its broadcasts but not the actual physical radio waves.

We are not committed however to attempting to reduce privacy rights down to merely property rights and right over one's person. Indeed, being sceptical of the moral legitimacy of the institution of private property itself means that we must look for a broader theoretical basis to take the place of privacy rights. It is not difficult to find such a basis in the literature of privacy. Edward Bloustein [24] has argued that respect for the values of individual dignity and integrity, personal autonomy and individuality, is the ultimate ground for our privacy claims. We can plausibly say that respect for these values determines which of our conversations is published, so spy devices such as the sound wave interceptor are <u>prima facie</u> immoral because of a violation of these basic values and not a right to privacy.

Judith Andre [25] has pointed out that knowledge of others has value, especially instrumental value, to us. The ability to limit other's knowledge about us also of value. In our opinion many privacy claims are concerned not so much with the fact that someone knows something about oneself but with the fact that such information can be <u>misused</u> or <u>abused</u>. People don't keep secrets for the sake of a right to privacy, but because they have something to hide and they have something to hide because disclosure of certain information could harm their interests or that of their associates. Industry and the military keep secrets for this reason, and so do ordinary people. We are not claiming that the right to privacy can be reduced to, or thoroughly understood by means of this notion, but it certainly offers a powerful and deep explanation of many privacy claims. We do not, for example wish to have our conversations monitored because this information could be abused, or in some way used to harm our interests. People don't like peeping Toms watching them have sex, because again they could be the undeserving object of humour and ridicule - or even blackmail.

Jeffrey Reiman [26] has argued that there is a fundamental interest, connected to personhood which provides the basis for a universal right to privacy. Reiman's idea is that <u>privacy</u> is necessary for the creation of selves out of human beings, as a self is a human being who regards aspects of his/her existence such as thoughts, action and their body, as their own. Reiman says:

> "<u>Privacy is a social ritual by means of which an individual's moral title to his existence is conferred</u>. Privacy is an essential part of the complex social practice by means of which the social group recognises - and communicates to the individual - that his existence is his own. And this is a precondition of personhood. To be a person, an individual must recognise not just his actual capacity to shape his destiny by his choices. He must also recognise that he has an exclusive moral right to shape his destiny. And this in turn presupposes that he believes that the concrete reality which he is, and through which his destiny is realised, belongs to him in a moral sense". [27]

Similar remarks have been made by C.K. Boone:

> The inescapable conclusion from a comparison of total and non-total communities is that privacy is a premier <u>condition</u> for personhood. In order fully to appreciate what this means, one need only imagine a society in which the instruments for total surveillance have been perfected such that people's thoughts as well as their actions are transparent to others. In this kind of society it is evident that people could no longer have their <u>own</u> thoughts, their <u>own</u> sentiments, their <u>own</u> inner lives. The distinction between self and other would become blurred as one's alienated identity merged into the great river of totalitarian group identity. True, one might still sense pain and pleasure as one's <u>own</u> in such circumstances, but this potential is not evidence of a sense of selfhood, as can be inferred from the fact that even animals can experience it. The capacity to have one's own thoughts and one's own life, and to <u>call</u> them one's own, seems essential for selfhood, and this is precisely what is threatened in a

totalitarian society. Since the capacity for selfhood is a principal condition for personhood, in the absence of minimal privacy, personhood is inconceivable because selfhood is inconceivable. Correspondingly, in the absence of adequate privacy, the development of personhood, and hence personal autonomy, is threatened. Thus it becomes quite clear why as the unanimous opinion of authorities on totalitarianism indicates, totalitarian societies must destroy the private sphere. [28]

This type of argument is unsatisfactory in our opinion. The idea of <u>ownership</u> presupposed by the concept of a person is this: that the human being in question recognises that his/her thoughts and actions are their own and not someone else's. The concept of <u>ownership</u> used here is nothing more than the existential capacity to individuate oneself from others, to be able to distinguish between the 'inner' and 'outer' worlds. Privacy however is a complex social practice that typically refers to the right of a person not to have personal information about him/herself known by others. It is logically possible that I may come to know, through the magical means that today's philosophers typically appeal to, everything about you. I know your wishes, fears, desires and hopes. Yet surely you wouldn't cease to be a <u>person!</u> Rather what you are is a <u>fully known</u> person but a person all the same. This thought experiment shows that Reiman's notion of existential ownership is unsatisfactory as a foundation for privacy claims.

The results of this discussion can now be summarised and their significance for bioethics noted. We have argued that there is nothing morally distinct about privacy claims and that privacy claims if they are justified can be adequately defended by use of other moral concepts such as <u>justice</u>, <u>freedom</u> and <u>personal integrity</u>. We believe that it is quite unlikely that we could find a universal moral basis to a right to privacy, because of the extreme diversity of privacy claims. We have examined some leading attempts to do this, and have concluded that these attempts are failures.

The position which we have defended here has direct significance for the question of <u>medical confidentiality</u>. Medical confidentiality is a topic typically concerned with the question of the "privacy" of information about a patient, but it is a topic which can be more satisfactorily investigated without reference to the issue of the right to privacy that has filled the literature.

We do not believe that the traditional justification of the principle of medical condifentiality based upon the right to privacy as a basic human right, is a satisfactory justification. The claim is frequently made that when the patient shares detailed information about his/her body and/or mind with a physician, the patient is letting the physician into a "special inner circle". If the physician in turn lets others into that circle without the patient's consent, then he has shown <u>disrespect</u> to that person. As far as we are concerned, this claim is nonsensical unless appeal is made to other qualities, such as the abuse of the information or some harm to the person is demonstrated as a result of the disclosure of the information. It is theoretically possible that a physician's disclosure of certain information, such as a person's courageous struggle against cancer or AIDS, would not show disrespect to the person, but rather serve to celebrate the moral fibre of the patient. The principle of medical confidentiality is therefore not an absolute principle, justified by a so-called basic human right to privacy.

It is more satisfactory to see the principle of medical confidentiality as a utilitarian principle. The preservation of medical confidentiality is important, because without this at all, the patient may not make a full disclosure of the symptoms and possible causes of his/her illness because of the fear of public disclosure. A Catholic priest for example may fear to seek treatment for a sexually transmitted disease which he caught in a moment of weakness of the flesh, because of the fear of public disgrace. The principle of medical confidentiality as such is socially useful and should be retained, although it must be noted that those who usually appeal to privacy claims typically have something to hide! It is <u>not</u> however an absolute moral principle and it can be morally overridden by stronger utilitarian considerations. The American Medical Association recognised this, when in 1912 it revised its code of ethics to add a new clause into the confidentiality section of its code, to legitimate the physician reporting infectious disease. [29] The justification appealed to here is that the value of protecting society from the spread of infectious disease overrides the value of medical confidentiality about a patient's disease. The California Supreme Court ruled in the 1976 case of <u>Tarasoff v. Regents of the University of California</u>, that therapists who know or should know that a patient poses a violent threat to an identifiable third party, then have a definite obligation to take reasonable steps to protect the endangered person. The Court noted "a doctor is liable to persons infected by his patient if he negligently fails to diagnose a contagious disease, or having diagnosed the illness, fails to warn members of the patient's family". [30] The moral reasoning underlying this legal conclusion, is in our opinion sound: the physician does not have a "duty to warn" as such, but a deeper duty, to protect the general public from health risks.

If this argument is satisfactory, then there seems to us to be no good moral reasons for maintaining medical confidentiality when this endangers the life of an innocent third party. Consider the classic thought experiment dealing with medical confidentiality, that of a physician and a young couple about to be married. The physician knows that the husband-to-be has an active AIDS infection from past confidential consultations. Should the physician warn the wife-to-be of this to save her health or life? (Suppose she is at present HIV antibody negative). On utilitarian grounds the answer must clearly be 'yes' because the healthier life itself of an innocent third party is more important in this context than mere confidentiality about a disease - upholding a confidentiality will lead to someone's (possible) death. Medicine, it may be said, is not concerned with making people honest, only making them well. Thus a doctor has a moral duty, when faced with the moral intransigent AIDS patients, to inform those <u>directly</u> at risk, subject to the following attitude described by Gillett:

> "In most cases it will be possible to guide the patient into telling those who need to know or allowing them to be told (and where it is possible to so guide him it will be mandatory to involve him in an informed way). In the face of an expressed disregard for the harm being caused to those others concerned, we will be morally correct in abandoning what would otherwise be a binding obligation. We should and do feel the need to preserve and protect the already affected life of the potential victim of his deception and in this feeling we exhibit a sensitivity to moral rectitude. Of course, it is only the active sexual partners of the patient who are at risk and thus it is only to them that we and the patient have a moral duty (in this respect talk of 'society at large' is just rhetoric). If it is the case that sexual activity, as Nagel claims, involves a mutual openness in those who have intercourse, one could plausibly argue that the cynical moral and interpersonal attitudes here evinced undermined the patient's sexual rights (assuming that people have such). The sexual activity of this individual is aberrant or perverted in the important respect that it involves a harmful duplicity toward or deception of his sexual partner." [31]

Gillett adds the qualification that HIV status should only be revealed to sexual partners, but not employers and friends (i.e. non-sexual interacting agents). Nevertheless, let us move away from our very simple thought experiment and consider the case of gay and heterosexual prostitutes who have an active HIV infection and do not use condoms (perhaps to obtain more money). A problem now arises which has been accurately described by Sheldon Landesman:

> "Any legally or socialy sanctioned act that breaches confidentiality or imposes additional burdens (such as job loss or cancellation of

insurance) acts as a disincentive to voluntary testing. Thus if all physicians were legally required to report HIV-positive persons to a health department or to inform sexual partners at risk from the HIV-positive person, no one would come forward for testing. This is especially true if the physician is known to treat many patients with AIDS and HIV infection. The public knowledge that such a physician has violated confidentialilty would result (indeed, has resulted in several cases) in a sharp decline of potentially infected persons seeking counseling and testing. Consequently, a growing number of persons would remain ignorant of their infectiousness as would their sex partners". [32]

Commenting on the notion that a mandated "breach of confidentiality" would destroy the integrity of the doctor-patient relationship, with the result that individuals would be deterred from seeking treatment, Annas offers this counter-argument based upon U.S. psychological experience:

"The argument that a potential "breach of confidentiality" would destroy the therapeutic relationship is apparently refuted by the present legal ability of therapists to warn potential victims of a patient's violent acts. The only difference in this case was that the warning is now being required as a _duty_ instead of being available as an _optional_ right. Since this "right" to warn currently exists for both medical and mental health practitioners, and has not apparently destroyed patient trust, the majority are content that this expansion will not be harmful either. Other commentators have gone further, noting that not only is psychotherapy flourishing in an age when there are many exceptions to the doctor-patient privilege, but many mental patients seek therapy with the hope that something will be done to curtail their violent actions. The issue, according to these commentators, is therefore not lack of confidentiality, but lack of trust. They make an analogy to group therapy, where it is known at the outset that no absolute guarantee of confidentiality exists, and suggest that to maintain trust the therapist inform the patient of this duty to disclose at the outset of the relationship." [33]

Nevertheless, Annas does not consider the _general_ social ramifications of such a programme, beyond the isolated cases. Professor Ian Gust, for example, senior adviser with the Australian National Council on AIDS (ANCA), said in June 1989 that health authorities be given the right to trace partners of infected people without facing legal sanctions for disclosing confidential medical information. He says "Ultimately you have to be in a position to provide that information to those who are at risk or restrain the person who is doing it. I think society would regard it as remiss if we didn't have those powers". [34] It has been argued earlier in this book that there is a need for legal thinkers to develop and for Parliament to implement a comprehensive body of AIDS anti-discrimination laws to prevent the possibility of any discrimination against HIV infected people. In any case, tracing contacts of an infected person against their wishes, should be the rare exception to the standard activities of health authorities, rather than the norm.

In conclusion, the principle of medical confidentiality is an important moral obligation, but it is not an absolute moral obligation. The conditions under which it can be overridden cannot be <u>mechanically decided</u> in our opinion because they are highly context dependent (as considerations of utility typically are), but these conditions usually involve considerations such as protecting the patient's own life, the life of an innocent third party or the health interests of society in general. Whilst we cannot fully investigate the entire spectrum of moral issues raised by the topic of medical confidentiality, especially in the context of AIDS, we have shown that this field can be more satisfactorily investigated if we abandon the idea of a fundamental and absolute human right to privacy.

7. Conclusion

In this chapter we have given a critical examination, from a "socialist perspective" of some of the most important privacy claims, and we have argued that most privacy claims are both confused and unjustified and incompatible with genuine socialist concerns. Central to our concerns here has been an analysis and critique of the most important privacy claim in capitalist societies: that of private property and private ownership. We then addressed two different but related questions (1) the problem of the criteria of <u>possession</u> of private property, and (2) the problem of the criteria of legitimate <u>acquisition</u> of private property.

We attempted to clarify the idea of private property with reference to that of public property. Public property, or the socialisation of property as we have described has two basic features: (a) the worker-collectivity of the owning subject; (b) the dimension of social responsibility, this being the constraint on owners by and for the interests of society, if not humanity at large. Relations of counter-responsibility are the basic features of the institution of private ownership; that is that the owned resource is available to the self-interested use and/or control of the owners, and that owners be able to pursue their own interests exclusive of a concern for others, with the owned resource.

We then subjected the implicit view of human nature behind the justification of this ideology to criticism. There are no good reasons to believe that "utilitarian economic person" is a timelessly true portrait of human nature. We have an alternative conception of human nature (however vague and sketchy), consistent we believe with the central insight of twentieth century anthropology, that there are no <u>substantial</u> unchanging elements of human being which are common throughout history, let alone outside of the socio-historical process. Human nature is most plausibly viewed, not merely in terms of attributes inherent for all human beings as tokens of a type, but in addition, in terms of tendencies and potentials, which vary in the degree to which, and in the form in which they are concretely realised, largely because of socio-historical structuring.

We then discussed the problem of the criteria of acquisition of private property. Our concern here has been to criticise the second major strategy for the ethical justification for the distributional features of private appropriation: "productive desert-ism". The principle is unsatisfactory as an ethical principle.

Finally we concluded our critique of privacy by an examination of the issues of individual privacy and medical confidentiality with respect to the typical AIDS thought experiment. We argued that there is nothing morally distinct about privacy claims, and when we examine the justifications given of privacy claims, these justifications typically make use of moral concepts such as freedom and justice that can be adequately understood and defended without any consideration of a <u>sui generis</u> right to privacy. With respect to a famous privacy principle, the principle of medical confidentiality, we argued that this principle offers only a <u>prima facie</u> obligation, not an absolute obligation. It can be overridden, like most moral principles, by considerations of greater importance to human welfare. Nevertheless, in the case of AIDS, because of its highly sensitive moral and political nature, if society does accept the notion of the necessity of forced disclosure of AIDS cases, <u>then a very comprehensive and powerful body of laws must also exist to protect AIDS infected persons from discrimination</u>. The philosophical problem of AIDS and privacy can we believe, only satisfactorily be solved by such a strategy.

NOTES AND REFERENCES

1. T. Parsons, <u>The Structure of Social Action</u> (Free Press, New York, 1964).

2. Legal writing on the concept of privacy is vast. A selective sample of references now follows: M.C. Dunlap, "Where the Person Ends, Does the Government Begin? An Exploration of Present Controveries Concerning the 'Right to Privacy'," <u>Lincoln Law Review</u>, Vol. 12, 1981, pp. 47-75; R. Gavison, "Privacy and the Limits of Law", <u>Yale Law Journal</u>, Vol. 89, 1980, pp. 421-471; J.A. Rohr, "Privacy: Law and Values", <u>Thought</u>, Vol. 49, 1974, pp. 353-373; A. L. Allen, "Rethinking the Rule Against Corporate Privacy Rights: Some Conceptual Quandries for the Common Law", <u>John Marshall Law Review</u>, Vol. 20, 1987, pp. 607-639; A. Libeu, "What is a Reasonable Expectation of Privacy?" <u>Western State University Law Review</u>, Vol. 12, 1985, pp. 849-858; J.T. O'Reilly, "Medical Privacy and Medical Research: Is Government the Problem or the Solution?" <u>University of Dayton Law Review</u>, Vol. 12, 1986, pp. 243-274; C.M. Cleaver, "Privacy Rights in Medical Records", <u>Fordham Urban Law Journal</u>, Vol. 13, 1984-85, pp. 165-204; J. Hirschleifer, "Privacy: Its Origin, Function and Future", <u>Journal of Legal Studies</u>, Vol. 9, 1980, pp. 649-664; E.L. Shapiro, "The Right of Privacy and Heroin Use for Painkilling Purposes by the Terminally Ill Cancer Patient", <u>Arizona Law Review</u>, Vol. 21, 1979, pp. 41-59; C.E. Blackburn, "Human Rights in an International Context: Recognizing the Right of Intimate Association", <u>Ohio State Law Journal</u>, Vol. 43, 1982, pp. 143-163; K. Wells and F.S. Merritt, "Individual Rights (1980-1981)", <u>Urban Lawyer</u>, Vol. 13, 1981, pp. 713-721; R.A. Posner, "Privacy, Secrecy and Reputation", <u>Buffalo Law Review</u>, Vol. 28, 1978, pp. 1-55; B.S. Markesinis, "The Right to be Let Alone Versus Freedom of Speech", <u>Public Law</u>, 1986, pp. 67-82; J.M. Vache and M.J. Makibe, "Privacy in Government Records: Philosophical Perspectives and Proposals for Legislation", <u>Gonzaga Law Review</u>, Vol. 14, 1979, pp. 515-557; D.J. Glancy, "The Invention of the Right to Privacy", <u>Arizona Law Review</u>, Vol. 21, 1979, pp. 1-39; W.L. Prosser, "Privacy", <u>California Law Review</u>, Vol. 48, 1960, pp. 383-423; E.J. Bloustein, "Privacy as an Aspect of Human Dignity: An Answer to Dean Prosser", <u>New York University Law Review</u>, Vol. 39, 1964, pp. 962-1007; H. Gross, "The Concept of Privacy", <u>New York University Law Review</u>, Vol. 42, 1966, pp. 34-54; S.D. Warren and L.D. Brandeis, "The Right to Privacy", <u>Harvard Law Review</u>, Vol. 4, 1890, pp. 193-220; K.L. Johnson, "The Sale of Human Organs: Implicating a Privacy Right", <u>Valparaiso University Law Review</u>, Vol. 21, 1987, pp. 741-762; A.R. Rubenfeld, "Today's Plague,

Tomorrow's Laws", *Human Rights*, Vol. 14, 1987, pp. 17-19, 52; M.L. Closen (et al), "AIDS in America: Death, Privacy and the Law", *Human Rights*, Vol. 14, 1987, pp. 27-29, 48-52; M.J. Radin, "Property and Personhood", *Stanford Law Review*, Vol. 34, 1982, pp. 957-1015; G. Negley, "Philosophical Views on the Value of Privacy", *Law and Contemporary Problems*, Vol. 31, 1966, pp. 319-325; H. Kalven, "Privacy in Tort Law - Were Warren and Brandeis Wrong?", *Law and Contemporary Problems*, Vol. 31, 1966, pp. 326-341; W.M. Beaney, "The Right to Privacy and American Law", *Law and Contemporary Problems*, Vol. 31, 1966, pp. 253-271; E. Shils, "Privacy: Its Constitution Vicissitudes", *Law and Contemporary Problems*, Vol. 31, 1966, pp. 281-306; G.J. Heaney, "The Constitutional Right of Informational Privacy: Does It Protect Children Suffering from AIDS?", *Fordham Urban Law Journal*, Vol. 14, 1985-86, pp. 927-969; S.L. Davie, "Casenote: Constitutional Law - Right of Privacy - the Privacy Interests of AIDS - Infected Blood Donors", *Cumberland Law Review*, Vol. 18, 1987/88,, pp. 267-280.

3. T. Gerety, "Redefining Privacy", *Harvard Civil Rights - Civil Liberties Law Review*, Vol. 12, 1977, pp. 233-296. Citation p. 274.

4. R. Lisle, "The Right of Privacy (A Contra View)", *Kentucky Law Journal*, Vol. 19, 1931, pp. 137-145. Citation p. 144.

5. W.H.L. Dornette, "Confidentiality Issues", in W.H.L. Dornette (ed.) *AIDS and the Law*, (John Wiley, New York, 1987), pp. 249-256. Citation p. 256.

6. cf. R.F. Hummel, W.F. Leavy and M. Rampolla (eds.) *AIDS: Impact on Public Policy*, (Plenum Press, New York, 1986); J.A. Girardi, et al., "Psychotherapist Responsibility in Notifying Individuals at Risk for Exposure to HIV", *Journal of Sex Research*, Vol. 25, 1988, pp. 1-27; M.M. Weldon-Linne (et al), "AIDS - Virus Antibody Testing: Issues of Informed Consent and Patient Confidentiality", *Illinois Bar Journal*, Vol. 75, 1986, pp. 206-213; C. Niland and T. Nguyen, "AIDS: Scapegoating, Confidentiality and Legal Aspects", in A. Carr (ed.) *Meeting the Challenge: Papers of the First National Conference on AIDS*, (Australian Government Publishing Service, Canberra, 1986), pp. 153-157; Privacy Committee (New South Wales), *Acquired Immune Deficiency Syndrome (AIDS): Guidelines for the Testing for Antibodies to the HTLV-III (AIDS) Virus*, February 1986; A.B. Shrank, "Is Testing for HIV without Consent ever Warranted?" *British Medical Journal*, Vol. 294, 1987, p. 445; C. Shepherd, "Confidentiality and AIDS", *British Medical Journal*, Vol. 295, 1987, p. 1567; D.O. Crompton, "AIDS and the

Ethics of Disclosure", *Medical Journal of Australia*, Vol. 147, 1987, p. 522.

7. S. Lukes, "Methodological Individualism Reconsidered", *British Journal of Sociology*, Vol. XIX, 1968, pp. 119-129.

8. A. Gouldner, *The Future of Intellectuals and the Rise of the New Class* (Seabury Press, New York, 1979).

9. R. Bhaskar, *A Realist Theory of Science* (Harvester Press, Sussex, 1978).

10. For an attack on the sociobiological theory of human nature cf. M. Harris, *Cultural Materialism: The Struggle for a Science of Culture*, (Random House, New York, 1979) and J.W. Smith *Reductionism and Cultural Being*, (Martinus Nijhoff, The Hague, 1984); for a useful recent collection of critical essays, see A. Montagu (ed.), *Sociobiology Examined* (Oxford University Press, Oxford, 1980).

11. C.B. MacPherson, *The Political Theory of Possessive Individualism* (Oxford University Press, London, 1962).

12. J. Robinson, "Capital Theory Up to Date", *Canadian Journal of Economics*, Vol. 3, 1970, pp. 309-317. Reprinted in E.K. Hunt and J.G. Schwartz (eds), *A Critique of Economic Theory* (Penguin, Harmondsworth, 1972).

13. An elaborate mathematical argument demonstrating the impossibility of an orthodox (utilitarian) economic theory involving general ranking methods has been given by Richard Routley: "On the Impossibility of an Orthodox Social Theory and of an Orthodox Solution to Environment Problems", *Logique et Analyse* (N.S.) vol. 23, 1980-, pp. 145-166. This result is based upon Routley's repair and extension of Arrow's Impossibility Theorem, cf. "Repairing Proofs of Arrow's General Impossibiity Theorem and Enlarging the Scope of the Theorem", *Notre Dame Journal of Formal Logic*, Vol. XX, No. 4, Oct. 1979, pp. 879-890.

14. The philosophical literature on privacy is vast and includes P. Weiss, *Privacy*, (Southern Illinois University Press, Carbondale, 1983); F. Schoeman, "Privacy: Philosophical Dimensions", *American Philosophical Quarterly*, Vol. 21, 1984, pp. 199-213; J.M. Grcic, "The Right to Privacy: Behavior as Property", *Journal of Value Inquiry*, Vol. 20, 1986, pp. 137-144; D. O'Brien, *Privacy, Law and Public Policy*, (Praeger Special Studies, New York, 1979); S. Goode, *The Right to Privacy*, (Franklin Watts, New York, 1983); S.D. Hudson and D.N. Husak, "Benn on Privacy and Respect for

Persons", *Australasian Journal of Philosophy*, Vol. 57, 1979, pp. 324-329; S.I. Benn, "Privacy and Respect for Persons: A Reply", *Australasian Journal of Philosophy*, Vol. 58, 1980, pp. 54-61; R.A. Epstein, "A Taste for Privacy? Evolution and the Emergence of a Naturalistic Ethic", *Journal of Legal Studies*, Vol. 9, 1980, pp. 665-681; B.V. Johnstone, "The Right to Privacy: The Ethical Perspective", *American Journal of Jurisprudence*, Vol. 29, 1984, pp. 73-94; R.N. Beck, "The Right of Professional Privacy", *Personalist*, Vol. 55, 1974, pp. 145-150; R. Wacks, "The Poverty of "Privacy"," *Law Quarterly Review*, Vol. 96, 1980, pp. 73-89; R.T. Stratton, "State Interference with Personhood: The Privacy Rights, Necessity Defense, and Proscribed Medical Therapies", *Pacific Law Journal*, Vol. 10, 1979, pp. 773-800; R.G. Glover, "The Right to Privacy", *Canterbury Law Review*, Vol. 2, 1983, pp. 51-67; B.L. Bellman, "The Paradox of Secrecy", *Human Studies*, Vol. 4, 1981, pp. 1-24; H.J. McCloskey, "Privacy and the Right to Privacy", *Philosophy*, Vol. 55, 1980, pp. 17-38; J.W. Decew, "Defending the "Private" in Constitutional Privacy", *Journal of Value Inquiry*, Vol. 21, 1987, pp. 171-184; W.A. Parent, "Recent Work on the Concept of Privacy", *American Philosophical Quarterly*, Vol. 20, 1983, pp. 341-355, and "Privacy, Morality, and the Law, *Philosophy and Public Affairs*, Vol. 12, 1983, pp. 269-288; R.S. Gerstein, "Intimacy and Privacy", *Ethics*, Vol. 89, 1978, pp. 76-81; K.R. Conklin, "Privacy: Should There Be a Right to It?" *Educational Theory*, Vol. 26, 1976, pp. 263-270.

15. cf. A. Westin, *Privacy and Freedom*, (Atheneum Press, New York, 1967. Westin says:

    "Privacy is the claim of individuals, groups, or institutions to determine for themselves when, how, and to what extent information about them is communicated to others. Viewed in terms of the relation of the individual to social participation, privacy is the voluntary and temporary withdrawal of a person from the general society through physical or psychological means, either in a state of solitude or small-group intimacy or, when among larger groups, in a condition of anonymity or reserve". (p.7).

16. cf. R. Parker, "A Definition of Privacy", *Rutgers Law Review*, Vol. 29, 1974, pp. 275-296.

17. cf. O'Brien op.cit., note 14. This classification is from Schoeman op.cit., note 14, p. 199.

18. Schoeman, ibid p. 199.

19. Grcic, op.cit., note 14, p. 139.

20. Other material on medical confidentiality includes J.S. Ellin, "Confidentiality in the Teaching of Medical Ethics", Teaching Philosophy, Vol. 8, 1985, pp. 1-12; T.F. Ackerman, "Why Doctors Should Intervene", Hastings Center Report, Vol. 12, 1982, pp. 14-17; S. Bok, "The Limits of Confidentiality", Hasting Center Report, Vol. 13, 1983, pp. 24-31; J. King-Farlow, "Confidentiality: Medical Ethics and Professional Morality", Philosophical Papers, Vol. 10, 1981, pp. 9-15; W.C. Starr, "Ethical Theory, Confidentiality and Professional Ethics", Metaphilosophy, Vol. 15, 1984, pp. 129-140; O.M. Ruebhausen and O.C. Brim, "Privacy and Behavioral Research", in T.A. Shannon (ed.) Bioethics, (Revised), (Paulist Press, New Jersey, 1981), pp. 569-599; A.P. Peter and H. Sanchez, "The Therapist's Duty to Disclose Communicable Diseases", Western State University Law Review, Vol. 14, 1987, pp. 465-478; G. Schwartz, "Confidentiality Revisited", Social Work, Vol. 34, 1989, pp. 223-226; A. Dubro, "Your Medical Records. How Private are They?" California Lawyer, Vol. 3, 1988, pp. 33-34, 36; M.D. Basson, "The Right to Privacy When Lives are at Stake", in M.D. Basson, R.E. Lipson and D.L. Ganos (eds.), Troubling Problems in Medical Ethics, (Alan Liss Inc., New York, 1981), pp. 239-240 with A.L. Caplan pp. 245-255, G.D. Abrams, pp. 257-268, M.D. Basson, pp. 269-271; S.E. Marshall, "Public Bodies, Private Selves", Journal of Applied Philosophy, Vol. 5, 1988, pp. 147-158; D.J. Kenny, "Confidentiality: the Confusion Continues", Journal of Medical Ethics, Vol. 8, 1982, pp. 9-11; D.F.H. Pheby, "Changing Practice on Confidentiality: A Course for Concern", Journal of Medical Ethics, Vol. 8, 1982, pp. 12-24; H.E. Emson, "Confidentiality: A Modified Value", Journal of Medical Ethics, Vol. 14, 1988, pp. 87-90; M.H. Kottow, "Medical Confidentiality: An Intransigent and Absolute Obligation", Journal of Medical Ethics, Vol. 12, 1986, pp. 117-122; I.E. Thompson, "The Nature of Confidentiality", Journal of Medical Ethics, Vol. 5, 1979, pp. 57-64; J. Havard, "Medical Confidence", Journal of Medical Ethics, Vol. 11, 1985, pp. 8-11.

21. J.J. Thomson, "The Right to Privacy", Philosophy and Public Affairs, Vol. 4, 1975, pp. 295-314; for comments on Thomson cf. T. Scanlon, "Thomson on Privacy", Philosophy and Public Affairs, Vol. 4, 1975, pp. 315-322 and J. Rachels, "Why Privacy is Important", Philosophy and Public Affairs, Vol. 4, 1975, pp. 323-333.

22. Grcic, op.cit., note 14, p. 138.

23. Schoeman, oplcit., note 14, p. 210.

24. E. Bloustein, "Privacy as an Aspect of Human Dignity: An Answer to Dean Prosser", New York University Law Review, Vol. 39, 1964, pp. 962-1007.

25. J. Andre, "Privacy as a Value and as a Right", Journal of Value Inquiry, Vol. 20, 1986, pp. 309-317.

26. J.H. Reiman, "Privacy, Intimacy and Personhood", Philosophy and Public Affairs, Vol. 6, 1976, pp. 26-44.

27. ibid p. 39.

28. C.K. Boone, "Privacy and Community", Social Theory and Practice, Vol. 9, 1983, pp. 1-30. Citation pp. 23-24. cf. also J. Kupfer, "Privacy, Autonomy and Self-Concept", American Philosophical Quarterly, Vol. 24, 1987, pp. 81-89; C. Fried, "Privacy", Yale Law Journal, Vol. 77, 1968, pp. 475-493.

29. cf. L. Walter, "The Principle of Medical Confidentiality", in T.A. Mappes and J.S. Zembaty (eds.) Biomedical Ethics, 2nd edition, (McGraw HIll, New York, 1986), pp. 148-151. Citation p. 149 and "Ethical Aspects of Medical Confidentiality", in T.L. Beauchamp and L. Walters (eds.) Contemporary Issues in Bioethics, 2nd edition, (Wadsworth, California, 1982), pp. 198-203.

30. Quoted from M. Winston, "AIDS and a Duty to Protect", Hastings Center Report, Vol. 17, February 1987, pp. 22-23. Citation p. 22.

31. G. Gillett, "AIDS and Confidentiality", Journal of Applied Philosophy, Vol. 4, 1987, pp. 15-20. Citation p. 19.

32. S.H. Landesman, "Commentary", Hastings Center Report, Vol. 17, February 1987, p. 23.

33. G.J. Annas, "Confidentiality and the Duty to Warn", Hastings Center Report, Vol. 6, 1976, pp. 6-8. Citation p. 8.

34. J. Allender, "Forced Disclosure of AIDS Cases 'A Necessity'," The Australian, Thursday June 1, 1989, p. 6.

6 AIDS, egalitarian justice and the allocation of scarce medical resources

WITH **RODNEY ALLEN**

1   Introduction

2   The Idea of Justice as Equality

3   The Principles of Equality

4   The Justification of Equality

5   Radical Egalitarianism and the Allocation of Scarce Medical Resources

       (a) Freedom or Self-Determination

       (b) Act-Utilitarianism

       (c) Meritocracy

       (d) Rawls' Justice as Fairness

       (e) Nozick's Libertarian Theory

6   Conclusion : AIDS, Egalitarianism and the Need for Revolution in Health Care

1. Introduction

The issue of the rational and ethical ordering of medical priorities and resources and in general social priorities and resources has not rated highly on the research agenda of bioethics, despite calls by both Joseph Fletcher [1], and Paul Ramsey [2] for increased research attention. This vacuum received a major scholarly addition by the publication in 1981 of Justice and Health Care edited by Earl Shelp. [3] However, there has been very little work done on the application of egalitarianism to health care, especially the health care of AIDS patients. [4] It is the aim of this chapter to present a contribution towards the correction of these omissions.

Egalitarianism has not been a "live" issue in Australian politics in the 1980's, as the very idea of a fair and even distribution of the nation's wealth, is very much contrary to all that the right wing Hawke Labour government and a generally libertarian Liberal party stand for. Both parties, despite their differences are committed to the sanctity of the private ownership of society's means of production, increasing population expansion largely through immigration and massive development and increasing economic growth. In this process, of the great game of international and national market economics, there must be winners and losers. Consequently egalitarianism, generally linked to a rejection of the private enterprise system itself, has not even been a topic of suitable debate. The "egalitarian" visions even of Whitlam belong to some shadowy past in the Australian political process, which our rulers hope is long buried under the sands of pragmatism and economic opportunism. Inequality, we are told, is the price of an efficient economy.

In an article in The Bulletin, David O'Reilly summarizes data from a five year study at the Australian National University and other recent research, which shows that the gaps between the advantaged and disadvantaged has never been greater. [5] More than 60 percent of Australia's wealth is owned by 10 percent of the population (a third of these assets belonging to the richest 1 percent), and one in eight households lives below the poverty line, despite efforts to improve social welfare administration. Prime Minister Hawke and Treasurer Keating have argued for many years that the new economic imperative is the national debt crisis, and that belt tightening and a general decline in living standards are inevitable under the circumstances. The economy is to be treated by a tight monetary policy, including increasing interest rates, to put a lid upon spending, usually of imported goods. The real issue of the disastrous effects of free trade, recognised by even conservative economists, is not addressed. [6] The deeper solution to the foreign debt crisis, derivable from a radical egalitarian theory of justice - which would involve increasing self-reliance and independence for Australia, and the development of appropriate technologies, industries and products for Australia and owned by Australia - is never examined within the newly painted walls of Parliament House. [7] Australia seems happy to be a small banana-republic-shaped gear in the US - Japan money machine [8], or at least according to politicians - 83% of Australians see Australia as becoming a "less-fair" society and only 13% of Australians in 1989 saw Australia as a "fair" society. [9] This perception is confirmed by research at the Social Welfare Research Centre at the University of New South Wales, that saw Australia as one of the least equal industrialized countries, a view also confirmed by a 1988 World Bank report. [10]

The issue of the predicament of youth with respect to suicide and drug abuse was mentioned previously. Closely related to those problems is the problem of youth unemployment. Whilst youth unemployment has fallen from 27 percent to 17 percent now in 1989 under the Hawke government, a youth unemployment rate of 17 percent means that around 100,000 teenagers are seeking full time employment. Whilst the Australian First Home Owners' Scheme has helped 300,000 middle and low-income people into homes, 40,000 people are homeless and sleep either on the streets or in emergency accommodation and the Burdekin Report found that 25,000 children are homeless. No doubt with sky rocketting interest rates, that have doubled loan repayments since 1983 so that on average more than 30 percent of the family income is spent on repayments, many more Australians will be forced into alternative accommodation or homelessness. There are 2.6 million households in poverty, including 440,000 children, meaning that one in every eight Australians is in poverty. These figures must be understood with respect to Australia's relatively small population, compared to the rest of the over-populated globe.

The problem of poverty in Australia is worth placing in juxtaposition with <u>Business Review Weekly's</u> survey of the two hundred richest Australians (May 12, 1989). Here is a litany of this affluence: Kerry Packer estimated net worth $1.8 billion; Maurice Alter $240 million; Franco Belgiorno-Nettis/Carlo Salteri, $240 million; Marcus Besen, $280 million; John Fairfax/ Vincent Fairfax, $350 million; Warwick Fairfax/Mary Fairfax, $200 million; John Gandel, $330 million; Abe Goldberg, $250 million; Bruno Grollo/Rino Grollo, $620 million; David Hains, $450 million; George Herscu, $300 million; Robert Holmes a Court, $700 million; Solomon Lew, $390 million; Theo Morris, $340 million; Richard

Pratt, $360 million; Harry Triguboff, $300 million; Alan Bond, $100 million; Lang Hancock, $120 million; Lee Ming Tee, $138 million; and so on. There are also many sad, less fortunate Australians in the under $100 million category; Bob Ansett, $35 million; Tristan Antico, $44 million; Frank Bannigan/Kevin Bannigan, $68 million; Neville Beville, $55 million; Joe Burstyn, $40 million; Daniel Chen, $88 million; John Elliott, $70 million; Giuseppe Emanuele, $95 million; Con Polites, $70 million; and so on ad nauseam.

In this economic climate it is not surprising to find statements in the Australian press along the lines that "health funding is in a shambles". In South Australia, both the Royal Adelaide Hospital, the Adelaide Children's Hospital, the Queen Elizabeth Hospital, Modbury Hospital and the Flinders Medical Centre suffer. Cost-cutting measures at the Queen Victoria Hospital are to try to off-set a budget over-run of up to $800,000. Parents of 15 premature babies were asked in early 1989 to transfer to other public hospitals. [11] The Adelaide Children's Hospital was over-running its budget by more than $3 million, Modbury Hospital up to $500,000 and the Queen Elizabeth Hospital needed $8 million for new equipment. In the case of the Royal Adelaide Hospital, financial cutbacks have the potential, according to the RAH Medical staff society spokesperson, Dr. Randal Butler, to have a long term detrimental impact upon medical standards in South Australia because the hospital is the University of Adelaide's teaching hospital. Wards closing in the hospital include specialties, like ear, nose, throat, gynaecology and much orthopedics. [12] The Flinders Medical Centre intends (May 1989) to shut 1 ward after a 1 1/2 million budget out-run. There has been a 6 percent increase in patient demand over the past year, but with only a 1.7 percent increase in budget. At the same time, some of our leading business men can spend over double and triple the trivial sum demanded by one state's health care crisis, on art acquisitions.

The problem of the allocation of medical resources with respect to AIDS, must be understood within the context of a general scarcity of health-dollars. In 1987, Whyte (et al) stated in the Medical Journal of Australia [13] that the total cost per patient based upon data collected at St. Vincent's Hospital, Sydney, about 39 patients solely treated by the hospital, was $22,352 (range $4,229 - $58,398) with the median cost at $18,667. In-patient costs accounted for 95 percent of the total costs, the average cost of in-patient care being $21,224 (range $3,532 - $58,398) with the median cost at $18,067. The mean cost for the sample of out-patients was $1,107 (range 0 - $4,778) with a median cost of $828. These researchers concluded their paper with these words: "... it is clear that cases of AIDS will demand an increasing share of Australia's hospital resources, in spite of the less intensive treatment and lower unit costs here than in the United States". [14] By November 1988, AIDS was costing Australia up to $100,000 for <u>direct</u> costs for every patient dying or dead from the virus (including all hospital and medical costs, drugs and treatment with AZT). The indirect costs for lost productivity, income and taxes reaches $900,000, making the cost to Australia for each AIDS death $1 million. According to Professor Tony Basten (scientific adviser for the Australian National Council on AIDS), in a media release, doctors will be treating a further 3,000 AIDS patients by 1991. By 1990, the AIDS-care bill will be well over $100 million. Basten said "These costs are enormous and raise the point whether the taxpayer can afford it". [15] This cost though is a drop in the ocean compared to the projected United States cost of providing health care services to AIDS patients, taken to be at least $8.5 billion (U.S) in 1991 with an indirect cost of $55.6 billion by 1991. [16]

Mainstream writing on the problem of the allocation of resources for AIDS programmes, within the context of economic rationalism, does not suggest any satisfactory response to this problem. Ken Donald for example says: "... we are going to have grave difficulty in getting enough fiscal resources. Health budgets are already heavily committed and we have a whole range of new clients and customers and none of the other diseases are going to go away". [17] Nor has the issue of dealing with long term costs of AIDS into the next century been seriously considered and solved by the <u>Report of the 3rd National Conference on AIDS</u>. [18] As far as we are aware, only the President of the Health Commission of the City and County of San Francisco, Philip Lee has ventured to give a global moral opinion on this topic. He says:

> "The failure of the Federal govenrment to meet its responsibilities in providing for an equitable system of health care financing does not eliminate the high costs of health care. Rather, it simply shifts those costs to other levels of government or to the private sector and to the individual citizen. If the AIDS epidemic does nothing else, it must underscore the urgent need for an adequate and just system of national health insurance". [19]

Lee is optimistic that national health insurance would be able to cope with the <u>long term</u> costs of AIDS; we are not, especially if AIDS is to be treated (as it must) as a global problem. [20]

In this chapter we believe that a socially deeper approach is needed to deal with the massive problem of health care funding that AIDS-care will require. We will maintain that to deal with a problem of human survival such as AIDS, society must be radically restructured along egalitarian lines - and ultimately the entire world needs to be restructured so that no individual and no nation posseses immense per capita wealth whilst others do not. This restructuring is vital if humanity is to deal effectively and justly with problems such as environmental destruction, famine and AIDS. To develop this argument will require more space and research time, than can be presented in this book, and certainly in this chapter. Nevertheless, with boldness of spirit, we now present our first sketch of an egalitarian theory of justice with respect to the basic goods of human life, especially health care, that is an important part in our image of an alternative world. This chapter develops the critique of the capitalist social order which we began in the previous chapter, and will continue in the final chapter of this book.

2. The Idea of Justice as Social Equality

The idea of social equality has fascinated people for centuries. An urgent concern with it arises as we have seen naturally from people's inevitable social involvements. People's social relationships necessarily confront them with some form of equality or inequality, so they have, by and large, been concerned to articulate and understand the idea of social equality, to adopt attitudes towards it, and to act on the basis of these attitudes. In other words, this idea has been one important and continuing focus for the operation of humanity's intellect, emotions and will. Yet for all this, there has been precious little agreement in approach. People have given different interpretations of this ideal. They have seen various and varying forms of it. Some have seen it (or some form or forms of it) as a value worth pursuing, while others have seen it (or some form or forms of it) as an evil and a threat to civilisation, social well-being, or even social justice. There have been, in short, widely varied estimates of the importance and value of this ideal.

Modern social and political philosophers, for their part, have approached the idea of equality with excessive caution, conservatism and timidity, perhaps partly because of the huge amount of human interest and emotion tied up in this area. They have, it seems, only been interested in describing as clearly as possible what is involved in the common notions of equality, in seeking out the "lowest common denominator" in the various common approaches to equality. So their conclusions have, for the most part, been trivial and unenlightening. We find the literature statements such as the following:

> "All social inequalities not necessary or justified should be eliminated" [21]

> "In its simplest form the ideal of complete social equality embodies the wish that everything and everybody should be as similar as possible to everything and everybody else." [22]

> "[There should be] equal consideration of human interests." [23]

It is not, we think, unfair to these "lowest common denominator" writers to summarise their views only by reference to their slogans, for their discussion of "justifiable inequalities" and "morally relevant differences" is, for the most part, mystifying, unclear, undetailed and frequently containing unsystematic references to such concepts as "need", "interest" and "desert" - but in the end, leaving us with nothing more substantial or helpful than the slogans. Their approach could perhaps best be summarised by an even more clearly vacuous slogan "Equality for Equals!"

Often, in modern philosophy, where there is some explicit awareness of the inadequacy of this "Equality for Equals!" approach, this has resulted simply in the adoption of an anti-egalitarian attitude, in the idea that equality is not in itself a value at all; that it is a trivial and unimportant value; or that an emphasis on questions of equality is only a confused way of emphasising something else which really is a value ("justice" or "freedom" or "humanity" for example) and which only requires some equality, whilst requiring or allowing much inequality. J.R. Lucas adopts a position something like the latter when he writes:

> "There are two sound principles of political reasoning, the principle of Universalisability and the principle of Universal Humanity, and each has been described as a sort of Equality... But they are not the same Equality, nor are they compatible, and they cannot be run in harness to lead to a full-blooded egalitarianism. Each, however, by itself can lead to some conclusions which an egalitarian would endorse. Though these conclusions are less, and necessarily less, than all that an egalitarian would wish, they represent the only Equalities that are obtainable and reasonable to seek". [24]

H.J. McCloskey adopts a somewhat harsher line, maintaining that the pursuit of equality as such is not at all worthwhile:

> "A State which concerns itself solely with liberty, or with the general happiness, or with justice, is one which does not commend itself to most of us. However there is a big difference between such states and one geared to equality. In the case of the former, we feel that a good is being realised but at the expense of many other goods. In the case of equality (which, as we have seen, involves unjustly treating dissimilars similarly, or levelling out all differences, personal and other, to achieve a dull uniformity and conformity) there

> is no evident good of any sort being realised
> through or in the equality itself, that what good
> such a state achieved would be due to equality
> coinciding with some other good such as justice,
> liberty, fraternity, happiness. In any case, the
> demand for equality seems more likely to collide
> rather than coincide with the demands for these
> other goods". [25]

In general, modern social and political philosophy has understood equality as either a triviality or an evil.

Of course there has been much more emphasis upon the ideal of equality in the socialist tradition of political thought than there has been within the liberal tradition. Radical socialists, at least have been overridingly concerned with social classes with respect to the means of transcending class - divided societies and creating classless societies. But even here, the main tendency has been to dismiss social equality as a mystifying concept, an element in the ruling ideology of bourgeois society, an element that could only serve the class interests of the bourgeoisie. There has been surprisingly little discussion and explanation of class and classlessness in terms of equality and social justice. [26] Marx himself had very little to say at all on the nature of classless society, and what he did say was extremely vague, unexplicated and not justified by carefully constructed ethical arguments. Among the things he did say, of course is this:

> "After the enslaving subordination of individuals
> under the division of labour, and therefore also
> the antithesis between mental and physical labour
> has vanished, after labour has become not merely a
> means to live but has become itself the primary
> necessity of life, after the productive forces have
> also increased with the all - round development of
> the individual, and all the springs of co-operative
> wealth flow more abundantly - only then can the
> narrow horizon of bourgeois right be fully left
> behind and society inscribe on its banners: from
> each according to his ability, to each according to
> his needs". [27]

Whilst we recognise Marx's writings themself to be theoretically inadequate on the question of exposition and justification of principles of equality, nevertheless we believe that Marx's view, including his sketchy hints concerning the nature of classless society or communism, are very important for development of a theory of equality.

Clearly then there is a need for a new, critical theory of social equality, a theory which goes beyond the mere uncritical description of what is already implicit in our everyday social practice and discourse, a theory which seeks to build up and evaluate a coherent and intelligible concept of equality. There is such a need regardless of whether one is inclined initially towards a pro- or an anti-egalitarian stance; for in either case, the large issues at stake must be intelligibly and critically articulated, not left submerged in a sea of vague slogans.

In this chapter we shall attempt to defend the thesis of <u>radical egalitarianism</u>: that people should be treated similarly in respect of the value of their lives for themselves, that is, in such a way as to secure for them an equal degree of satisfaction of their real interests. We shall structure our discussion around three related sets of questions concerning social equality. First, what is social equality? What principles articulate (or are constitutive of) a coherent and intelligible conception of equality? Second, is social equality justifiable? That is, is social equality justifiable as a <u>social value</u>, an end worth pursuing by social action. Finally, we shall consider some of the general problems raised by considering the application of the principle(s) of social equality to the concrete social situation of the distribution of scarce medical resources with respect to the AIDS crisis. This situation has generally been regarded as a counter-instance to radical egalitarian principles: we show that this is not so.

3. The Principles of Equality

We believe that there are two complementary principles which together spell out, in normative terms, a viable and radical conception of social equality. One of these is relatively formal and trivial, the other relatively substantial and important.

The first of these we shall call the <u>formal principle of equality</u>. It is not a new idea; nor is it a rare one in either recent or classical philosophical writing on the theme of equality. Indeed, many variations on it, some slightly less formal and trivial than others, have been the primary concerns and conclusions of the protagonists of the "Equality for Equals!" approach. It may be expressed thus:

> (EE) People should be treated similarly unless there is sufficient reason for treating them differently in certain respects, i.e. for differentiating between them in respect of certain aspects of their social lives and the social conditions of their well-being.

Clearly, this principle by itself, just considered in abstract isolation, does not provide any account of what are, and what are not, reasons justifying similarity or difference in social treatment. It does not specify any criteria of relevance; i.e. criteria specifying the sorts of considerations which are relevant as justifying reasons to propose similar or differential treatment in the social sphere. Thus, the formal principle of equality considered in isolation is incomplete: it requires for completion a specification of criteria of relevance, by a substantive account of the sorts of considerations which count as reasons for and against certain lines of social action. And furthermore, if we are to have a coherent concept of social equality at all, we must be able to specify complementary criteria of relevance for the formal principle of equality which are themselves constitutive of the concept of social equality. Another way of putting this point is to say that it is substantively meaningless to speak of equality as simply uniformity of similarity without specifying criteria according to which any two things (for our purposes, social situations of individuals) are to be counted as the same or different; i.e. without specifying a sense for "sameness", a respect in which two things might be the same. Despite this legitimate need for criteria of relevance, the "Equality for Equals!" philosophers have more or less stopped short their account of social equality as such with the nugatory assertion of the formal principle of equality.

By itself, this principle only lays down that actions directed towards other people, social actions, ought to be based upon reasons, and it abstracts the idea of "reason" from considerations to do with what are good and bad reasons for social actions. Consequently, it leaves us with only an "evaluatively-neutral" or "value-free" idea of reason in this area; an idea of reason abstracted from any substantial considerations of justification and relevance.

In any case we have already said that the formal principle of equality is relatively trivial. Would it however be satisfied by any clear example of social injustice? Is it in this sense absolutely trivial? We think not. To see this, consider two different types of injustice, each or both of which could characterise the operation of a particular legal system. First, the laws themselves might be unjust - for example, laws requiring certain forms of racial discrimination. Second, the laws might be administered or applied unfairly, independently of their content. For example, judges may be susceptible to bribes, or some may show bias towards, and impose stiffer penalties upon, say, defendents appearing with long hair or no hair at all. Now the formal principle of equality can be construed as an insistence upon the rule of law, or at least in principle. Therefore, it does in fact rule out the second sort of injustice - i.e. capriciousness, selfish partiality or malicious bias in the application of laws or principles. Berlin brings out this point clearly when he writes:

> "This type of equality derives simply from the conception of rules as such - namely, that they should allow of no exceptions. Indeed, what is meant by saying that a given rule exists is that it

should be fully, i.e. equally fully obeyed by those who fall under it, and that any inequality in obedience would constitute an exception, i.e. an offence against the rules. Insofar as some minimum degree of prevalence of rules is a necessary condition for the existence of human societies - and insofar as morality, both personal and political, is largely conceived in terms of rules, the kind of equality with which obedience to rules is virtually identical, is among the deepest needs and convictions of mankind. In this sense, equality is co-extensive with morality as such - that is, to the degree to which social morality is conceived as a system of coherent sets of rules. A plea for equality in this sense is therefore a plea for life in accordance with rules as opposed to other standards, for example the ad hoc orders of an inspired leader or abritrary desires. In this sense, then, to say that inequality is wrong is in effect to say that it is wrong to obey no rules in a given situation, or to accept some rule and to break it; and a situation in which some men, for no stated reason and in accordance with no rule, consistently get more than other men with the same, or sufficiently similar, relevant characteristics (however this is determined) is then described as being unfair". [28]

We have now an argument for what for Williams was intuitively clear. It seems therefore, that although the formal principle of equality EE, is very largely trivial, it is not absolutely trivial. It does rule out "rule-less" behaviour.

Nevertheless, as we have already indicated, the formal principle EE is logically incomplete as a principle of social equality. It requires completion by the specification of criteria of relevance for similar or differential treatment, or (what comes down to the same thing) by criteria of "sameness" and "difference" in social situations. So now the question may reasonably be asked of us: what is your substantial and important principle of social equality? It will, we believe, be helpful to answer this question in two steps. Our first step can be expressed by this principle (which will be elaborated further in the course of the argument):

(EV) People should be treated in such a way as to secure for them <u>equal value</u>.

Hence a society characterised by social equality, would be a society the lives of whose members would have equal value for themselves, insofar as this can be determined by social action and arrangement.

Most writers on this subject have noticed that there is

a difference between "inequality" and "difference"; that although social inequality must consist in some sort of difference between people, not all differences between people (indeed, not all social differences) amount necessarily to social inequalities. Some differences between people in a society (e.g. some differences in occupation) might be systematically correlated with social inequalities without being what these inequalities consist in *essentially*. So any adequate theory of equality must provide an answer to the question: what sorts of social differences between people *necessarily* amount to social inequalities. Our first step makes a start towards answering this question. It is to maintain that the sort of difference which necessarily amounts to social inequality, is a socially-determined difference in the value of peoples' lives to themselves (i.e. the quality of their lives).

There is, in fact, a very well-worn anti-egalitarian line of argument which goes like this:

(AE) It is obviously not morally justifiable to treat everyone in an absolutely uniform way. For example, it would not be morally justifiable to treat a cripple in exactly the same way one would treat a non-cripple. People have different needs and capacities, and they exist in different circumstances. All these differences must be taken into account when considering the justification of actions and arrangements involving them. Therefore complete or radical social equality is morally indefensible.

Argument AE does not establish the moral indefensibility of radical egalitarianism. It is in fact based upon a false premise: equality is uniformity *simpliciter*. Equality for us is not a boring - or an irrational state of uniformity, but rather *equality of value* - *uniformity of value*. More accurately, it is uniformity in the value of people's lives to themselves, in the quality of their lives insofar as it can be socially determined. Clearly, a standard of social equality so conceived would require a wide variety of differences in the treatment of individuals - all those differences that would be required in order to secure equality of value in differing circumstances, for example, a cripple and a non-cripple would need different treatment in order to secure for each the same value in life.

4. The Justification of Equality

We now turn to a consideration of the issue of the justification of social equality. It has already been stated that a substantial principle of equality may, in a preliminary fashion, be expressed as follows: people should be treated in such a way as to secure the *equal value* of their lives for themselves, insofar as this can be socially determined. Interpreted in the light of the account of value previously discussed in this book, this principle may be stated as follows:

> (ESI) People should be treated in such a way as to secure for themselves an equal degree of satisfaction of their real interests, insofar as this can be socially determined.

Roughly speaking, this means that people should as far as possible be given equal shares in the conditions of human happiness.

It should be realised that this "equal satisfaction of interests" principle is <u>not</u> to the effect that the "felt" or conscious wants of all people ought to be equally satisfied. For the conscious wants of people do not necessarily coincide with what is of value for them. People may, and in fact do, want things which are not in their interest, and do not want things which are in their interest. Thus the equalizing of degrees of conscious want satisfaction need not result in the equalizing of value. It is <u>equality of value</u> which is essential for social equality. This is why it is important in this connection to speak of "interests" rather than "wants" or "desires".

There are some further brief points which can be made here. First, the idea of equality as the equal satisfaction of interests must be distinguished from that of equality as the equal consideration of interests. Equal consideration may be given to people's interests even though some people rather than others have their interests - their real interests - frustrated, on the basis of their own individual merits. By contrast, the "equal satisfaction" principle requires that each person's real interests be given as far as possible equal satisfactions, irrespective of their merit as so far achieved: <u>it is not compatible with a "meritocratic" distribution of goods</u>. Again, we shall have more to say on this point later.

Second, it will be quite justly thought that so far we have discussed social equality only abstractly; that we have said nothing about the concrete social ramifications of egalitarianism, about the methods and problems of concretely achieving it. We shall not discuss these important problems in detail in this work. For the present, though, it is worth noting that this "equal satisfaction" principle is a very radical idea in our contemporary circumstances of advanced capitalism or "late" capitalism. It is an expression of the slogan: "To each according to his/her needs" (provided that "need" is <u>not</u> interpreted as "basic need", i.e. what one needs merely to survive). Capitalist industrial societies seem to be governed by the ideal, though certainly not the reality of: "To each according to her (and perhaps "her") merits" rather than": "To each according to her/his needs".

In hard reality, capitalist societies are based on an exploitative productive mechanism which inevitably results in systematic inequalities throughout the entire social structure. The "equal satisfaction" principle is nowhere concretely realised to any significant extent. Consider, for example, income. Income is, quite uniformly in today's industrial societies, a condition for the satisfaction of interests. Social equality, therefore, requires that it be, in general, uniformly distributed. Yet today, all over the world, the dominant tendency is for income differentials to be maintained, and even expanded.

Finally, it will be recalled that we have so far distinguished <u>two</u> principles of equality, one being formal and incomplete, the other being relatively substantial and significant. Now these two principles are both consistent and complimentary (at least we have discovered no counter-instance which would establish such an inconsistency). The formal principle (the idea that people should be treated similarly unless there is a reason for treating them differently) merely specifies a necessary condition of there being any social arrangements at all. The substantial "equal satisfaction" principle specifies the sort of social arrangement which counts as egalitarian (namely, one which contributes significantly to <u>equality</u> in the degree of people's interest satisfactions) and the sort of social arrangement which counts as inegalitarian (namely, one which contributes significantly to <u>inequality</u> in the degree of people's interest satisfactions). Thus the substantial principle specifies what counts as a reason <u>in terms of equality itself,</u> for treating some people differently from others. Such a reason must be a reason for supposing that a certain difference in treatment will contribute to the achievement of <u>equality of value</u> for the people concerned, i.e. an equal satisfaction of their interests.

We must now move on from a general consideration of the question "What is social equality?" to the not unrelated questions: "Can social equality be justified as a social value?"; "Is social equality a value in itself, intrinsically?"; "Ought people act and be treated in accordance with the principle of social equality?" We need to understand in what way, if any, social equality is a social value, and how, if at all, it may be grounded or justified as a value. In this section we shall argue that social equality is a justifiable social value, albeit one amongst a number of other socially applicable values. Clearly on our account, equality could not be a <u>basic value</u>, since we have explicated it in terms of other values. Therefore it presupposes other values.

It should also be recognised that whilst it is true that people do share certain general characteristics - e.g. the capacity to feel pain, the need for food and shelter, the need for respect and affection in one's own right, some intelligence and reasoning ability, some moral capacity, etc. - and while it is important because of these facts, all this does not amount to a social equality in the sense which we have specified, nor *a fortiori* to a justification of it. Catering for common or shared humanity is perfectly compatible with inegalitarian social policies, for it is a matter only of providing a *mininum* of needs and capacities, those that are shared by everyone else; in other words, for the *lowest common denomination* of each individual's needs, wants and capacities as they presently stand. There is plenty of room for inegalitarian treatment once shared basic human characteristics are catered for. It is in this way that an argument purporting to justify equality can degenerate into one merely for the provision of a basic minimum of social welfare upon which inegalitarian structures may be constrainedly built.

Since catering for common humanity is compatible with inegalitarian arrangements, it is compatible with a systematically meritocratic distribution of goods. In fact, the argument from common humanity as so far stated may be used in support of meritocracy. For: while it is true that all people share, in some form and degree, the characteristics of intelligence and rationality, nevertheless they possess these characteristics, many have claimed, in widely differing forms and degrees, and precisely because of this, some people *deserve* more social benefits than others. Again: while it is true that all people share, in some form and degree, moral capacity and activity, nevertheless they possess these characteristics in widely differing forms and degrees - and, once again, it may well be argued that precisely because of this, some people *deserve* more social benefits than others. It is in this way that an argument purporting to justify equality may be inverted into one justifying inequality. Hence one more crucial point about the argument from common humanity as so far stated is that it fails to distinguish between (a) the fact that very nearly all people share certain very general human characteristics in common, and (b) the fact that people share these same common characteristics in different forms and to different degrees.

At the bottom of it all lurks the simple fact that people are not equal in any respect over and above that of being people. Social equality is not out there in the world, waiting to be discovered by keen observers. It is not a presently existing aspect of either the social or natural world. It is neither a social nor a natural fact. On the contrary, it must be struggled for, actively sought and created by and from concrete social movements. Insofar as it is progressively approached as a social fact, *it must be realised and sustained by self-conscious social activity*.

Where do we go from here, in our argument, if equality is to be regarded as a value? We cannot give up the attempt to ground the value of equality in human nature and its circumstances, for that would be to retreat to intuitionism, super-naturalism or some other untenable theory of value. The value of equality requires a grounding in human reality. However, this grounding need not take the simple form of postulating a corresponding fact for the guiding ideal of social equality. Social equality may be related to human nature in less direct ways. So what we propose to do now is (a) show that our idea of equality is essentially bound up with a general, very plausible and very widely accepted conception of morality and (b) show how these conceptions are given intelligibility and applicability by human nature and its circumstances.

The concept of morality which we have in mind is a form of thought and human endeavour which is essentially distinguished from <u>self-interest</u>; which requires an interest in the interests of all people alike as ends in their own right. From the standpoint of the individual agent, morality is primarily and necessarily concerned with the satisfaction of the interests of <u>other</u> people. In large part, it gains its significance as morality by way of contrast with mere self-interest (and partial-group interest). Now our principle of equality lays down a manner of treating all people's interests as ends requiring satisfaction in their own right. Consequently, it is a moral principle essentially bound up with the deepest roots of the human ethical enterprise itself. And if it were not construed as a moral principle, we would lose our conceptual grip on morality as something distinct from self-interest. The principle of equality articulates one way of extending our concern for ourselves into a concern for other people as ends in their own account, rather than as mere means to our own satisfactions: <u>therefore</u> it is a <u>morally</u> justified principle.

The principal fact about human beings which relates to their moral claim to equality, is <u>that they all have interests</u>. They do not, at every level, have the same interests, but they are all the same in that they have interests. These interests are not purely determined by and in people's consciousness; they are not identical with "felt" wants and desires. We may not be conscious of many of our interests. We may have our interests brought to our consciousness, by ourselves and other people: this we believe is both an important and widely experienced aspect of human social life. Our consciousness may contradict our interests - i.e. we may consciously desire that which is not in our interest. Nonetheless, if we did not have conscious wants, we would not have any interests. As we've already said, a human interest is a potential want of a human being, the satisfaction of which would at least not be self-defeating or frustrating or should contribute to the full human development or flourishing of the person concerned. Human interests are the interests of objective human nature, which may be (and has been) much less than adequately realised in

various social forms and historical epochs. Interests are
<u>not</u> purely subjectively determined.

Now, although not everyone has at the same level, the
same interests, everyone does have interests, and moreover
everyone alike has an interest in the satisfaction of his/her
interests. This "second-order" interest is the same for
everyone. For: while it makes sense to speak of any person
having more of an interest in say mountaineering than
another, it makes no sense to say that one person has more of
an interest in the satisfaction of his/her interests than
another. It is this truth which lies at the basis of the
value of social equality. Everyone has an equal interest in
his/her full human development, though not individually equal
capacity for it. We can help each other towards it, through
co-operative social action. Hence equality makes sense as a
guiding ethical standard.

Furthermore, while people do not share the same
interests at every level, nevertheless the ideas of "human
interest", "human nature" and "human development" presuppose
that <u>at a general level</u> there is a significant uniformity in
human interests. There must be more common interests than
simply the abstract interest in the satisfaction of
interests, in order for the idea of human interest itself to
make sense. And indeed there are such general common
interests, which take differing forms for different people in
different concrete circumstances; among these interests we
include health, safety, knowledge, friendship, cooperation,
pleasure, creative-activity, love, truth-seeking and so on.
Not only is it strictly logically impossible to seek to
consistently frustrate all of one's interests (since this
"frustration-interest", even if it is taken as a meta-
interest is still an interest of this person which must
itself be subjected to frustration, entailing in turn that
such a task would itself be frustrated), but one could not
seek to frustrate, or indeed have many of one's interests
frustrated without various mental and physical illnesses
occurring - and consequently living a life which is poor,
brutish and short.

Therefore, there is something right in the attempt to
ground equality in common human nature after all. We cannot
safely assume that there is a very significant identity in
the characteristics and capacities possessed by human beings
in their flesh-and-blood actuality. But we can say that
there are general and significant common human interests. We
can say that there is potentially a state of human
flourishing, of full human development which contains common
elements for all human beings. We can say that humanity has
in general the capacity to approach progressively full human
development through co-operative action. It is in these
facts that the value of equality can rightly be grounded -
not in some hopefully assumed uniformity in the capacities
and characteristics of flesh-and-blood individuals. The

common human nature we seek resides in the nature of human interests. This "objective human nature", this human potential, is foreshadowed in and based upon the "facts" of human nature as it has currently evolved; but it is not reducible to them.

5. Radical Egalitarianism and the Allocation of Scarce Medical Resources

Bernard Williams has distinguished three ways in which goods may be scarce or limited; he has written:

"... some desired goods, like positions of prestige, management etc..., are by their very nature limited: whenever there are some people who are in command of prestigious positions, there are necessarily others who are not. Other goods are contingently limited, in the sense that there are certain conditions of access to them which in fact not everyone satisfies, but there is no intrinsic limit to the numbers who might gain access to it by satisfying the conditions: university education is usually regarded in this light nowadays, as something which requires certain conditions of admission to it which in fact not everyone satisfies, but which an indefinite proportion of people might satisfy. Third, there are good which are fortuitously limited, in the sense that although everyone or large numbers of people satisfy the conditions of access to them, there is just not enough of them to go round; so some more stringent conditions or systems of rationing have to be imposed to govern access in an important situation." [30]

In general then, we can distinguish between (1) accidental, (2) contingent and (3) necessary limitatons of desirable goods and services. Here we will consider the case of the fortuitous limitation of certain medical resources by constructing a situation which seems to preclude any use of radical egalitarian principles of resource allocation.

Suppose that there is a hospital containing twenty young, equally desperately ill patients with AIDS, and only enough AZT or some new anti-AIDS drug for ten patients. These numbers are arbitrary, and may be much higher. In other words, there can be no clinical choice made between these patients based upon a particular patient having a better chance of survival. [31] Suppose also that each patient needs, in order to continue to survive, virtually full use of his/her ration of the drug taken continuously to repress HIV biochemical activity. There is no doubt that this sort of desperate situation may arise at present in Africa in treating AIDS patients and it could possibly arise in the West if the number of AIDS patients continue to rise at an alarming rate. This is the classical moral problem of distributing a limited and crucial medical resource, formulated as one might find on a television programme such as "Hypotheticals".

Now firstly, how, if at all, can our principles of equality be applied to this situation? This question is distinct from: what ought to be done in this situation? For it might be the case that, even if we can treat these AIDS patients equally, nevertheless in the final analysis we ought not to do so. We shall raise the latter question shortly, but first we must take up the problem of what, if anything, counts as equality in such a situation.

It might conceivably be urged that the only way of treating these AIDS machines patients in accordance with our stated ideals of equality is to let them all (equally) die. Such a situation is utterly morally counter-intuitive, and if a critic could establish by reasoned argument that our position is committed to such claims, we would surely be committed to accepting an unreasonable moral theory. However, our principle of equality cannot be criticised on this ground for the simple reason that the principle itself is a way of distributing satisfactions which is consistent with treating people as ends in their own right. The reference to satisfactions, rather than frustrations, is essential to an adequate grasp of the principle. Therfore, an application of the principle which yields universal frustration contradicts the very point of equality. While the idea of equalising satisfactions must also involve that of equalising burdens or frustrations, nevertheless it cannot, without becoming self-defeating, require the equalisation of burdens to the point where no meaningful satisfactions are possible at all.

Should we then conclude that there is no way of treating our AIDS machine patients equally? No - for we believe that we must consider the claim of random selection to be counted as a mode of equality in this and like situations. The use of random selection, to be sure, is a very frequently used strategy of moral philosophers in dealing, even in part with such thought-experiments. It may come as some surprise to readers to be asked to consider methods of random selection as modes of equality. There has been one plausible reason for this: the use of random selection would result in a discrimination favouring some individuals rather than others - seemingly without good moral reason at all - and hence it could not be an egalitarian procedure at all. Once more it would seem that our principles of equality break down at a crucial point.

In reply to this objection, we maintain that random selection is selection without morally relevant grounds, as the critic notes, but it is a way of not discriminating between the people concerned, according to any rule, meritocratic or otherwise. On this point it is similar to a straight forward application of the egalitarian principle. Therefore, we believe that random selection may be viewed as a form of equality, but only in relation to certain sorts of imperfect circumstances; those in which straight forward egalitarianism would not result in any meaningful interest satisfactions at all, and probably many of these where straight forward egalitarianism yields an unnecessary and wasteful multiplication of burdens. This is not a counter-example to our position because the AIDS patients example raises the same difficulty for meritocratic moral principles, since one can define the thought-experiment in such a way that no patient has any more merit (beyond being a person in need of medical treatment) than any other. The defender of some meritocratic moral principle may well be able to interpret modes of random selection as a device for achieving (imperfectly perhaps) meritocracy: this remains an open question. Our claims here are not to produce any alleged counter-instance to meritocratic moral principles, in the present context, but to point out that random selection is a device which in the circumstances, reasonably approaches equality; that it is an imperfect mode of equality, nonetheless appropriate to this sort of imperfect situation.

The use of methods of random selection as a basis for a reasonable selection system has been discussed previously in the ethics literature dealing with the problem of the allocation of scarce medical resources. [32] Rescher has argued that any acceptable selection sytem is essentially non-optimal. Allowing random selection, and hence the element of chance avoids the problem of basing life-or-death decisions upon imperfect selection methods. The use of random selection also has other advantages that Rescher lists. It makes matters easier for the rejected patient, who like all of us is conditioned to accept the workings of chance, but who like most of us, would object to decison making which is ultimately based upon subjective judgement. In a fair lottery one at least has a chance, and the rejected patient may at least draw some consolation from this, because life itself is contingent like a lottery. Finally, the use of random selection relieves some of the burden of responsibility that faces adminstrators. Consequently there is much to recommend the use of random selection in a selection system for the allocation of scarce medical resources.

Even if we agree that random selection would count as equality for our HIV infected patients in their highly imperfect circumstances, there still remains the questions: "ought these patients be treated equally?" and "what, in the final analysis, ought to be done?" From the stand point of the hospital doctors and management, there are a number of general types of answers that can be given to these difficult questions. One is that the patients ought to be treated equally, as equally as is meaningfully possible in the circumstances (i.e. random selection of the patients who are to use the drugs or scarce resources). The remaining general types of answers will be discussed under the following headings (a) Freedom or Self-determination; (b) Act-Utilitarianism, (c) Meritocracy (d) Rawl's Justice as Fairness and (d) Nozick's Libertarian Theory.

(a) **Freedom or Self-determination**

It may be urged that the reasonable thing to do is to allow the patients themselves to decide freely, without external coercion and in full knowledge of the facts, who is to use the machines and who is not. This will produce no problems if volunteers are produced. However, the problem with this answer, granting the latter point, is that it evades the question of moral justification. Allowing the patients themselves to decide does not solve their problem, it merely places it squarely in their hands. If they are not to give up reasoned decision making for a free-for-all, they presumably must decide on some ethical principles to which they must appeal to justify their decision. It is such principles which are here at issue. Therefore the self-determination answer is mistaken.

Moving for a moment to a general plane, the widespread idea that freedom and autonomy as social values are somehow in essential conflict with equality is a very misleading confusion, which deserves at least some consideration from us before we consider act utilitarianism. It is a useless and trivial truth that egalitarianism, just like any other social arrangement, must restrict freedom in the abstract absolute sense of the term; that it must cut out some of what are abstractly possible courses of action for an individual. Thus for freedom to be an intelligible social value, it must be represented as an intelligible human interest in concrete social conditions; it cannot be thought of as a bare unrelated abstraction. Without going into the task of explicating freedom as a social value here, it is still clear that equality requires and presupposes such freedom, for insofar as it is a human interest, equality requires its satisfaction equally for all people. Furthermore, social freedom essentially involves equality. For societies which are tyrannical, autocratic, oligarchic, and hierarchic, not only violate many peoples' freedom, they also distribute the satisfaction of this human interest unequally. Moreover, whether or not the development of human freedom hinders the development of social equality in particular concrete situations will depend upon the conditions under which, and the purposes for which, the freedom is used. Thus freedom as an intelligible social value and equality do not necessarily contradict each other; on the contrary, each is a condition of the full development of the other. [33] This is not to deny that in particular circumstances, an emphasis on equality may yield different results from an emphasis on freedom; that they <u>may</u> conflict in practice. When they do, we suggest that equality should be given <u>prima facie</u> greater weight than freedom, for the reason that it is only on the basis of equality that other potentially social values can be rendered actually and genuinely social, rather than the property of a particular class or group. But again this is not to deny that considerations of freedom cannot outweight those of equality in particular practical contexts. Unfortunately, we don't believe anything more precise can be said in abstraction from concrete analyses of particular situations.

Remembering our dying AIDS patients, we consider the next general type of solution.

(b) **Act-Utilitarianism**

Act-utilitarianism, in its simplest and probably most plausible form, is the idea that a particular act morally ought to be performed, only when its peformance will bring about the greatest amount of good, where "good" is understood to be some type of non-moral value (so the principle is non-trivial). Utilitarianism conceives of this principle as the supreme regulative and overriding principle of morality. Clearly then, there will be as many different forms of act-utilitarianism as there are theories concerning the nature of non-moral values. The most widespread forms are hedonistic and eudaimonic utilitarianism which identify non-moral value with, respectively, pleasure and happiness.

Now there are some common objections to simple act-utilitarianism, and the one which is most relevant to a concern with equality, is that while enjoining the maximisation of good, it neglects considerations of distribution. It is compatible with any mode, in particular with seriously unjust modes of distributing maximum good. Moreover in particular cases, it may be possible to maximise good only at the serious expense of some of the people involved. The happiness of many may be built upon the extreme misery of a few. And the very great happiness of a few may be build upon the relative misery of many. Both these general types of situation seem compatible with simple act-utilitarianism.

To see the basic point clearly, consider for example two possible actions A and B, which affect only two people, X and Y, but in such a way that A produces 100 units of good whilst distributing them extremely unequally, whilst B produces 70 units of good and distributes them equally. The simple act-utilitarian criterion would require the choice of A, whilst equality, and it seems to us, intuitive moral consciousness would require the choice of B, provided that the concrete circumstances are not <u>extremely</u> unusual in a way that bears upon the choice. Of course, the criticism of act-utilitarianism advanced here may perhaps be countered by the utilitarians' claiming that <u>equal distribution</u> is itself one of the goods to be realised through the use of the act-utilitarian principle. The trouble is, however, that this move trivialises act-utilitarianism, and severely comprises it as (a) a single and unambiguous supreme principle of morality, and (b) a doctrine which defines moral rightness wholly in terms of non-moral value. It is clear, though, that applying the utilitarian criterion to concrete circumstances may yield results which clash with those yielded by an application of the principle of equality stated here.

Looking at last at our AIDS patients, act-utilitarianism requires that in their situation, whatever is done be such that it produces the greatest possible quantity of good throughout <u>all</u> the social ramifications of the possible courses of action. Equality requires random selection. The two principles could only coincidently coincide in their determinations for this type of situation. Other things being equal, act-utilitarianism would yield that ten patients be selected to survive - those who would contribute most in the future to the promotion of human happiness. Given certain elaborations of the circumstances, other results are possible for the act-utilitarian. It may be that none of these patients should be allowed the use of the drugs, since they are unlikely to promote human happiness, or it may be that the ten least worthy patients from act-utilitarian viewpoint should be selected to survive, for perhaps the relatives of these ten have planted a bomb in the hospital which they will explode if their demands are not met. In any case, random selection is an unlikely outcome of simple act-utilitarianism applied to this sort of situation.

In this sort of situation equality, even where it unavoidably takes the form of random selection, is morally to be preferred to act-utilitarian outcomes, provided that the surrounding circumstances are not such that this course rather than the act-utilitarian one will produce comparatively <u>extreme</u> suffering or fail to produce a comparatively <u>enormous</u> expansion of happiness. Admittedly this last qualification leaves the matter vague. However we cannot believe that act-utilitarianism must be overridden by equality or any other moral principle in all circumstances, however extreme - if, for example, we were obliged to balance the destruction of the whole world against the sacrifice of one innocent life. Generally, and unfortunately vaguely, we believe that every practical situation should be viewed from an act-utilitarian angle <u>amongst others</u>; that utility should be pursued where this is reasonably consistent with other moral principles such as equality; but that utility should be pursued at the serious expense of such other moral principles as equality <u>only</u> when the benefits of so doing (not just from the standpoint of aggregate utility itself but also from that of the "long-term" promotion of equality, justice and universal human dignity) are comparatively <u>very great</u>. On our view, the simple principle of act-utilitarianism is one moral principle, <u>partially</u> underpinning and characterising less fundamental ones - however, it is not in isolation the one supreme regulative principle of morality, and by itself it is often overridden by other considerations. In matters of morality, as in matters of epistemology, foundationalism seems untenable and we have no mechanical decision procedure to decide right from wrong.

All this, does at least mean that our HIV infected patients should not, on our view, be treated in a simple act-utilitarian fashion. But why not? So far we had just stated a position on this (albeit, we believe a very plausible one from an intuitive point of view) without argument. By way of argument for the normal moral priority of equality over utility, we can only refer back to what is, besides utility itself, an equally fundamental moral principle (but not necessarily a "foundational principle" as this has come to be understood in philosophy, since as we stated above, in some circumstances any particular general moral principle may be overridden) - this is the idea that <u>people should be treated as ends rather than as mere means</u>, the principle of universal respect, universal human worth, universal human dignity. Now: what happens when utility is pursued at the expense of equality is that some people are being treated primarily as means to the satisfaction of others, their interests are being sacrificed in the name of an abstraction, the <u>general</u> happiness. Thus, to allow utility to always predominate over equality is to allow systematic violation of the principle that people are ends in themselves; it is consequently, to rob utility of its character as a <u>moral</u> consideration. For utility to operate as a moral principle, it must be systematically modified by, systematically interrelated with, equality and other modes of treating people as ends rather than means. Even when utility should predominate - when, that is, the stakes are very high - it still should be qualified by equality as one of the desirable ends to be maximally realised in the long run. Utility is not an isolated self-sufficient moral principle: rather, it is an aspect of an internally inter-related and developing field of evaluative and other concepts. Since this is so, it cannot - especially in abstract isolation - be granted general moral priority over equality.

(c) **Meritocracy**

It may be urged that our AIDS patients be treated meritocratically; that the ten most meritorious, the ten most deserving of them, be selected for survival. Now, deserts or merits may take many different forms. We can speak of an individual's merits in the sense of his potential or capacity for contributing to social well-being, to human betterment or to his own development in moral, creative and intellectual dimensions, to self-realisation. These individual capacities can be treated as <u>forward looking</u> merits. Alternatively, we can speak of <u>backward-looking</u> merits, an individual's past achievements in moral, creative and intellectual dimensions, or even his original or past potential for such achievements. And we can speak separably of an individual's moral merit, his intellectual merit, his merits in all sorts of creative and semi-creative activities and roles - as, for instance, motor mechanic, farmer, parent or political strategist. With so many forms of merit to choose from, even if we decided that our AIDS patients should be treated meritocratically, we would still face the problem of determining which forms of merit are relevant, and their proper priority, in this situation.

However, a prior question is whether, given so many possible forms of merit, it even makes sense to speak generally of treating people meritocratically; whether any general distinction can be drawn between treating people on their merits and treating people according to their needs and interests. We believe that it is possible to draw such a general distinction, and that it is an important one. We shall attempt to draw it via two related points.

(1) To speak of an individual's merits is to speak (implicitly) comparatively. It is to rank him not only in terms of some standard of human worth, but also <u>in comparative relation to his fellows: against his fellows</u>. Thus to treat persons on their merits, is to treat them proportionately to the <u>differences</u> between them and others in respect of merit. Assessment of merit (whatever sort of merit) is essentially a matter of differentiating between individuals. So treating people on their merits is essentially a matter of handing out differential rewards, and differences in merit can always be found between any two individuals, since merit, like length is infinitely divisible. Meritocratic treatment, then, is necessarily inegalitarian, necessarily a matter of discriminative distribution of satisfactions and frustrations. Treating people according to their interests on the other hand, is necessarily egalitarian; people can and do have similar general interests (e.g. pursuit of truth, love, happiness, security, health), and then this principle requires that these interests equally be satisfied, whereas the merit principle would require that these interests be satisfied proportionately to the comparative ranking of the individuals concerned on some scale of worth.

(2) To speak of an individual's merits is to consider him/her non-socially, individualistically, as a concrete individual in a particular place with empirically given achievements and capacities as of a particular time. It is to judge an individual, comparatively, on the basis of what is peculiar to him, on the basis of what characterises him/her as that individual - it is not to

consider the social dynamics of his/her situation, the social possibilities, the possibilities of social development by this individual. To speak of an individual's interests, on the other hand, is to consider him/her not just as he/she now is, but as the individual he/she might and should become: it is to consider him/her socially, in the light of how social action and changing social conditions can develop him/her; it is to consider him/her has a member of humanity, in the light of the general capacities and potential of human kind; it is to consider him/her dynamically as a developing social being, not statically as the individual he/she now is. Thus, to treat people according to their interests is to attempt to provide for them the conditions for self-development, for change beyond the confines of their individuality as it now, statically is. By contrast, to treat people according to their merits, or according to their desserts, is to reward or punish them proportionately to the state of development, they, as individuals ranked against other individuals, have presently reached.

Looking again at our AIDS patients, to treat them meritocratically would be to rank them on some scale of merit, and then to select the ten most meritorious of them for survival, i.e. to treat of their interests as far as possible in proportion to their merits. To treat them in this way whatever form(s) of merit are used, would, we believe, be wrong. There are a number of arguments that can be offered in support of this contention.

First, it seems that the basic nature of morality as a concern for all people's interests as ends in their own right must preclude (as far as possible) the deliberate frustration of some people's basic needs, i.e. the conditions of their continued survival, simply on the basis of their merits. We could not claim to be treating persons as ends unless we allowed them all, equally (as far as possible) the conditions for continued survival. However, the best we can achieve with this argument, is to establish the priority of equality over merit in the area of basic needs.

Second, it may reasonably be argued that people should not have their interests deliberately frustrated on the basis at least of those individual merits for which they are not, at least for the most part responsible, which are not outcomes of their own unconstrained choice and effort (intellectual ability, creative ability etc.) In the area of criminal punishment, it may be urged, we do not and should not punish everyone equally for one man's crime, nor should we punish randomly; rather, we should punish only those who are morally responsible for crimes. Our AIDS patients, however, we assume cannot be held morally responsible for their disease, nor for the social burden of curing them - hence it can be concluded, none of them should be "punished" via the device of treating them meritocratically.

Third, and most importantly, there is a general line of argument for the moral priority, in general, of equality over merit where the satisfaction of human interests is significantly at stake. At the outset it must be admitted that the principle of treating people on their merits is a moral principle albeit one generally subordinate to equality. It does have its proper applications - e.g., in the selection of competitive football teams (although thorough-going Socialists might well want to question the moral worth of such sports). It also seems that in many cases, merit considerations would clearly override egalitarian concerns - for example where one patient's life and contribution to society is greatly needed, so much so, that not to save his/her life would significantly frustrate the interests of a great many people, and make their lives much poorer. Of course here, careful weighing of the respective costs and benefits must be given for each specific case, so once more it is difficult to be more precise than we were previously with respect to related issue arising from the principles of utilitarianism: benefits must be <u>very great</u>. Granted this point, we also point out, that this style of counter-example does not tell against our principles of equality, since it seems here that an explicit appeal is being made to the satisfaction of the interests of a large number of people.

To put this point perhaps more clearly, whilst we grant that to treat people on their individual merits is not in itself a way of treating them as means purely to others' satisfaction and consequently remains one way of treating them as ends in their own right, we maintain that to treat any class of people meritocratically is <u>necessarily</u> to frustrate some relative to others, for it is to discriminate between people in respect of interest satisfactions on the basis of their individual merits. Treating people on their merits, then, essentially involves at least the relative frustrations of some individual's interests. Equality on the other hand, does not <u>necessarily</u> require the relative frustration of the interests of any individual. Now, as we have already argued, the basic principle of evaluative reasoning (qua human ethics, ignoring ecological considerations <u>in this context</u>) is simply this: the satisfaction of human interests as such is good, and the frustration of human interests as such is bad. We must, therefore conceive the objective of morality as being the promotion (under the above qualification), universally, of the satisfaction of human interests. Thus the merit principle, insofar as it essentially involves some frustration of human interests, contradicts, to that extent, the very point of morality as we view it. This does not mean that it cannot be a moral principle at all, but it does imply that in general, merit must be suborindate to equality as a moral principle.

(d) **Rawls' Justice as Fairness**

John Rawls' influential book <u>A Theory of Justice</u> was written to supply a superior moral theory to utilitarianism. Rawls also took his theory to provide a concise set of principles of justice which both underlie and explain the reasoned moral judgements of social life - a condition which he felt utilitarianism was unable to meet. In summary the principles of justice which Rawls offers to us are as follows: [34]

(1) The principle of greatest equal liberty: the principle that each person should have an equal right to the most extensive system of basic liberties, compatible with a similar system of liberty for all;

(2) The principle of equality of fair opportunity: offices and positions are open to all persons under conditions of equality of fair opportunity. This is to say that persons with similar abilities and skills are to have equal access to offices and positions;

(3) The difference principle: social and economic institutions are to be arranged so as to benefit maximally the worse off.

Principles (1), (2) and (3) are ranked in terms of <u>lexical priority</u>, that is, (1) is lexically prior to (2) and (2) is lexically prior to (3), but (3) is <u>not</u> lexically prior to (1). To say that principle (1) is lexically prior to principle (2) is to say that the conditions of (1) must be satisfied before the conditions of (2) are satisfied. Hence in situations where these principles conflict decision making is made by reference to the lexical priority ranking. These principles specify the basic conditions for the just distribution of <u>primary goods</u> or goods every rational person wants because of their important use in any rational life plan. Principle (1) regulates the distribution of basic liberties such as freedom of speech, freedom of conscience, freedom of political participation and so on; principle (2) regulates the distribution of power and authority and principle (3) regulates the distribution of the other primary goods such as wealth and income.

Rawls does not include any right to health care among his principles of justice. Nevertheless a Rawlsian could argue with some plausibility that health care is a primary good covered by the difference principle because it is only rational to want to care for one's health. Rawls' theory is concerned with macrosocial questions of justice of distribution regulating the basic structure of society as a whole, so caution must be taken in mechanically applying his principles of justice at the microsocial level - in for example the case of our problem of the distribution of scarce medical resources. If we suppose that the Difference Principle is directly applicable to our AIDS patients, then we must claim that the primary good of health care is to be distributed so as to maximally benefit the worse off. In other words give access to AZT to those patients that need it the most. Unfortunately we had assumed that *all* of the AIDS patients were *equally* ill. Therefore a decision based upon the Difference Principle cannot be made.

We should not be surprised to find that Rawls Difference Principle does not aid us in solving our target problem of the allocation of scarce medical resources. For Rawls the rightness or wrongness of particular actions or decisions is dependent upon the nature of the entire institutional structure of society, and is not the other way around. Hence whilst it has been necessary to discuss Rawls' theory here for the sake of completeness, our discusson has led us to a dead end. Unfortunately, the same conclusion can also be drawn, as we shall see, about the applicability of Nozick's Libertarian Theory to our target problem.

Before passing onto a discussion of Nozick's position, we wish to point out the relationship between our own theory of justice and Rawls' and why we do not feel that a point-by-point critique of *A Theory of Justice* is in order here. First, if we are right in our argument that social equality is a fundamental social value, and that freedom or liberty and equality are essentially linked so that having an equal right to the most extensive system of basic liberties is only possible in an egalitarian society, then Rawls' position collapses into our own. In other words, radical egalitarianism can account for and justify all three of Rawls' principles of justice, in an explanatory unified and parsimonious fashion without making use of any lexical priority principle at all. The principle of greatest equal liberty and principle of equality of fair opportunity follow immediately from the position of radical egalitarianism because liberty and fair opportunity can be considered the objects of human interests, important objects which satisfy interests and add to a flourishing life. On the radical egalitarian position the Difference Principle is given an almost trivial justification. If it is the case that society consists of a group or class of persons that are worse off than other groups in terms of the basic goods of life, then that society is simply not a radical egalitarian society. For social and economic institutions to be arranged so as to benefit maximally the worse off, means for the radical egalitarian, that society must be changed so that these very class differences themselves are eliminated. John Rawls though interprets the difference principle to mean that economic inequalities are just, if they make the worst-off people better off then they would be under any alternative scheme. Now we cannot see and nor would any other fair mind see that societies with the massive socio-economic inequalities that presently characterize western capitalist nations can seriously be described as just even if they do make the worst-off people at least slightly better off in real income terms than they would be under any available alternatives. Large inequalities morally distort entire societies. They become societies of envy and hatred, of polarization and alienation, rather than co-operation and solidarity. In unequal societies the wealthier classes set the standards of desirable, mainstream life. The poorer classes usually cannot afford to meet these standards, so they tend to be excluded from the mainstream of social life. They become fringe dwellers of an affluent society. Production is skewed towards the demands of the rich. For instance, the Western capitalist nations notoriously have huge public housing problems, because their building industries prefer the profitable business of erecting expensive condominiums and office towers to the provision of cheap good quality houses for the poor. Life at the bottom of an unequal society is qualitatively impoverished to a degree not redeemable by the possession of a few more consumer goods than would be available in more egalitarian circumstances.

In any case, it is not true that the present unfettering of acquisitiveness is making the poorer people better-off. The living standards of the bottom people throughout the West are falling. In Australia, Professor Ronald Henderson (who headed the National Income Inquiry in the 1970s) has estimated that the proportion of people living in poverty has doubled between 1975 and 1987, from 8% to 16%. In the United States, the share of total income of the bottom fifth of American families declined from 5.6% to 4.7% between 1959 and 1984. In the same time the share of the top fifth rose from 40.6% to 42.9%. The decline at the bottom does not look like very much; but in fact it amounts to a loss of one-sixth of the tiny share this group previously had. It's just not credible that the worsening conditions of the poor could not be improved by increased public welfare spending, and the consequent restricting of the freedom to amass personal weatlh.

(e) **Nozick's Libertarian Theory**

Robert Nozick in <u>Anarchy, State and Utopia</u> [35] has produced a widely discussed and frequently criticised defense of Libertarianism. The basic elements of his position can also be concisely summarised. Central to his position is the fundamentality of the right to private property. Individuals have a property right in their persons and through that which they come to hold in accordance with two principles:

(1) the principle of justice in (initial) acquisition;

(2) the principle of justice in transfer.

According to principle (1) a person may come to justly own a previously unowned thing without violating anyone else's ownership rights provided that it is <u>justly acquired</u>. An item is justly acquired providing the unowned item has been "mixed with one's labour" or improved by one's work. This is largely the account of ownership presented by John Locke (the 'Lockean Proviso'). In acquiring such items the conditions of others should not be made worse by creating a situation where they can no longer freely use what they previously could, or if one's appropriation does result in this, then adequate compensation is provided.

Once one has justly acquired a holding it may be justly transferred by sale, trade, bequest or even gift. A person is in other words, morally justified in having the exclusive control over private property obtained through a just initial acquisition subject to the Lockean Proviso, and he/she is justified in transferring this property to any person of his/her choosing. The principle of justice in initial acquisition specifies the justified ways of acquiring private property, whilst the principle of justice in transfer specifies the justified ways of distributing private property.

Nozick's theory is essentially concerned with prevention of violations of Libertarian rights. These rights are basically rights against interferences rather than rights for something. Indeed the idea of any right to health care, let alone equal rights to health care, is a fundamentally unjustified right. The consistent Libertarian will maintain that no one has a right to health care (which they have not acquired in accordance with the 'Lockean Proviso') and neither may anyone be rightly forced to help any of our AIDS patients. A Libertarian may feel pity for such patients and may because of social conditioning wish to help them, but there is no moral reason for offering aid. Questions of the maximisation of utility and the conditions for the freedom, happiness and flourishing of people are irrelevant questions as far as the issue of justice is concerned, the Libertarian maintains.

What can be said about the satisfactions of this solution to our target problem of the allocation of scarce medical resources? In our opinion Nozick's position is so highly counter-intuitive that the above consequence constitutes a <u>reductio ad absurdum</u> of the theory. This consequence follows because Nozick nowhere provides any satisfactory rational justification for his basic Lockean rights principles, and as far as we are concerned, being radical egalitarians and critics of the institution of private property itself, we are by no means willing to allow Nozick the unargued assumptions upon which his entire theory is based. In our opinion the idea of accepting as an article of faith the fundamentality of the right to private property is a fundamental error. This logical generosity is nowhere found in other areas of philosophy, such as epistemology, and we see no reason for allowing it to occur in ethics. Further, after the lengthy critique of privacy claims, seen in the last chapter, we conclude that there is no satisfactory rational justification for the institution of private property itself. Unlike our assessment of Rawls, we can see no merit in Nozick's position at all as an aid in understanding our target problem.

In conclusion, after examining a number of competing theories of justice, we conclude that radical egalitarianism presents the most satisfactory response which we know to the problem of the allocation of scarce medical resources.

6. CONCLUSION: AIDS, Egalitarianism and the Need for Revolution in Health Care

We wish to now make another point about the relationship between egalitarian principles and health care in the context of discussing Charles Fried's paper "Equality and Rights in Medical Care". [36] Fried argues that any right to health care does not imply a right to equal access, a right that whatever is available should be available to all. Indeed, equal access to health care is a "dangerous slogan" which could only be realised by "intolerable government controls of medical practice or a thoroughly unreasonable burden of expense". [37] One of Fried's arguments involves the case of the future development of an artificial heart. He says:

> "...if the right to health care is taken to mean the right to whatever health care is available to anybody, and if this entails that it is a right to an equal enjoyment of whatever care anyone else enjoys, then what are we to do with respect to the artificial heart? Might we decide not to develop such a device? Though the development and experimental use of it involves an entirely tolerable burden, the general provision of the artificial heart would be an intolerable burden, and since if we must provide it to any we must provide it to all, therefore perhaps we should provide it to none". [38]

Fried is not putting forward a callous defense of the rich, rather as he in fact says, he is making the analytical point that to insist upon a right to equal access to health care without a general social commitment to equality is highly problematic. [39] As he says, if American society tolerates inequalities in wealth and income, it is anomalous to single out health care as a sphere where equal access should reign. [40] In this chapter we have turned this proposition on its head, by first arguing for the general philosophical acceptability of radical egalitarianism, and <u>then</u> arguing for egalitarianism in health care with respect to the allocation of scarce medical resources. In short then, we see the task of justifying a radical egalitarian approach to justice in health care as a part of the larger task of the justification of radical egalitarianism as a general principle of distributive justice for modern society.

It is a consequence of the radical egalitarian position on social justice, that a society where 60 percent of its wealth is owned by 10 percent of the population (a third of these assets belonging to the richest 1 percent) is a moral obscenity. It is our view that an egalitarian society which socializes and rationalizes wealth, so that the areas most needing funding and constitutive of general human social interests such as health care, housing and education is an infinitely better society than our present one. Western governments today, and increasingly intellectuals who have long abandoned the Socratic idealism of their youth have joined with business in an unprecedented celebration of acquisitiveness and greed. The new-breed conservative governments of the West are busy creating 'entrepreneurial cultures', perhaps to be housed in a Japanese backed multifunctional polis, unshackling market forces, backing wealth creation by private accumulators, privatizing industries and starving public sectors of the economy.

This exclusive preoccupation with money for money's sake cannot sanely figure as an important value in social life. For healthy people, money is merely the means that enables worthwile activities to take place - producing things, providing services, helping people, developing skills and knowledge. Yet many big players in today's business scene seem to have forgotten that there is any point to life besides money itself. They do not any longer simply invest in factories and machines that produce things, for that is not profitable enough; instead they reach for enormous profits through the trading of financial assets, through merger and takeover artistry, and through the playing of equity and futures markets.

The more serious objection to the drive for personal wealth concerns social justice. The desire to become rich is a desire for a superior position in an order of economic and social inequality. It is in effect a desire for social injustice. The fourth century Archbishop of Milan, Ambrose, stated this criticism more eloquently than modern left-wing economists can, with torrents of statistics from their ever-ready computers. "Think you", he inveighed, "that you commit no injustice by keeping to yourself alone what would be the means of life of many? It is the bread of the hungry you cling to; it is the clothing of the naked you lock up; the money you bury is the redemption of the poor".

We have already given reasons, in our discussion of John Rawls, to believe that the poorer classes are not better off in the present new conservative entrepreneurial culture than they would be if there were less emphasis on the amassing of personal riches, and more social appropriations of wealth.

Those Western governments (including Australia's) that are applauding and encouraging private acquisitiveness, and attempting to create a social climate in which it will flourish, are making all of us worse off. They are destroying the public life, the public cultures, the public resources of their nations. They are cutting back public expenditure, privatising public institutions, or else trying to turn them into commercial or semi-commercial enterprises - all in order to provide more room for private enterprise, more opportunities for private wealth accumulation.

The whole range of public services and institutions is becoming atrophied - health services, schools and universities, public transport services, public utilities, environmental pollution and conservation agencies, welfare organizations, public broadcasting services. Our governments are exacerbating the sort of situation that J.K. Galbraith once described as 'private affluence, public squalor'. The sphere of State-sponsored and taxpayer-subsidized public activity, of work for public benefit rather than profit, is diminishing. The voices of responsibility for society as a whole are being silenced. We are all being sucked into the maelstrom of commercial brawling. The result will be ramshackled public institutions, derisory educational and cultural standards, increasing poverty, and the neglect of society-wide problems - in short, the impoverishment of public life.

It is the thousands of people who work for the ideals of public service rather than profit, in governmental and other non-profit organisations, who are the expression of social concern and the bearers of the public interest. They, at least sometimes, respond to people's needs rather than their money. They should be supported and encouraged; not starved of funds and excoriated as unproductive waste. It is a tragedy that, for example, in Britain the National Health Service (NHS) is being so financially squeezed that it cannot adequately meet the demands made on it. For it is the institutional expression of the moral right of sick people to high quality health care regardless of means.

Another important dimension to the question of the justice of personal wealth is the international context. We now live in an economically interconnected world; where the economies of the richer nations are structurally linked with, and often adversely affect, those of the less developed countries. Throughout this world there are millions of starving or chronically undernourished people. and many more of those lives are blighted by a desperate day-to-day struggle for survival. In fact, 35,000 people die from starvation every day. In these circumstances the possession of immense personal wealth is simply a moral obscenity. All the inhabitants of the richer nations have some share in this obscenity - especially when, as camera-laden tourists clad in designer jeans, they step over the bodies of the dying in the streets of Bombay or the villages of central Africa. There is, however, something particularly insensitive and obnoxious about people who devote their whole lives to becoming rich through such activities as merchant banking, advertising, real estate speculation and stock market manipulation.

The market is a morally defective mechanism. [41] It is an efficient mechanism for distributing scarce resources among rival claimants; but its efficiency derives from the fact that it recognises only one type of claim - wealth. This is why the market will cater to every whim of the rich, while neglecting the needs of the poor. This is why the world contains Hilton hotels with every imaginable luxury, overlooking squalid slums where people suffer from malnutrition. Captialism is basically unjust.

Our point is really an old and fairly familiar one; that <u>laissez-faire</u> capitalism causes serious moral distortions. The present emphasis on the freeing of market forces, and on giving the acquisitive drive its head, is a large step backwards. Capitalism must be moderated by social interventions in the public interest, and by significant levels of social appropriation and redistribution of wealth. Social intervention in the operation of advanced market economies is morally essential. There is no "Invisible Hand" that automatically translates private acquisitiveness and greed into public benefits and social justice. High levels of government spending, and of taxation, are not marks of declining societies, they are, rather, some of the few hallmarks of civilization and social responsibility that are possible in the capitalist world.

All of these points, and many more are advanced and discussed in detail by Ted Trainer in <u>Abandon Affluence!</u> [42] - especially with respect to Third World poverty. It will be appropriate to explore these ideas in more detail in the final chapter of this book where it will be argued that to deal with growing environmental crisis a radical restructuring of not only individual nations, but of global economic and political relationships. AIDS is a very important part of a matrix of problems that threaten the health, and indeed, the very possibility of long term survival of the human species itself.

Anticipating the growing crisis AIDS presents to health care funding, noting that the spirit of the times is towards economic rationalization, utilitarianism and the cult of entrepreneurism, but recognizing that there is to some degree a "seesaw" in history [43] our aim here has been to describe (albeit briefly) the principles of social justice that will ultimately have to be adopted if society is to remain to any degree just and humane.

NOTES AND REFERENCES

1. J. Fletcher, "Ethics and Health Care Delivery: Computers and Distributive Justice", in R.M. Veatch and R. Branson (eds.), Ethics and Health Policy, (Ballinger Publishing Co., Cambridge, 1976), pp. 99-109. Citation p.102.

2. P. Ramsey, The Patient as Person, (Yale University Press, New Have, 1970), p.268.

3. E.E. Shelp (ed.), Justice and Health Care, (D. Reidel, Dordrecht, 1981).

4. On egalitarianism in health care cf. G. Outka, "Social Justice and Equal Access to Health Care", Journal of Religious Ethics, Vol. 2, 1974, pp. 11-32 and R.M. Veatch, "What is 'Just' Health Care Delivery?", in R.M. Veatch and R. Branson (eds.), Ethics and Health Policy, op.cit., Note 1, pp. 127-153.

5. D. O'Reilly, "Retreat Australia Fair", The Bulletin, April 25, 1989, pp. 52-58, 60.

6. T. Sykes, "How Free Trade Damages Australia", Australian Business, March 15, 1989, pp. 42-44.

7. cf. H.E. Daly (ed.), Economics, Ecology, Ethics: Essays Towards A Steady - State Economy, (W.H. Freeman and Company, San Francisco, 1980).

8. T. Trainer, "What Ails Australia: The Alternative View", Social Alternatives, Vol. 6, 1987, pp. 17-20. Trainer sums up the economic situation of Australia (and according to the talks given in Australia by David Suzuki 1987 and 1989, Canada as well) with penetrating truth and clarity:

> "Giving market forces free reign is the surest ticket to banana republic status for Australia. Consider our trade and industry situation. Over the last ten years we have allowed market forces to cut our manufacturing capacity in half, to shift it to South East Asia where the wage rate is one-tenth as high. Previously we allowed market forces to build us into dependency on mineral and agricultural exports, and now their prices have dropped. We have a massive trade deficit national debt largely because we have to import lots of things we could be producing for ourselves, and once did. Not so long ago nations only traded surpluses; now we all have been drawn into trading necessities, which means that when the global economy doesn't want your bananas or wheat you have had it. Now we must

frantically search for the 'sunrise' industries that might enable us to earn the export income necessary to go on buying all the things we could be making for ourselves had we developed the right industries... In other words, the only recipe conventional economics has, is for us to compete more fiercely in the global market to win back some sales of something, anything. But even if we succeed, this just means that other people in other countries lose those sales. We are all locked into a zero - sum game where salvation for Australians can only come at the expense of damnation for others.

9. Opinion poll quoted by O'Reilly, op.cit. Note 5, p.53.

10. ibid, p.55.

11. B. Hailstone, "QVH Moving Babies to Cut Costs", The Advertiser, (Adelaide), Tuesday April 18, 1989, p.9.

12. "Hospital 'will take months' to Recover", The Advertiser (Adelaide) Thursday, May 11, 1989, p.1.

13. B.M. Whyte (ed al), "The Costs of Hospital-Based Medical Care for Patients with the Acquired Immunodeficiency Syndrome", Medical Journal of Australia, Vol. 147, September 21, 1987, pp. 269-272.

14. ibid, p.272.

15. "Each AIDS Patient 'costing us $1m'", News (Adelaide), Thursday November 17, 1988, p.25.

16. A. Scitovsky and D. Rice, "Estimates of the Direct and Indirect Costs of Acquired Immunodeficiency Syndrome in the United States, 1985, 1986, and 1991", Public Health Rep. Vol. 102 (1), 1987, pp. 5-17; R.J. Buchanan, "State Medicaid Coverage of AZT and AIDS - Related Policies", American Journal of Public Health, Vol. 78, 1988, pp. 432-436.

17. K. Donald, "Priorities in Allocation of Resources for AIDS Programs", in A. Carr (ed.) Meeting the Challenge: Papers of the First National Conference on AIDS, (Australian Government Publishing Service, Canberra, 1986), pp. 72-74. Citation p. 73.

18. Department of Community Services and Health, Living with AIDS Toward the Year 2000: Report of the 3rd National Conference on AIDS, (Australian Government Publishing Service, Canberra, 1988).

19. P.R. Lee, "AIDS: Allocating Resources for Research and Patient Care", <u>Issues in Science and Technology</u>, Winter 1986, pp. 66-73. Citation p. 73.

20. J.M. Mann, "AIDS": A Global Strategy for a Global Challenge", <u>Impact of Science on Society</u>, Vol. 38, 1988, pp. 159-170.

21. H. Bedau, "Radical Egalitarianism", in H. Bedau (ed.) <u>Justice and Equality</u>, (Prentice Hall Inc., Englewood Cliffs, New Jersey, 1971), pp. 168-180. Citation p. 168.

For a detailed discussion of the socio-political ramifications of the ideal of equality cf. B.S. Turner, <u>Equality</u>, (Tavistock Publishers, London, 1986) and M. Walzer, <u>Spheres of Justice: A Defense of Pluralism and Equality</u>, (Basic Books, New York, 1983).

Walzer's view is that no person should be dominant in one sphere of human good such as wealth, because of dominance in some other sphere, such as political power : "... personal qualities and social goods have their own spheres of operation where they work their effects freely, spontaneously, and legitimately". (p.19) More revealing Walzer says:

> "To convert one good into another, when there is no intrinsic connection between the two, is to invade the sphere where another company of men and women properly rule. Monopoly is not inappropriate within the spheres. There is nothing wrong, for example, with the grip that persuasive and powerful men and women (politicians) establish on political power. But the use of political power to gain access to other goods is a tyrannical use ... In political life - but more widely, too - the dominance of goods makes for the dominance of people" (p.19).

The problem with Walzer's form of egalitarianism is that it is highly doubtful whether the spheres of goods are distinct. Fame and wealth tend to go hand-in-hand as do social influence and wealth. Even if they did not, if Walzer really believes that "the dominance of goods makes for the dominance of people", then there is no good reason to allow dominance within one sphere. That is to say, the sort of argument used by Walzer to reject the morality of dominance of more then one sphere, can with only a little imagination be applied to the dominance of one sphere. If the radical egalitarian position argued here is correct, then Walzer's position is demonstrably inadequate. cf. also M.W. Howard, "Walzer's Socialism", <u>Social Theory and Practice</u>, Vol. 12, 1986, pp. 103-113.

22. I. Berlin, "Equality", <u>Proceedings of the Aristotelian Society</u>, Vol. LVI, 1955-56, pp. 301-326, Citation p. 311.

23. S.I. Benn, "Egalitarianism and the Equal Consideration of Interests", in H. Bedau (ed.) <u>Justice and Equality</u>, op.cit., Note 21, pp. 152-167, Citation p.157.

24. J.R. Lucas, "Against Equality", in H. Bedau (ed.) <u>Justice and Equality</u>, op.cit., Note 21, pp. 138-151, Citation p. 142; A. Weale, "An Anti-Egalitarian Fallacy", <u>Philosophy</u>, Vol. 52, 1977, pp. 352-354.

25. H.J. McCloskey, "Egalitarianism, Equality and Justice", <u>Australasian Journal of Philosophy</u>, Vol. 44, 1966, pp. 50-69, Citation p. 58.

26. An exception to this is the work of Kai Nielsen, c.f. "Marx, Marxism and Egalitarianism", <u>Ratio</u>, Vol. 28, 1986, pp. 56-68, "Class and Justice", in J. Arthur and W. Shaw (eds.) <u>Justice and Economic Distribution</u>, (Prentice Hall Inc., Englewood Cliffs, New Jersey, 1979), pp. 225-245; "On the Very Possibility of a Classless Society":, <u>Political Theory</u>, Vol. 6, 1978, pp. 191-207; "Radical Egalitarian Justice: Justice as Equality", <u>Social Theory and Practice</u>, Vol. 5, 1979, pp. 207-226; "Impediments to Radical Egalitarianism", <u>American Philosophical Quarterly</u>, Vol. 18, 1981, pp. 121-129.

Other articles of interest on egalitarianism include H. Frankfurt, "Equality as a Moral Ideal", <u>Ethics</u>, Vol. 98, 1987, pp. 21-43; A. Levine, "Towards a Marxian Theory of Justice", <u>Politics and Society</u>, Vol. 11, 1982, pp. 343-362; T. Honderich, "The Question of Well-being and the Principle of Equality", <u>Mind</u>, Vol. XC, 1981, pp. 481-504; F.E. Oppenheim," Egalitarian Rules of Distribution", <u>Ethics</u>, Vol. 90, 1980, pp. 164-179; E. Gellner, "The Social Roots of Egalitarianism", <u>Dialectics and Humanism</u>, Vol. 6, 1979, pp. 27-43; J. Raz, "Principles of Equality", <u>Mind</u>, Vol. 87, 1978, pp. 321-342; T. Nagel, "The Justification of Equality", <u>Critica</u>, Vol. 10, 1978, pp. 3-27; C. Ake, "Justice as Equality", <u>Philosophy and Public Affairs</u>, Vol. 5, 1975, pp. 69-89.

27. K. Marx, "Critique of the Gotha Programme", in K. Marx, F. Engels and V. Lenin, <u>On Historical Materialism: A Collection</u>, (Progress Publishers, Moscow, 1976), pp. 159-173. Citation p.165.

28. Berlin, op.cit., Note 22, p. 306.

29. cf. Benn op.cit., Note 23 and D. Locke, "The Principle of Equal Interests", *Philosophical Review*, Vol. XC, 1981, pp. 531-559. In this context cf. also B.M. Landesman, "Egalitarianism", *Canadian Journal of Philosophy*, Vol. 13, pp. 27-56.

30. B. Williams, "The idea of Equality", in Bedau (ed.) *Justice and Equality*, op.cit., Note 21, pp. 116-137. Citation pp. 130-131.

31. We consider here a more difficult statement of the problem of priorities in the allocation of scarce medical resources than that considered by K.M. Boyd and B.T. Potter, "Priorities in the Allocation of Scarce Resources", *Journal of Medical Ethics*, Vol. 12, 1986, pp. 197-200 and most other writers.

32. cf. N. Rescher, "The Allocation of Exotic Medical Lifesaving Therapy", *Ethics*, Vol. 79, 1969, pp. 173-186 (Rescher advocates the use of random selection only after utilitarian and other judgements have been made); R. Young, "Some Criteria for Making Decisions Concerning the Distribution of Scarce Medical Resources", *Theory and Decision*, Vol. 6, 1975, pp. 439-455; J.F. Childress, "Who Shall Live When Not all Can Live?" in T.A. Shannon (ed.) *Bioethics*, (Paulist Press, New Jersey, 1981), pp. 501-515.

33. P. Spicker, "Why Freedom Implies Equality", *Journal of Applied Philosophy*, Vol. 2, 1985, pp. 205-216; J. Exdell, "Liberty, Equality and Capitalism", *Canadian Journal of Philosophy*, Vol. 11, 1981, pp. 457-471.

34. J. Rawls, *A Theory of Justice*, (Harvard University Press, Cambridge, 1971); N. Daniels (ed.) *Reading Rawls*, (Basic Books, New York, 1975).

35. R. Nozick, *Anarchy, State and Utopia*, (Basic Books, New York, 1974).

36. C. Fried, "Equality and Rights in Medical Care", in T.L. Beauchamp and L. Waters (eds.) *Contemporary Issues in Bioethics*, 2nd edition, (Wadsworth Publishing Company, California, 1982), pp. 395-401.

37. ibid, p. 395.

38. ibid, p. 395.

39. ibid, p. 398.

40. ibid, p. 399. The radical egalitarian position with respect to the problem of the allocation of scarce

medical resources holds that human life (at least) is priceless. This means in medical contexts (ignoring ecological considerations) only human lives can be balanced and traded against other lives, that no amount of money and goods and services could equal the value of a human life, including an infinite amount of money and goods and services. This is to say that human life is of <u>primary</u> value or intrinsic value, whilst the value of goods and services is only of <u>secondary</u> value, having value only because of the existence of primary valuers. The value of a human life is <u>incommensurable</u> with the value of goods and services. Social radicals who speak of "people before profits" would seem to presuppose precisely this sort of moral principle to justify their criticisms of the status quo. Ecologically sensitive people may say that ecosystems, animal and plant life are priceless in the same sense of not being able to be replaced by something else as its equivalent, but here let us restrict our attention to human beings. It does not logically follow from the doctrine of the pricelessness of life that all lives are of equal value. All the doctrine entails is that human lives in general can't be morally weighed up against, and traded against bundles of goods and services.

Michael Bayles ("The Price of Life", <u>Ethics</u>, Vol. 29, 1978, pp. 20-34) has argued that it is both rational and morally permissable to place a price on one's own life and that there is a method of using this price to determining various social policies. Bayles believes that whilst it does not prove that morally human life has a price, there is strong evidence to show that society does price human lives. In building skyscrapers for example, it is common knowledge that few if any skyscrapers are built without the loss of life of some construction workers and these workers are given danger money because they are engaged in a hazardous occupation. Isn't this placing a price upon human life: we choose to have skyscrapers and cars which are far less than being totally safe, knowing full well that some innocent people will die? How can this be justified if human life is priceless? Perhaps this shows that human life is not priceless.

Some writers such as Morton Kaplan ("What is a Life Worth"? <u>Ethics</u>, Vol. 89, 1978, pp. 58-65) feel that all these considerations show is a pricing of statistical risks. In a discussion of the skyscraper example Kaplan points out that if a worker does get his foot caught in a rope and dangles precariously from a girder, attempts are made to save his life. This shows, Kaplan believes that the building of a skyscraper is not traded against the lives of construction workers at all. To vary the example, a platoon of soldiers may be sent to rescue an encircled few soldiers, even though up to a certain vaguely defined threshold, more lives may be lost than if the encircled soldiers were left to die. The reason for this Kaplan describes as follows:

> "These situations symbolize the obligations that we think bind all men to each other within a moral community and they emphasize the features that define us as human beings with a claim upon one another that transcends the instrumental. The dramatic juncture affects the social reinforcement process in the absence of which our immediate conflicts of interest inevitably would drive us into isolation. Damage at this symbolic level bleeds out into the larger symbolic patterns of society, which are connected in webs in which the meaning of the elements depends on the characteristics of their neighbourhood and not on deductive chains in which the elements, such as a particular death, have fixed values independently of their placement in context". (p.60)

Another way of dealing with Bayles' example of the skyscraper is to bite the bullet and claim that skyscraper construction should be made as safe as is technically possible, even though it is unrealistic to demand absolute safety. It is unreasonable to demand absolute safety because no product, including a lead pencil, is absolutely safe - it is possible that one may prick oneself with the pencil and die of poisoning. We are not pricing human life if we do all that is practically and technically possible to minimize risks to people in the workplace.

Examples of the pricing of life also occur in medical contexts, Bayles points out. He claims that if it is permissable to forgo livesaving treatments because of cost, then life has a monetary value. Pricing of live also allegedly occurs in the existence of economic limits on the amount of money to be spent upon lifesaving technologies. An even better example is given by John Harris in his description of the British government's "euthanasia" programme (<u>The Value of Life: An Introduction to Medical Ethics</u>, (Routledge and Kegan Paul, London, 1985, pp. 85-86). Due to cutbacks in health funding people have died who could have lived. The <u>Guardian</u>, a British newspaper, reported on the 6th January 1984 the following description of this problem: "Heart patients at Wythenshawe Hospital, Manchester, who could have been saved by open heart surgery, are dying because of a shortage of nurses and beds, caused by the crisis over hospital funding... Six patients waiting for surgery died within four weeks just before Christmas (ibid, p.85). These sorts of examples, which very easily could be multiplied strongly supports Bayles' view that life is often given a monetary price. Nevertheless these examples do not show that this is a morally good thing. On the contrary, that people who could have led normal lives die because life-saving operations cannot be performed due to lack of funds is evil - especially in a society that seems glad to spend millions on lavish royal weddings.

It may be argued that it may be rational to trade one year of one's life for a vast sum of money, provided one is relatively young and healthy. If a year seems too long, then make the time one day. Live one day less and receive one million dollars. Would you do it? Most people I think would, provided they had no reason to believe that they would die soon. If you do this are you pricing a part of your life? I don't believe that one is.

If life has a price, then life is a commodity and the placing of a monetary value upon it indicates that there are purchasable goods and services of an equivalent value. However, if someone swapped a day of his/her life for a million dollars, it would still be a mistake to therefore say that 1 day of life equals $1 million. The mere fact of the swap does not demonstrate any such equivalence: the same person would probably also swap a day of his/her life for 2 million dollars and upwards as well. But what then is the price of life? It could be anything, even one dollar. A person dying of thirst would surely swap one day of life for five cents, if this could buy a glass of cool water. The swapping argument, if sound, therefore shows that one day of life may have any price at all, depending upon the context. This is totally unlike any other commodity and it is fair to say that if the price of life could be anything, then it is absurd to say that life has a price at all. Finally, the point should be made again that the practice of people pricing their lives no more shows that they are morally permitted to do so, then the fact that slave traders have sold slaves and women have hired their bodies to men for sex, shows respectively that slavery and prostitution are morally justified.

What is the source of the pricelessness of human life? Kenneth Henley, "The Value of Individuals", Philosophy and Phenomenological Research, Vol. 37, 1977, pp. 345-352, has argued that the value of individuals arises because they are irreplaceable. Human individuals are irreplaceable because they are unique. Whilst this is true it doesn't show that individuals are therefore priceless or of any positive value whatsoever. It is not self-contradictory to suppose that individual x is both unique and worthless even though this may be a false claim. Nor does it show that it is incorrect to suppose that something of equivalent or greater value might be exchanged for x (Bayles, op.cit., p.24). My approach to the problem of the source of the pricelessness of human life is entirely different from Henley's approach. Human life is of intrinsic value and of fundamental value, because our goods and services only are of value insofar as they satisfy human interests and enrich human life. The case of swapping a year or a day of life for a quantity of money only has initial plausibility because one feels that the quality rest of one's life would be enriched by this sacrifice. This exchange however only makes sense because we have already given life a prior value irreducible to money. Indeed money only has value because life itself has value: there is simply no more basic value to ground the value of money in. In a society such as contemporary Australia, where the really important decisions are ultimately based upon the recommendations of some narrowly educated evaluatively myopic economists, this is an important lesson to learn.

41. For technical discussions of the limits of market rationality and mainstream economics cf. A. Buchanan, Ethics, Efficiency and the Market, (Clarendon Press, Oxford, 1985), A. Etzione, The Moral Dimension: Towards a New Economics, (Free Press, New York, 1988); for ecological limits of mainstream economics cf. W.R. Catton, Overshoot: The Ecological Basis of Revolutionary Change (University of Illinois Press, Urbana, 1982) and H.E. Daly (ed.), Economics, Ecology, Ethics: Essays Toward a Steady - State Economy, (W.H. Freeman and Co., San Francisco, 1980).

42. F.E. Trainer, Abandon Affluence! (Zed Books, London, 1985).

43. G. Blainey, The Great Seesaw: A New View of the Western World, 1750-2000, (Macmillan, Melbourne, 1988). On AIDS Blainey says "If AIDS should become a devastating cause of death in the last decade of this century, it could dominate one end of the seesaw. Indeed in the short term, it has more potential for terror than the fear which occupies the opposite end of the seesaw, the fear of nuclear war" (p. 308).

7 AIDS, the environmental crisis and beyond: a study of global catastrophes

1. AIDS in the Context of the "Crisis of Civilisation"

    (1) Nuclear Warfare and Nuclear Energy

    (2) The Destruction of Soil and Agricultural Land

    (3) The Destruction of Natural Diversity

    (4) Our Poisonous Planet

2. The Critique of Industrialism, Capitalism, Consumerism and Economic Rationalism : The Limits to Growth and to Economic Rationality

3. Against the Economists : Towards a Moral Economy

4. Towards a Sustainable Future

"... I find myself unable to see anything at the end of the road we are following with such self-assured momentum but Samuel Beckett's two sad tramps forever waiting under that wilted tree for their lives to begin. Except that I think the tree isn't going to be real, but a plastic counterfeit. In fact, even the tramps may turn out to be automatons ... though of course there will be great programmed grins on their faces". [1]

"This age is not utterly insalubrious for philosophy. Our problems are so great and their sources too deep that to understand them we need philosophy more than ever, if we do not despair of it, and it faces the challenges on which it flourishes". [2]

1. AIDS in the Context of the "Crisis of Civilisation"

Most discussions of AIDS have failed to understand the significance of AIDS as both a global and local problem of how AIDS fits into what has been called the "crisis of civilisation" [3] - but fortunately not all discussions are guilty of this. At the Fifth International Conference on AIDS, in the context of the WHO'S claim that 9 times as many adults would develop AIDS during the 1990s than had done during the 1980s, President Kenneth Kaunda of Zambia made a plea to the superpowers to abandon nuclear weapons and devote the saved resources to dealing with AIDS and other diseases. He described AIDS as being like a "soft nuclear bomb" in its effects upon society. [4] Robert Ornstein and Paul Ehrlich in their new controversial book <u>New World New Mind</u> [5] relate the AIDS pandemic to global socio-economic conditions:

"For decades now humanity has been setting itself up as the progressively ideal target for a worldwide epidemic. The combination of rapidly increasing numbers of malnourished people, who live in conditions of poor sanitation and with impure water, with ever-more-rapid transportation systems has been making the human epidemiological environment ever more precarious. We have created a giant, crowded, "monoculture" of human beings, millions of whom are especially vulnerable to disase and among whom carriers can move with unprecedented speed". [6]

Along with this situation there are evolutionary possibilities that only biologists are daring to contemplate:

"It is even therefore conceivable that humanity will sooner or later have to deal with strains of

AIDS that can be transmitted by the bites of arthropods (perhaps by the bites of mosquitos that were interrupted while feeding on someone carrying the virus). Worse yet, a variety of AIDS virus might evolve that can be transmitted by relatively casual, non-sexual physical contact or even by inhaling droplets sneezed into the air. The odds of it happening seem very small, but the consequences if it did occur would be, to say the least, daunting. With millions virtually certain to die in Africa, the possibility that the virus, if uncontrolled, could result in extremely high death rates in the developed countries should not be overlooked". [7]

Although Ornstein and Ehrlich do not go on to argue that above point through, it is quite conceivable that new strains of AIDS, or even more lethal disease entities, may evolve in the twenty first century. According to the neo-Darwinist theory of evolution, the biochemical engine of evolution is mutation, with environmental selection of mutants occurring by the process of natural selection. Mutations are often caused by heat, radiation (natural or man-made) and chemicals. It is precisely these elements which are increasing in quantity in our polluted world. Now if you accept that today's living organisms got here by evolutionary processes, there is no reason at all for believing that evolutionary change has stopped. In an increasingly toxic world it is a very bad bet to suppose that evolutionary change will favour the vitality of the human species over disease organisms. It is well known that in a nuclear war, it is the beetles and insect species which are most likely to survive not humanity; it is also well known that certain strains of bacteria can receive severe damage to their DNA only to immediately begin to repair it. It takes only a modest amount of radiation to kill a human being.

AIDS as a global problem is closely interconnected with other well known environmental problems. Professor Margaret Kripke of the University of Texas hypothesizes that increased doses of ultra-violet (UV) radiation, due to depletion of the ozone layer may weaken the human immune system. It is hypothesized, but not empirically demonstrated, that the progression of AIDS may be hastened in individuals with an active infection. Given the increase in the incidence of skin cancers and eye cataracts expected from increased doses of UV radiation, it is again a safe bet, that human health will not be improved by depletion of the ozone layer (the thesis of <u>biotic impoverishment</u>). [8]

It is the aim of this chapter to move beyond the AIDS epidemic to consideration of the wider global environmental problems threatening human existence. This is not a random change in interest but an important consideration as the above arguments show. Further, writers must now begin to consider AIDS within the context of the "crisis of civilisation" if for no other reason than the fact that any programme dealing with the AIDS problem must compete for limited research resources with programmes dealing with environmental problems. In addition to this, I have argued that an adequate response to AIDS requires social programmes that will involve striking at the heart of the problem, for example dealing first hand with the IV drug problem. This radical argument gains considerable strength placed in the context of the global environmental crisis.

In the Australian context (1989), especially after the results of the Tasmanian election, it is believed that the Green-environmental vote is enough to decide the result of a federal election. [9] Environmental issues reach the cover stories of financial magazines such as <u>Business Review Weekly</u> [10] which talk about business "survival", and editorials in conservative newspapers which speak about human survival and the survival of life on earth itself:

> "The signs have always been there. From primitive stages we have been destroying our resource base. A belief that developed through the ages - humanity's supremacy and ability to solve every problem - helped to obscure this knowledge from us. Indeed, it still does. Many people avoid thinking about the dangers to our common future by believing science, technology or some other human ingenuity will deliver solutions without our having to make serious sacrifices...
>
> The human-centred world view will no longer suffice. Even humanity's survival depends on our making the environment our first concern; the planet we have ravaged is teaching us to broaden our consciousness or pass like dinosaurs to our extinction, along with everything else we value, and many more things to which we failed to assign value until it was too late. [11]

These words could easily have been from Ehrlich, Suzuki, Capra or Illich, as could these words from an article in <u>New Scientist</u>:

> "It is more or less official: much of the activity we call development destroys the topsoil, fresh water, atmospheric systems and genetic resources upon which human progress must be based. It is hard to say just when it became official. Perhaps it happened in London on the night of 3 March, when David Hopper, vice president of the World Bank for policy, planning and research explained how and why the bank often spent large sums to ruin good agricultural land". [12]

It is not the aim of this section to give a comprehensive examination of the savage terrain of the environmental crisis; rather the following is a Cook's tour of the principal trouble spots. [13]

(1) <u>Nuclear Warfare and Nuclear Energy</u>

Whilst there is welcome talk of global <u>perestroika</u>, and widespread belief that the environmental issue will replace the Cold War on the stage of international affairs, the nuclear issue can hardly be dismissed as unimportant. Daniel Ellsberg, by obtaining previous classified information has shown that the Americans have known that they have had a nuclear superiority to the Soviets throughout the 1950s and 1960s. There were apparently explicit nuclear threats made by several American presidents during this period of nuclear superiority which the public never heard of. This is worth reflecting on. Several American presidents, who were elected to supposedly serve the American people and not to function as God-like dictators, had contemplated initiating a nuclear war. The idea of a nuclear first strike means killing milions of people of a nation, mega-genocide. What sane purpose would this serve America if it did destroy the Soviet Union? How can ruling elites contemplate mega-genocide and expect to be able to rule their own people? [14]

Critics have argued that the threat of a new arms race, this time with space based technologies, will be initiated by the Strategic Defense Initiative (SDI). They have argued that at best SDI could protect only nuclear weapons, not people and that it will be perceived by the Soviets as an attempt to achieve U.S. first-strike capability. [15] The Soviets could always add missiles to obtain any former balance, at much less cost than any American space defense - the total U.S. bill could be over $600 billion, and the Soviets could neutralize the system at one tenth of the cost. Economics and sanity suggest that it would be more reasonable for the U.S to use economic means as a method of defense - to attempt to get the USSR economy so dependent upon the U.S economy that any nuclear attack would become an act of economic suicide. This is not the only threat of nuclear warfare as Capra notes (keeping in mind that only 10-20 pounds of plutonium is required to make a bomb, and a nuclear reactor produces 400-500 pounds of plutonium a year):

> "Nuclear technology is now being promoted especially in the Third World. The aim of this promotion is not to satisfy the energy needs of Third World countries, but those of multinational corporations extracting the natural resources from these countries as fast as they can. Politicians in Third World countries often welcome nuclear technology, however, because it gives them a chance to use it for building nuclear weapons. Current American sales of reactor technology abroad

guarantee that by the end of the century dozens of countries will possess enough nuclear material to manufacture bombs of their own, and we can expect those countries not only to acquire the American technology but also to copy the American patterns of behaviour and use their nuclear power to make aggressive threats.

The potential of global destruction through nuclear war is the greatest environmental threat of nuclear power. If we are unable to prevent nuclear war, all other environmental concerns will become purely academic". [16]

Even a limited, but intense nuclear exchange, raises the horrors of nuclear winter and mass starvation. [17]

The fear of misuse constitutes a powerful argument against the development of the nuclear energy option as a response to the greenhouse effect. Another equally powerful argument developed in the literature is that because there is no threshold level below which radioactivity is safe (theoretically one alpha particle could cause a DNA mutation; less than one-millionth of a gram of plutonium is carcinogenic), the nuclear option must be proved to be safe. Chernobyl showed that it is not - no technology can be foolproof. [18] Storage of tons of high level nuclear waste is a massive problem; plutonium for example is dangerous for at least 500,000 years, the half-life of plutonium being 24,400 years. Any storage place must be geologically stable for millennia. Ironically, Right wing supporters criticize environmentalists who worry about the greenhouse effect because of the uncertainities of climatic models - how much more uncertain must geological models be that deal in such time spans! The geology of the Earth is not a fixed inert structure - it is over such time scales, dynamic. Finally, electricity production accounts for only 30% of fossil fuel use and nuclear power provides only 15% of global electricity supply - it cannot solve the problem of the greenhouse effect. To support the global electricity supply by 100%, hundreds, if not thousands of billions of dollars would have to be spent, with a nuclear power station commissioned every 2.4 days for at least the next 38 years. The cost would be out of the reach of all Third World countries, and arguably all but a few developed countries. [19]

(2) <u>The Destruction of Soil and Agricultural Land in the Context of Population Increases</u>

The number of Mayans in the lowlands of Guatemala had doubled on average of every 408 years since the time of 800 B.C. reaching by A.D. 900 about five million. Then within decades the population fell to one-tenth of this level. Deevy [20] suggests that this was due not to outside invasion but to population-induced environmental stress, especially the destruction of the topsoil. Lester Brown says "... world population is expanding at nearly 2 percent per year, and in many countries the rate is 3 percent or more. The ultimately disastrous rate of increase among the Mayans appears almost leisurely in comparison". [21] Indeed at the growth rate of 1.7% it is estimated that there will be 6.3 billion people by the year 2000. There is a decline in the overall rate of population increase in the world. Nevertheless by the time the world reaches a replacement level of reproduction by the year 2020 the population of the world will be around 11 billion. Population increases not only create a demand for more cropland, pushing agriculture onto more fragile soil, but also creates an increased demand for converting agricultural land to urban use. Leggett describes this enormous destruction as follows:

> "The geologists at Interlaken compiled a graphic catalogue of man's impact on the planet. He scrabbles 50 billion tonnes of minerals from the ground each year, in so doing shifting the equivalent of three times the sediment moved each year by the world's rivers. This process leads to inevitable leakage from the minerals-to-goods cycle, causing an exponential rise in toxic metals in seas, lakes and soils. He mines and burns billions of tonnes of coal each year, so venting a further Pandora's box of wastes, including carbon dioxide, the principal (current) contributor to the greenhouse effect.
>
> Feeding himself with carelessness typical of his tenure, he causes the erosion of 25 billion tonnes of soil each year, 0.7 per cent of the total farmable soils which took thousands of years to form. He lays down 30 kilograms of fertiliser per person each year to increase his crop yield, so polluting the water he must drink. His accidents and spillages leave their imprint everywhere. Dioxins from his chemical industries find their way into the tissues of polar bears. Radioactive particles from his nuclear bombs and reactors accumulate at the South Pole within days of their release". [22]

The following facts speak for themselves [23]:

- 20 million square kilometres of lands are at risk of, or are undergoing desertification; the deserts expand by an area twice the size of Belgium every year.

- One third of the world's cropland may disappear by the year 2000 if present trends continue.

- Erosion is resulting in the formation of a new island in the Bay of Bengal from soil washed away from the Himalayan Valleys.

- Without forests, the monsoon cycle in Southeast Asia will result in enormous erosion.

- 4 million tons of topsoil are lost per year in the United States. In Illinois, for every bushel of corn produced, 2 bushels of topsoil wash/blow away.

- Prime farmland in USA and Canada of more than 1.2 million acres disappears under concrete and roads each year.

- There will be a doubling of water use for irrigation by the year 2000 with problems of soil salinization and loss of productivity. Damage to farmland by salt costs Australia $500 million a year. Soil salinity and acidification affect about 2.7 million sq.kms of Australian farming lands or 54% of the total productive rural land.

- The total cost of land degradation for Australia is about $2.1 billion a year which is more than 4% of this country's total export earnings.

(3) The Destruction of Natural Diversity

- African Congo, Amazon River basin and the forests of Southeast Asia are being destroyed at rates of between 600 and 700 square kilometres per day. [24] Space satellites have detected as many as 8,000 separate fires in a single day; in 1988 an area of 112,880 sq.km. bigger than Scotland, Wales and Northern Ireland was burnt. The Governor of Amazonas, Mr. Amaxonino Mendes handed out 2,000 free chainsaws in 1988 and in 1989 still continues to do so.

- By the year 2000 if present trends continue, China may lose more than a quarter of its already scarce forests; 5 billion tonnes of soil are lost each year; 7 million hectares of China's 100 million hectares of farmland are plagued by salinity problems; construction destroys 8.5 million hectares of farmland a year. [25]

- Wild species, apart from being of intrinsic value in themselves (deep ecology), are a storehouse for numerous chemical compounds for use in medicine and for breeding new strains of agricultural crops (more than 40% of drug prescriptions in the United States alone depend upon natural biological resources). A lethal blight on any of the world's main food crops of rice, wheat, corn and sorghum would mean that more than half of the world's food producing agricultural lands would fail, resulting in the greatest famine in human history. Wild strains, essential for pest-resistance breeding programmes are being lost by the expansion of monocultures; once extinct, the genetic diversity cannot be recovered by any technological method (genetic recombination presupposes that one has "raw" genetic materials to start with.) [26]

- "At the beginning of this month (November 1988), a cargo ship carrying 11,000 cubic metres of logs began unloading at the Japanese port of Kitakyushu. The logs were from the Amazon rainforest, a new source of material for Japan's timber industry, the world's largest consumer of tropical hardwoods. A further 27,500 cubic metres will arrive in December; next year, the shipments should be running at the rate of 40,000 cubic metres per month. About one-fifth of the timber will end up as wooden boards for shaping concrete on building sites, and will be discarded after a few uses". [27]

- "The regional and global consequences of human activities may undermine the ability of natural ecosystems to recover. ... Air and water pollution can poison species and hinder their reproduction. The global warming trend expected to result from rising atmospheric carbon dioxide levels will alter the distribution of plants and the animals that depend on them. A depletion of stratospheric ozone, induced by the use of chloroflurocarbons in industrial countries, could permit enough damaging ultraviolet light to reach earth's surface to damage plant leaves and cause skin cancers and immune system problems among animals and humans alike. The cumulative effects of such changes can alter ecosystems in ways that increase the vulnerability of plant and animal species to extinction. Scientists call the process "biotic impoverishment" - a series of changes that leave soils less fertile and vegetation less productive, favor outbreaks of pests and diseases, and require costly adjustments from humans trying to raise food in the midst of a biologically depleted landscape". [28]

- "<u>Almost two-thirds of Central America's lowland and lower montane forests have been cleared or severely degraded since 1950. Much of the land had been cleared to make way for ranching schemes to supply the United States and other western countries with cheap beef for hamburgers</u>". [29]

(4) <u>Our Poisonous Planet - Toxic Chemicals, the "High Tech Holocaust" and Acid Rain</u>

It is not news that multinational corporations, and even national level corporations are immensely powerful, often having budgets that exceed the Gross National Products of many nations. A strong tendency therefore exists for multinationals to be laws unto themselves, to meddle in the internal affairs of countries, to get laws changed to favour them and to walk with heavy boots over international conventions. Perhaps the most infamous example of this meddling is the role played by the multinationals ITT, Kennecott and Anaconda with the CIA to topple the democratically elected government of Salvador Allende. [30]

Multinational and giant national chemical companies have also been responsible for chemical accidents that have killed thousands of people and polluted the environment. Some examples are spills in 1986 from Ciba-Geigy, Sandoz and BASF in Western Europe, Basel Switzerland, the Sevesco dioxin spill and the Bhopal disaster. Multinationals though are not the only villains, as the Chernobyl nuclear disaster in April 1986 showed.

Nor for that matter, is Soviet industry clean and ethically responsible. The Soviet Aral sea, one of the world's largest inland seas once covering more than 64,000 sq. kms., now hardly receives river outflow water, but receives instead defoliants, pesticides and fertiliser residues, a product of the cotton industry. Tens of thousands of people have died as a result of this pollution. Two thirds of the population of the Karakalpak region suffer from a wide variety of diseases including cancer and 11% of all babies die before they are one year old. [31]

The death toll however from the accidents by multinational chemical companies is unacceptable. In Bhopal, 3-4 December 1984, methylisocyanate (MIC) killed more than 2,000 people and injured or disabled up to 200,000 people. [32] The Union Carbide plant in Institute USA, a little later, leaked an ultra-toxic gas aldicarb oxime; the plant manager delayed informing emergency services because he did not believe that the toxic cloud would harm the community! These incidents of what Bellini calls "high tech holocausts" [33] reveal elements of covering up, delaying tactics, veils of secrecy and obfuscation and a failure of corporations to face public responsibility, continuing to act with the attitude that they are a law unto themselves.

A recent report by the U.S. Environmental Protection Agency stated that at least 1.1 billion kilograms of deadly chemicals are emitted into the air annually from the United States alone, including 60 cancer causing agents, the highly poisonous gas phosgene and methylisocyanate, the same gas which devastated Bhopal. [34] The chemical industry responded to the report denying that the EPA established a health risk because it was unknown from the raw data what were the amounts and concentration of exposure to the chemicals. This demand for absolutely conclusive scientific proof as a weapon to protect environmental polluters is seen with respect to all humanity's environmental crises - destruction of the ozone layer, the greenhouse effect, acid rain, forest destruction and so on. [35] However it is philosophically doubtful whether <u>conclusive</u> scientific proof is ever possible for any proposition. Presumably we are never to act until it is too late; the USA is to keep pouring 1.1 billion kilograms of poisons into the air for hundreds of years. But of course, long before that the ecosystem will be massively polluted and life as we now know it will be degraded or extinct. [36]

This environmental degradation is not the exclusive fault of big business: consumers are a major contributor to an unsafe world. Consider for example the rubbish disposal system of a large city such as New York. Land fill at Fresh Kills, a 1200 ha site, receives the one tonne of annual rubbish that each New Yorker produces; it has received 100 million tonnes of garbage to date and gets 24,000 tonnes more each day. Perhaps symbolically, given present trends, by 2005 the pile of waste will be 155m, 70m higher than the Statue of Liberty. [37]

<u>Acid rain</u> (and associated phenomena such as acid snow, mist and dry deposition) derives from two sources: human sources such as coal-burning power plants, motor cars and ore smelters and natural sources such as volcanoes. [38] The acid rain and soil phenomena that troubles the ecologist is due to emissions of sulphur dioxide and nitrogen oxides, although other emissions such as hydrochloric acid, ammonia, and other organic compounds also influence acidity. [39] Normally the nitrates and sulphates can be returned to their basic forms by natural breakdown processes. The difficulty comes when through the burning of coal, the rate of oxidation of sulphur exceeds the breakdown capacity of ecosystems. It has been argued that sulphur oxides attack brickwork and metals in buildings (the Taj Mahal may be eventually ruined by these effects) and depositions on fields stunts the growth of plant life, destroys forests and creates lethal smogs (as seen in London in 1952, where more people died than during the cholera epidemic of 1866). Pearce gives a dramatic picture of the effects of acid rain:

> "The skies above Europe are poisoned. Toxics are carried on the breezes from power stations and autobahns across the most polluted continent on earth. When the poison falls to the ground it chokes the pores of leaves on trees from the Alps to the Urals; it eats away at stone and brick, paper and rubber; it destroys soils and flows into rivers where it kills fish by disrupting the operation of their gills. It kills humans too". [40]

The argument of books on acid rain published in the mid-1980s was that the solution to acid rain was sulphur dioxide control and that the technologies for its control already existed - the problem was who pays. Lester Lave, in a review of three books on acid rain all published in 1988, agrees that lakes and forests have died (this is an observational fact), but claiming that acid rain is principally caused by sulphur dioxide emissions is too simplistic. [41] L.J. Kulp for example believes that ground level ozone (a strong oxidizing agent) along with a multitude of other pollutants may account for the death of European forests. He cautions us against believing that merely cutting down sulphur dioxide is an adequate response to what is shaping up to be a multidimensional environmental problem. [42] This is not to say that sulphur is not the driving force behind the chronic acidification of surface waters such as lakes, but rather to recognise as well the actions of oxidants such as ozone and hydrogen peroxide. Acid rain appears to be a complex unwanted by-product of the industrial process itself.

This brief Cook's tour of the environmental crisis has not included any discussion of the greenhouse effect [43] or the depletion of the ozone layer, [44] for the reason that these "sexy" topics have had enorous exposure by the media and are perhaps the best known environmental problems. Other problems such as the destruction of the soil, are less "sexy" and receive less media attention. Nevertheless, any one of these problems is sufficient to destroy the ways of human life as we know it, and obviously enough, all of these problems are interrelated. The greenhouse effect for example may produce higher than expected sea level rises if the bulk of the rain forests of the world are completely destroyed. The humus in the soil will oxidize and add significantly to the carbon dioxide in the atmosphere.

The aim of good science is to give simple but powerful explanations for a diverse range of activity. Boyle is correct when he says that the "problem of global warming is us. Industrialization, the extension and intensification of agriculture, and the rising demand for fossil fuels as populations grow rapidly in the developing world". [45] More precisely the root "cause" of the environmental crisis is multidimensional. This interacting and synergetic system comprises a set of exploitative and utilitarian practices between humans and between humans and nature and a metaphysical world view or ideology. The ideology and the social and ecological practices, interact and mutually support each other. It is the task of the bulk of this chapter to destroy the alleged rational credibility of this ideology.

2. The Critique of Industrialism, Capitalism, Consumerism and Economic Rationalism: The Limits to Growth and to Economic Rationality

In the light of the global crisis of civilization one would hope that the Australian nation's intellectual leaders, sheltered and nurtured by the great universities of the country, under the leadership of their Vice-chancellors, would be undertaking a critical review of the direction of Australian society in particular, and Western civilization in general. One would hope to find the best thinkers from both the Left and the Right debating fundamental value questions in an intellectually "exciting", but socio-ecologically frightening climate. In the past, both Left and Right intellectuals, saw their task as being the Socratic conscience of society [46] - today in Australia however, economic rationalism has firmly gripped these institutions. Vice-chancellors act now like company managers as many academics pursue profits through research for industry and private sector businesses, rather than truth and the critical examination of their society. Of course, it is well known that even in the socially tempestuous time of the 1960s and early 1970s the bulk of our universities' scientists and intellectuals were not acting as the Socratic consciences of their society, but working in research time on military, police or business projects. What is surprising today is the depth of penetration of economic rationalism into Australian intellectual life and its openness to such a degree that the following comments can be found in an editorial in a right-wing newspaper such as The Australian:

"Mr. Dawkins' real problem is his inability to grasp that university education is about thinking more than training and about culture more than future employment. Australia's real tragedy is that his legions of academic critics are often little better. The minister and the Vice-chancellors are unable to discuss higher education except in terms of economic benefit or bureaucratic empire-building. There must be more to a university education than finding a good job - although this is an important aim. There must be more to university teaching than securing one's quota of "equivalent full-time students" and "refereed papers per equivalent full-time member of staff". [47]

The intellectual battle in the Australian universities is paralleled by a broader conflict of world views: between what O'Riordan has called technocentrism and ecocentrism or what Alwyn Jones has called the industrial growth model and the deep ecology/ecosystems model. [48] Technocentrism divides into two camps, the "Accommodators" and the "Cornucopians". The "Accommodators" believe that economic growth can continue, providing effective environmental management occurs. The "Cornucopians" are super-optimists, believing that pro-growth goals define the rationality and value of a project and that any ecological problem can be solved with enough investment and technology. There are no inherent limits to growth, technology or science. Not even the sky's the limit, because beyond the earth is outerspace and its riches. Some Cornucopians even believe that humanity will one day control the structure of space-time itself, not merely playing God, but being God. (Once they have achieved this, one wonders what other horizon can be found!)

Ecocentrism is characterized by: (1) a lack of faith in large scale technologies because of their anti-democratic nature; (2) rejection of materialism, consumerism and economic growth for their own sake; (3) emphasis on small scale work that is integrated with the rest of one's life and the needs of the community; (4) community and social values rather than self-interest. Deep ecocentrism stresses not only the importance of nature for humanity, but the <u>intrinsic value</u> (in many cases the ideal equal value of non-human species and ecosystems cf. Table 1). Despite these differences, there is a unifying theme as Hugh Stretton observes in <u>Capitalism, Socialism and the Environment</u> "a repentance widely felt by many people of all social classes - a revulsion from mechanism and materialism, a nostalgia for more natural and neighbourly styles of life, and a genuine willingness to live on less". [49] J. Porritt in <u>Seeing Green: The Politics of Ecology Explained</u> sees the following as minimum criteria for being <u>Green</u> or ecocentric:

> "... a reverence for the Earth and for all its creatures; a willingness to share the world's wealth among <u>all</u> its peoples; prosperity to be achieved through sustainable alternatives to the rat race of economic growth; lasting security to be achieved through non-nuclear defense strategies and considerably reduced arms spending; a rejection of materialism and the destructive values of industrialism; a recognition of the rights of future generations in our use of all resources; an emphasis on socially useful, personally rewarding work, enhanced by human-scale technology; protection of the environment as a precondition of a healthy society; an emphasis on personal growth and spiritual development; respect for the gentler side of human nature; open, participatory democracy at every level of society; recognition of the crucial importance of significant reductions in population levels; harmony between people of every race, colour and creed; a non-nuclear, low-energy strategy, based on conservation, greater efficiency and renewable resources; an emphasis on self-reliance and decentralized communities". [50]

There is a large body of literature produced during the last twenty five years supporting these crucial theses. [51] Thinkers such as Sale [52], Routley and Routley [53], Bahro [54], Roszak [55], Pausacker and Andrews [56], Gorz [57] and Capra [58] would no doubt agree with the following comments of Ted Wheelwright, with the qualification that industrial "socialist"/state capitalist societies are just as guilty of the following evils:

> "... if you wanted to design a socio-economic system which would exploit and despoil the environment, create industrial pollution and enormous cancerous cities, you would design the capitalist system. You can fiddle with it here and there, alter a few prices, and tax various sorts of behaviour. You will probably improve it quite a bit; but as usual those who profit from it will manage to pass on most of the costs to those who profit least. It is unlikely you will get to the root of the problem which is the very system itself - based on <u>irresponsible exploitation of nature and man [woman] for private gain</u>". [59]

It is the aim of this section to support this proposition by developing a critique of economic rationalism and growthism from a socio-ecological position. The general thrust of my argument for dealing with the AIDS pandemic is to engage in a radical transformation of society. There is no doubt that this book conflicts with the spirit of economic rationalism and the cultural relativism of the times: hence the need for this critique. An excellent place to begin is at the base of social scientific thought itself.

Dunlap and Catton [60] argue that the social sciences have largely been anthropocentric and operated with an oversocialised conception of humanity. [61] The conditions of rapid growth and progress since the Enlightenment has created the illusion that humans are <u>completely</u> free from environmental constraints. Consequently social processes are exclusively to be understood by reference to social, cultural and technological variables, rather than ecological variables. As well, the social sciences have tended to be ecologically optimistic, rejecting any thought that humanity may fail to be able to adapt to changing environments - including an environment influenced by the polluting toxins of modern industry. Although Dunlap and Catton's cited works were written before the AIDS pandemic, it is clear that AIDS has presented a severe challenge to the technological optimism of modern molecular techno-medicine. [62]

Nevertheless Dunlap and Catton's view is only half correct in my opinion. Blame for the gulf between ecology, biology and the social sciences must also be placed in the lap of the ecologists and biologists. The attempt by neo-Darwinist biologists to understand human-ecological relationships has typically been in a strongly reductionistic fashion, ignoring completely the possibility of culturally and socially emergent properties and entities, that are non-reducible to bio-genetic entities and properties. In <u>Reductionism and Cultural Being</u> [63] I placed this trend within the context of the materialist - physicalist

TABLE 1: **Two Competing Modern World Views** (Modified from Jones (1987) and Sale (1980, 1985) with additions)

Social Indicators and Factors	Technocentrism/ Industrio-scientific Growth Paradigm	Deep Ecology/Deep Green Ecosystems/ Bioregional Paradigm
Social Scale	State Nation/World Internationalism	Region or Bioregion Community National Self-reliance
Economy	Increasing economic growth, quantity of consumer goods over quality profit motive meritocracy development progress global economy competition maximizes	Steady-state, sustainability and qualitative growth in problem-solving social need egalitarianism conservation stability national and community self-sufficiency cooperation satisizes
Politics	centralization ruling elites, class structure and status groups	decentralization, direct democracy, no class structure, no status groups
Society/ Institutions	external, hierarchical power structure, uniformity	community based, egalitarian power structure, diversity
Technology	bigger is better, industry and consumer based, all high tech is good, technology and science have no essential limits	"small is beautiful" need-based appropriate technology, not all high tech is good - technology must serve human **and** ecosystem interests, limits of technology and science
Nature	humans detached, controlling, managing or exploiting; interference is automatically justified	humans integrated, responsible, conserving, reverence, respectful, interference requires justification
Ethics	human centred, only humans are of intrinsic value, nature counts only with respect to human values	various positions: biospheric egalitarianism to biospecies impartiality all hold nature of intrinsic value, not not only humans are objects of value

Weltanschauung (or as it is called by Capra, the "Cartesian" reductionist programme). [64] The strongest challenges facing the physicalist Weltanschauung have come from physics itself - with the difficulties of developing a realistic quantum mechanics, and the impossibility of denying the stratification of the world and of emergent properties. [65]

Along with this is the development of alternatives to the essentially utilitarian gene-centred models of biological processes used by mainstream neo-Darwinist biologists. [66] None of these developments show that there are no limits to growth, that humankind can treat the environment as they please without consequence. On the contrary, the rejection of atomism and utilitarianism has led to the resurgence of holistic, systems models of humanity and nature that emphasise mutual interdependence. Within this context extreme biological reductionist theories such as sociobiology and extreme cultural theories such as post-structuralism and deconstruction, can be seen as not only deeply theoretically flawed, but as largely irrelevant to understanding our global ecological and social crises. Extreme responses produce more extreme counter-responses; that seems to be the illogic by which much of academic social science has advanced.

The propositions of a new ecological sociology (NEP) are these:

1. Whilst humans are culturally and technologically an exceptional species they are still an interacting part of global ecosystems, dependent upon other species for their survival.

2. Human life is heavily influenced by socio-cultural factors, but human life is also influenced by the biophysical environment - climate changes, pollution and so on.

3. Constraints or limits to human life are dictated by the biophysical environment; humanity is not autonomous.

4. Technological developments cannot override ecological and physical laws, such as the second law of thermodynamics. There are limits to growth and limits to technological and scientific achievements.

Indeed the fourth proposition has received support from post-empiricism philosophy of science. Although the work of writers such as Paul Feyerabend has been seen as supporting relativism, irrationalism and nihilism, another interpretation of the state of modern technical philosophy, is that there are essential limits to science and rational understanding. In my own published writings in logic, metaphysics and the philosophy of science, I have tried to show that whilst there are truths and rational beliefs (i.e. scepticism is false), human understanding is limited. The way in which this is done is by showing that there is no satisfactory resolution to the <u>paradoxes</u> in any field of study -logic, quantum mechanics and even sociology. This establishes a <u>theoretical</u> limit to science, and since technology is applied science, a theoretical limit to technology. [67]

Abstract theoretical limits are however not of much interest to our exuberant social scientists and the new breed of brash environmentalists who hope to patch up the system with a technological fix. There is however another argument which decisively refutes the thesis that technology can solve all human problems. Barry Jones in <u>Sleepers, Wake!</u> [68] recognizes that every technological change has an <u>equal</u> capacity to enrich or degrade the quality of life, depending upon its use. There is in my opinion no doubt whatsoever that many technological advances have been objectively beneficial - consider anesthesia for example. However, very many technological advances have brought new social problems with them - IVF technology for example, whilst others are simply evil - nuclear, chemical and biological weapons for example. Nor are technologies completely value free, a society using primarily nuclear energy imposes, as Gorz points out "a centralized, hierarchical police-dominated society". [69] David Ehrenfeld in <u>The Arrogance of Humanism</u> [70] argues that the idea that all human problems can be given a technological fix is absurd because most technological inventions are capable of doing social and technological damage, and by "Murphy's Law", rewritten as Ehrenfeld's Law - if a technology can be used for the worse, then it will be.[71] This need not even be conscious, as two examples will show. First, Illich has stated that the typical American spends four hours a day either driving, paying for or caring for his/her car. Dividing the number of hours per year into the number of miles travelled, gives a figure in miles per hour on average (regardless of individual driving speeds) that is equivalent to the average speed on foot. [72] Second, for each unit of food energy produced in Australia, about five units of energy are expended, with chain store packaging using 28.6% of the total energy. [73] Both of these examples are illustrations of ecological irrationality, but alleged techno-capitalistic enrichment. Thus one technological fix may give birth to another problem, requiring another technological fix, and so on in infinite regression. If technology in itself produces problems of living, which it does, then it follows that not all human problems can be solved by technology.

Another argument for the general limits to growth was given by Hirsch in <u>Social Limits to Growth</u>. [74] He argued that status style goods become relatively more important with increasing affluence, but satisfaction does not commensurately rise because others are now enjoying what was once a privilege. This argument is a useful counter-argument to Pareto optimality conditions. [75] It was however earlier noted by Karl Marx in <u>Wage Labour and Capital</u>:

> "A house may be large or small, as long as the surrounding houses are equally small it satisfies all social demands for a dwelling. But let a palace arise beside the little house, and it shrinks from a little house to a hut". [76]

The best known ecological argument for the limits to growth is Meadows (et al) <u>The Limits to Growth.</u> [77] This work employed computer modelling to predict when various resources would run out, and the report was clearly incorrect in many areas. For example the prediction that aluminium would be exhausted in 31 years was surprising given that 15% of the upper 16 kilometres of the Earth's continental crust is aluminium oxide. <u>The Limits to Growth</u> was <u>too</u> technologically pessimistic and too simplistically Malthusian in its argument to be widely accepted. Nevertheless, even if the world does not run out of mineral resources, such resources as we shall see, are still finite (not infinite) and fixed. Mining resources will be subjected to diminishing returns and increasing relative costs at each technological level.

The Australian writer Ted Trainer in <u>Abandon Affluence!</u> [78] has reworked the original argument of Meadows (et al) arguing that the whole world cannot live at the standard of the middle and ruling classes of the U.S., Japan, Europe and Australia. Contrary to David Pepper's remarks about limits-to-growth thesis leading to Malthusian right wing ideology, "ecofascism" and scientific racism, [79] Trainer along with most socio-ecologists does not accept global inequality as an inevitable fact of life and believes that the West should abandon its affluence, adopt "sustainable" conserver lifestyles and redistribute massive resources to the Third World. If the school of thought, deriving from neo-Marxist writings on economic imperialism, is even partially correct - that the advanced nations are advanced <u>because</u> (causally) of exploitation of the Third World - then the moral case for abandoning affluence and achieving global equity of wealth is decisive. Not only that, but we would achieve, as Trainer argues, a much safer world with minimal risk of nuclear annihilation. As P.E. O'Sullivan puts it "Deep ecology adopts in human affairs, an anti-class posture and advocates social justice within developed societies, and between them and the Third World". [80]

An alternative vision to today's consumer, growth-based economies is the conserver society or steady-state economy. In essence the conserver society has a lower rate of material output, is less dependent upon the exploitation of natural resources - especially non-renewable, is keen to re-use and recycle, and rejects growth-oriented demands artificially created by advertising techniques. [81] Daly, following John

Stuart Mill's writing in his chapter "On the Stationary State" in his *Principles of Political Economy*, lists the following definitive conditions:

(1)   A constant population (approximately)

(2)   A constant population of physical wealth.

(3)   (1) and (2) are such that a good life is lived by the members of the population, and it is sustainable.

(4)   There is the lowest feasible rate of throughput of matter and energy to maintain the human population and wealth; "birth rates are equal to death rates at low levels so that life expectancy is high; and production rates are equal to physical depreciation rates at low levels so that durability or 'life-expectancy' of artifacts is high". [82]

The steady-state economy would be neither capitalist nor "socialist". Whilst having decentralized market decision making, there would be maximum income and wealth limits, no monopoly class ownership of the means of production, and no sustained drive to accumulate. The steady-state economy is defined in ecological terms, implying nothing about GNP; GNP is itself seen as an inadequate concept:

> "The problem with GNP is that a large part of it is cost masquerading as benefit. The flow of new production (and associated depletion and pollution) required to maintain and replace the existing stock of assets is clearly a cost, albeit a necessary one. For any given stock of assets the less new production is required for maintenance and replacement the better. But GNP counts replacement as benefit - the faster things wear out or become obsolete, the greater the production flow and the higher GNP. Also, the extra expenditure required to protect ourselves from the undesired "side effects" of growth, such as extra medical bills resulting from pollution-induced illness of which cancer is a prime example, are added to GNP. The relevant question then becomes - which part of GNP is growing faster, the cost part or the benefit part? The question is evaded by claiming ... that GNP is just an index of economic activity, not of welfare, while continuing to treat it at a policy level as if it measured welfare". [83]

Why would people wish to limit economic growth, the mainstream economist asks? [84] The basic arguments for the steady-state economy are based upon <u>finitude</u> and <u>entropy</u>. The finitude argument is well known but it is probably the weakest argument for the limits to growth. Daly believes that the most serious problem relates to renewable rather than non-renewable resources due to: (1) high rates of pollution; (2) the non-sustainable expansion of population and consumption that has occurred through use of non-renewable resources - this is currently greater than that which could be supported by renewable resources alone. With increasing growth, there is a danger of 'overshoot' when non-renewable resources run out or become uneconomic.

The real limit to industrial growth is not necessarily a shortage of minerals or of energy, but the abundance of entropy produced at the end of consumption. Nicholas Georgescu-Roegen, an expert on the relationship between economic processes and thermodynamics, sums up this argument concisely:

> "Every time we produce a Cadillac [or Toyota] we irrevocably destroy an amount of low entropy that could otherwise be used for producing a plow or a spade. In other words, every time we produce a Cadillac, we do it at the cost of decreasing the number of human lives in the future. Economic development through industrial abundance may be a blessing for us now and for those who will be able to enjoy it in the near future, but it is definitely against the interest of the human species as a whole, if its interest is to have a lifespan as long as is compatible with its dowry of low entropy. In this paradox of economic development we can see the price man (woman) has to pay for the unique privilege of being able to go beyond the biological limits in his (her) struggle for life". [85]

According to the Second Law of Thermodynamics the entropy of a closed system continuousy increases towards a maximum; a closed system exchanges no matter and no energy with its environment. Entropy is a measure of the amount of energy no longer capable of conversion into work. An entropy increase means a decrease in "available energy"; pollution itself is a form of entropy. Rifkin [86] develops many of the social implications of Georgescu-Roegen's work.

Recycling cannot be the complete answer to the pollution-entropy problem. Pollution is the sum total of the available energy of a process transformed into unavailable or dissipated energy (matter is after all a form of energy). Recycling involves the expenditure of energy, is far from 100% efficient, and with respect to exponential industrial growth, can only increase the entropy of the environment. Although recycling is not the complete answer to the environmental crisis, it can buy time for the necessary social changes. Nor can this problem be solved by the development of a so-called post-industrial information society, as long as it still requires exponential economic growth:

> "... the faster information is generated by the computerized society, the faster those sense data are used by the society's transformers to collect and convert available energy. The increased energy flow-through, in turn, creates greater disorder, a faster depletion of the existing energy base, and a greater concentration and centralization of the society's economic and political institutions. The very purpose, then of the computer is to provide more sense data, more rapidly, in order to facilitate the faster conversion of available energy through the system". [87]

Nor for that matter, in Rifkin's opinion would a totally efficient solar technology support indefinely a highly centralized industrial technological society:

> "... we would continue to witness the exponential increase of entropy here on earth as solar energy is used to convert more and more of our limited terrestrial energy resources (matter) into the production process, transforming them from a usable to an unusable state. It is not, then, just the form of energy a society uses that is critical, it is also the amount of energy. If solar energy actually could flow in highly concentrated forms for industrial use, we would experience many of the same economic and social dislocations that result from our high energy use now. That's because <u>the</u> use of solar energy cannot be divorced from the stock of fixed terrestrial matter that it interacts on and converts. In living and in industrial processes, solar energy must always be combined with other terrestrial resources in order to produce a product. That conversion process always results in the further dissipation of the fixed stock of terrestrial resources on the planet". [88]

The obvious objection to the thermodynamic argument is that the earth is not a closed system because whilst no matter is significantly exchanged with its environment, significant amounts of energy reach the earth from the sun. As well, living things exhibit an increase in complexity over time - all of this seems hard to make consistent with the law of increasing entropy. It can however be done with some careful thinking about what a closed system is. If the above criticism was correct, then there would be no reason at all for taking the second law of thermodynamics as the "arrow of time". Yet regardless of quantum mechanical complications, we never observe the ash turning back into the unburnt wood, the broken glass reassemble itself. We do observe order and self-organisation, or to use Prigogine's term, "dissipative structures", but this does not logically conflict with the second law of thermodynamics. [89] Whether or not we follow Sheldrake and maintain that received physics has not explained "form", we can accept that self-organisation and increasing biological complexity can occur by whatever mechanism one likes, as long as a thermodynamic price is paid, with an increase in entropy of the environment. At this point we can see that Rifkin's argument is essentially correct. Receiving solar energy from the sun does not in itself necessarily mean that the entropy of the earth is not increasing. The sun still shines over areas of the Amazonian and Asian rain forests that have been cut down even though the entropy of the area has increased. Without the biological conversion mechanism of photosynthesis, to transform solar energy into chemical energy, the incoming solar energy merely heats the soil and air and is ultimately lost.

More technically, Prigogine's "dissipation structures" occur in far-from-equilibrium situations which have not been shown to occur in macroscopic economic processes. Futhermore, the equation of neg-entropy and order, and entropy and disorder is in my opinion mistaken. To show this, we accept Prigogine's own problematic, that there has been increasing complexity of structures since the beginning of space-time-matter in the big bang. It follows then that the big bang atom, a compression of all matter and energy, and space and time would have a less complex structure than the universe today. By the second law of thermodynamics, the big bang atom has maximum neg-entropy. It follows then that neg-entropy and order cannot be equated, although they are related.

Neoclassical economics in many respects confirms this position, for scarcity and limitation is built into the very foundation of the theory itself. For example, almost all neo-classical economic texts accept that scarcity is a fundamental fact of social life. Even if basic physiological needs are met, consumers are said to have potentially infinite wants. Resources are however finite and limited. Therefore the production of various commodities with respect to a limited resource base requires a choice between relatively scarce commodities. The so-called "production-possibility" or "transformation curve", expresses the idea that in any economy there is a trade-off assuming that resources can be transferred between industries, producing more of one good, means producing less of another. The increments of some good obtained by foregoing successively greater quantities of some alternative commodity represents the <u>social opportunity cost</u>. If we are concerned with maintaining a military state with ever-increasing stockpiles of weapons, then we cannot simultaneously produce a simultaneous maximum capacity of consumer goods. Along with this, the law of diminishing returns (first formulated by David Ricardo) is viewed as one of the most fundamental economic laws: it states that in physical economic processes, there is a tendency for successively lesser extra outputs to be gained from adding equal increments of a variable input to some constant amount of a fixed input. In the case of agricultural production, inputs are not, fortunately, always fixed, for to avoid diminishing returns the conditions of production are changed by technical advances. Nevertheless, in a fashion similar to the standard application of Godel's theorem, diminishing return will operate at that level with that given state of technology. The standard economics textbooks point out that the decline in extra returns follows because the addition of the varying resource (such as labour) does not receive proportionate increases in other factors. The texts fail to prove _why_ this "observed fact" should hold in reality. The answer we have seen lies in the second law of thermodynamics. It is noteworthy that technology itself, being the product of human beings with finite physical brains, may be subjected to diminishing returns as Brown explains:

> "Investment in scientific research - long the answer when productivity lagged - may itself be experiencing diminishing returns. Within agriculture, for example, cereal hybridization and the discovery of chemical fertilizer required relatively small investments of time and money, but comparable future advances in food production may be harder to realize. In physics, splitting the atom and developing solid-state physics were landmark breakthroughs, but comparable seminal gains may require the lifetime efforts of thousands of highly trained physicists.
>
> In retrospect, Ricardo appears to have been ahead of his time. Diminishing returns were postponed by expanding geographical frontiers and advancing technology. Now the frontiers are gone and technology is not always able to offset or postpone diminishing returns. To be sensible, national economic and demographic policies must be responsive to the new Ricardian realities." [90].

It is not possible to escape the impact of the law of diminishing returns within the framework of neo-classical economics by appealing to the law of diminishing marginal utility as putting a "break" upon the infinity of wants of rational economic men and women. The reason for this is that diminishing marginal utility may apply to the consumption of any good such as beer or chocolate, but the _number_ of potential wants for distinct commodities, even if each distinct commodity in its consumption undergoes diminishing marginal utility - is _infinite_ (or potentially infinite). Moreover it is possible to conceive of goods that may violate the law of diminishing marginal utility for exceptional individuals (such as increments of wealth for the ultra-greedy, or increments of knowledge for Plato) because this law is based upon psychological reality and hence human nature. The law of diminishing returns, based upon physical thermodynamic properties is more fundamental. This however means that the most <u>basic</u> considerations of economics are <u>not</u> utility considerations, supply and demand considerations or even central plans - but as we have seen, <u>thermodynamic</u> considerations. Economics by definition must be based upon physical ecology, although I will argue, it has a <u>moral dimension</u> which means that it is not purely a physical science.

It has not been realized by mainstream economists that the central assumption of the infinity of wants of rational economic men/women conflicts with the popular meta-system value-judgement that economic growth is a good thing. The point of economic growth, they say, is to satisfy an ever-increasing number of human wants. Economic growth and consumerism may create new wants, but the hope is that another increase in economic growth can satisfy those wants. However, let us look back at this whole process and ask whether individuals are actually becoming more satisfied by this process. The global or total satisfaction or utility of an economic individual may be defined as the ratio or satisfied wants SW to the unsatisfied reservoir of actual and potential wants PW. Now the fraction $SW/PW = n/\infty$ which is equal to zero for any finite positive natural number of wants n. If we become a little more mathematically sophisticated and speak about limits instead of an actual infinity, then we will say that the global satisfaction of an individual tends towards zero for any finite n, PW is said to increase without bound, whilst SW at any time t is always bounded by some finite positive natural number. Thus we cannot say that increasing economic growth necessarily increases global satisfaction or utility of an individual, as long as we have the endless growth of wants and desires of economic men/women. But surely then, the process of economic growth as a mechanism for satisfying infinite wants and tastes, by contrast to finite needs, is logically pointless and self-refuting. If this result is thought to be paradoxical and intolerable, then the argument should be taken as a <u>reductio ad absurdum</u> of the core assumption that the very point of economics is to somehow rationally deal with the human condition of scarce resources, finite commodities and <u>infinite wants</u>. This problem cannot be dealt with in any logical way without some critical examination of wants - especially a social, legal or moral limitation of wants and desires. This is precisely the limits to growth.

Finally, according to neo-classical economics, increased growth is economically rational if and only if the marginal benefits of growth exceed the marginal costs. Now even if this was true at present, the law of diminishing marginal utility and the law of increasing marginal costs mean that eventually, the costs of economic growth will be too high - in respect to pollution, the development of vicious cycles of satisfaction and frustration and so on. Thus even received economics must accept that beyond some point, growth is uneconomic, and irrational. Growth must have social opportunity costs.

R.G. Lipsey (et al) [91] maintains that the limits-to-growth advocates assume constant technology, which they do not for they consistently make use of economics' own concepts of scarcity. Finite resources Lipsey believes violate the law of conservation of mass-energy, which is outlandishly false, and in any case irrelevant since our argument is based on the second law of thermodynamics. Bell [92] and Kaysen [93] reject outright the idea that there are ecological limits to growth, but they do it without argument. A more interesting criticism of this position was given by the journalist P.P. McGuinness [94] who tells us that ecologists dismiss economists. He also tells us that economics shows that environmental protection has a cost. He asserts (without proof) his basic religious faith that the free market price system will produce a solution. The very idea of any social green reform of society for McGuinness, and almost all of The Australian writers, is the most evil of evil thoughts, for it denies freedom of choice to individuals. (He never demonstrates that capitalism promotes freedom of choice or justifies the slide from political freedom to free markets.) Thus for McGuinness, it is not right to radically change society to reduce pollution levels (this would interfere with consumerism) but instead one should "sell" the rights to pollution at a price which either makes it economically necessary to either stop or reduce pollution levels. The shallowness of McGuinness' position is revealed by merely a little thought about this. Since the idea of social regulation of private enterprise is evil, who sells the right to pollute? What is the cost of threatening not only the genetic diversity of life on earth, but risking the extinction of the human race for the consumerist values McGuinness accepts?

The only way to attribute a price to an irreproducible object (such as non-toxic drinking water and "clean" air) is to have absolutely every one bid on it, to avoid parochial bids. But irreproducible resources are like that: future generations are not present at today's markets and cannot bid against us. Thus there is no such thing as the cost of irreplaceable resources or of irreducible pollution. On this reasoning no economic considerations could justify cutting down the Amazonian rainforests - certainly not for Japanese, American and European parochial interests. [95]

What then is wrong with McGuinness' position, apart from its omission of mention of the vast scholarly objections to the neo-classical economic position, is its mistake in taking dollars or yen as the only measure of value. It can be proved that life itself cannot be reduced to a money equivalent; money is a modern concept that exists as a mechanism for managing the financial affairs of human life. Money therefore cannot be itself of more fundamental value than human life. Ehrlich's point is that the industrial-consumerist system with its desire for increasing affluence, more throw-away goods, expanding populations and massive immigration programmes, had led us to an environmental crisis that may lead to the extinction of the human race. It is the values of the system that McGuinness and millions of other intellectuals defend with their empty talk of "freedom of choice", which is problematic. Freedom of choice is not to be understood as freedom to develop higher moral values and ecologically sane life styles - it is understood as freedom of choice of goods on a supermarket shelf, many of which are open to moral and ecological critique.

Even in terms of mainstream economics, McGuinness' response is inadequate. To every social and environmental problem he says: increase the price. For example to deal with the increased greenhouse gases he suggests increasing the price of petrol (which in itself is not unreasonable) and having worse roads. Now whilst price increases may solve some isolated problems in this fashion, to deal with every environmental and social problem (there are so many they fill volumes of books) in this way would result in virtually infinite inflation and the collapse of the capitalist economic system (an interesting thought). The conclusion is therefore evident: free market forces themselves cannot adequately deal with the global ecological crisis.

Another argument that can be used against McGuinness' position is based upon Hardin's "The Tragedy of the Commons". [96] This often reprinted argument is essentially this: consider a common pasture, with herdsmen/women who are rational selfish egoists seeking to maximise their gain. The utility of adding one more animal to any individual's herd has a positive component of approximately +1, receiving all the proceeds from the sale of the additional animal. The negative component arising from the additional over-grazing created by one more animal is shared by all herdsmen(women), so the negative utility is a faction of -1. Thus utility is maximised by adding another animal to the herd, and so on - a decision reached by each of the individual herdsmen/women. The result is ruin of the commons. The commons here, need not be a pasture, and we need not consider only herdsmen/women. The commons could be any environmental resource at all; the thought experiment can be easily generalized. Hardin accepting the cardinal rule of neo-classical economics: never ask a person to act against his/her own self-interest (self-interest being independent of the interests of others), believes that individuals pursuing their own self-interest in a society that believes in the freedom of the Commons, leads to the ruination of all - that is, each individual. Accepting economic egoism Hardin goes on to argue for a design of institutions based on the assumption that people will act selfishly. At no point does he realise that without any logical difficulty whatsoever his argument can be turned on its head: it is not the Commons which is a problem but his selfish individuals who lack social responsibility. We simply cannot solve environmental problems by denying that there is a Common-environment as pollution (e.g. acid rain) does not stop at the boundaries of the nation state. We can, and should deny that a Commons should be free, in the sense that individuals can do with it as they like. But once we do this, Hardin's cardinal rule of neo-classical economics must be abandoned. More importantly, what Hardin has shown is that utilitarian considerations are not merely insufficient, but often in contradiction with the social interest of undeniable universal goods. Most critics of Hardin have found his conclusions repulsive, and criticized the assumptions of his argument such as egoism, or criticized the myth as lacking historical foundation. In doing this they have failed to see, as Hardin himself fails to see, that the argument is a <u>reductio ad absurdum</u> of the cardinal rule of neo-classical economics, for it means that utilitarian egoism is logically inconsistent. Acting as an utilitarian egoist may lead to consequences directly conflicting with any concept of the satisfaction of self interest, despite utility maximization. Acting altruistically, is in many instances the best thing a purely rational egoist could do. [97]

3. Against the Economists: Towards a Moral Economy

I argued in the previous section that there is a solid core of mainstream or neo-classical economics that is very close to an ecological-thermodynamic position. This position does not appeal to any epistemologically weak psychological foundations for scientific study such as profit maximization, utilitarianism, revealed preference or consumer sovereignty. Its theory of rationality is not narrowly restricted to the maximization of individual self interest, but is wide enough to include all methods of reasoning and evaluation that have been available since the dawn of philosophy. Given that there is an extensive body of literature criticizing the logic and scientificity of much of the neo-classical paradigm, it is necessary to look elsewhere for a philosophical foundation for socio-ecology. [98]

Our first port of call is classical Marxism. Now I have argued elsewhere that two of the moral positions associated with Marxism - the critique of privacy and radical egalitarianism -are substantially correct on moral grounds. This does not commit me to accepting the bulk of Marxist sociology and economics, and fortunately so, for there are challenging problems and major dilemmas threatening what we may call "fundamentalist Marxism". [99] Fundamentalist Marxist economics is a position which sees a set of inexorable laws of motion of capitalism, following from the labour theory of value. [100] An example of such a law, is the tendency of the rate of profit to fall. This view contrasts with a social theory of economy which sees prices and wages as a product of class conflict.

Marx's argument for socially necessary labour-time as the basis of the value of any commodity is this:

(1) Under pure and perfect competition, every market exchange must be the exchange of two equal values.

(2) The value in (1) must be given by something contained in each commodity (<u>Capital</u>, Vol. 1)

(3) This must exist in equal quantities common to both.

(4) Therefore the two things must be equal to a third thing, not identical to either thing exchanged.

(5) This common thing cannot be a natural property of commodities, hence by elimination it must be socially necessary labour time.

This argument, accepted without question by fundamentalist Marxists, begs the question against those who view prices and wages as the products of class conflicts and human relationships. It assumes via premise (2) that value is a metaphysical <u>property</u> of commodities, rather than a social <u>relationship</u>. If value is a relational phenomenon, then Marx's argument is unacceptable. In any case, Marx's argument as it stands does not prove that labour is the common denominator of commodity value: the neo-classicals could accept all of Marx's premises and conclude that it is <u>utility</u> that is the common denominator.

The labour theory of value is necessary for the basis of Marx's critique of capitalism via the concept of exploitation. The worker's labour is embodied in the final product: profit or surplus value is the difference between the necessary value to pay for the worker's subsistence and the value of the product. Sherman [101] has argued that under capitalism, workers who have only their labour to sell, work for a real wage that is less than the real output - but wages are determined by class conflict and the conditions of supply and demand:

> "Price, wages, and profits reflect a system in which workers are paid a certain wage, but the entire product is sold by the capitalist at whatever price it can command in the market. Consumer demand is based on the class income and class behaviour of those receiving labour income and property income. The very meaning and amount of prices, profits, wages are given by these relations, not merely by technical conditions. For example, the cost of production of a product in South Africa will be lower than in the United States - even with the same technology and machinery - because unions are suppressed, prejudice divides workers, and the State is used to

oppress the majority of workers ... So the prices of products, wages of workers, and profits of capitalists are the result of a certain set of class relations, certain rules of the game, certain social institutions - and not merely the technical conditions of production". [102]

Sherman's point can be supported by another example which also challenges the labour theory of value. Consider the production of commodities by robots controlled by tenth generation computers. Suppose that these computers and robots were themselves constructed by other computers, and so on (this is a projection of trends that already exist). We could imagine that this chain stopped with a set of technicians who built the first self-generating computers in the chain, but who were given a "fair" wage to set up the system. Here we have a system of production where the labour theory of value does not come into place and where products may be sold for great profits. All of this is consistent with massive unemployment, degradation, environmental destruction and alienation in the surrounding society. So the labour theory of value is not a timelessly true theory of value, nor is it a satisfactory critical foundation for a theory of all forms of capitalism. Something more is needed, and that is a <u>moral critique</u> based upon a theory of economic ethics and social justice. [103] Let us now consider work which leads us in the direction of a moral economy.

One recent argument for abandoning 'value-free economics' and introducing a moral dimension into economies is given by Amitai Etzioni's <u>The Moral Dimension: Toward a New Economics</u>. [104] The mainstream utilitarian rationalistic-individual epistemological foundation for neo-classical economics is rejected by Etzioni in favour of a view of human nature, as individualistic in the sense that they do advance their self or "I", but within a moral framework derived from a community that is perceived as a "We" rather than a cold dominating "They" or "Them". The "I" and "We" is in creative conflict by contrast to the essentially negative conflict between "I" and "Them" in received economics; thus Etzioni calls this paradigm the "I" and "We" position. It is directly opposed to the view of neo-classical economics that exclusively sees wants as centred on self-satisfaction or self-happiness. Etzioni points out that actors whilst indeed seeking pleasure and self-interest satisfaction, still seek to abide by their moral commitments: they are still moral agents. Further, moral values cannot be necessarily regulated by price. The reason for this in Etzioni's opinion, is that moral values (and these are for him essentially deontological concepts of rightness, duty and obligation) set the context in which the utilitarian orientations of the neo-classical economist operate. There is, as Durkheim before him recognised, a moral foundation to the economy which is ignored by the neo-classical economist when the discipline is methodologically defined. Nevertheless key elements of the neo-classical model are not abandoned.

> "The self-oriented, rational behaviour "modelled" by neoclassicists is assumed to occur within the context of personality structure and society. These, in turn, are perceived not merely as reflections of the aggregation of individual acts but as being formed to a significant extent by forces and dynamics that are fundamentally different ... from those assumed by the neoclassical paradigm. That is, rather than abandon neoclassical concepts and findings, they are viewed here as dealing with subsystems within society (markets) and personality (in which rational decision-making is circumscribed, substituted <u>and</u>, on occasion, supported by emotions and values). In other words, the approach followed here is one of <u>codetermination</u>. It encompasses factors that form society and personality, as well as neoclassical factors that form markets and rational decision-making". [105]

Thus Etzioni's position sets the general context through which the great play of neoclassical forces is acted. The position is interesting as a revision of the neoclassical position, but it is essentially tinkering, not an entirely new direction as Etzioni thinks. The neoclassicalist could accept unselfish behaviour and irreducible moral behaviour, as special complications to an essentially sound abstract model. Etzioni is in a dilemma here: if he completely rejects utilitarianism (and revealed preference) the derivation of demand curves has been eroded. With respect to the long standing question of the value freedom of the social sciences and economics, Etzioni's position is quite consistent with the mainstream economic view of values, concisely expressed by Keith Hancock:

> "... when the economist takes it upon himself to say what <u>ought</u> to be done he moves into an area where his professional competence deserts him; and if he speaks to the world as if his prescriptions are derived from his Economics he is, wittingly or unwittingly, defrauding the public". [106]

Hancock's view, following Lionel Robbins', is that economics is concerned with facts, not values, and that there is a logical gap (the is-ought gap) between factual statements and evaluative statements. Now most distinctions in philosophy are vague and the is-ought gap is no exception. Under naturalistic ethical theories, the gap can be bridged by accepting that some factual statements are evaluative. In my opinion, nothing of significance hangs on this old debate. The <u>justification</u> of methods of inferring facts from facts, by either induction or deduction, depends as we have seen upon values. Even Hancock admits that value-free economics is itself based upon a value-judgement - i.e., do not conceal alternative courses of action from the public, do not knowingly mislead. However, economic theory makes presuppositions about the nature of social reality that involve normative evaluations, so neo-classical (and Marxist) economic theory involves fundamental evaluative judgements. C.A. Hooker has argued this point through with respect to the neo-classicists's acceptance of the market as the fundamental distribution mechanism in capitalist society and the resulting commodification of much of society. Hooker points out that the

> "market dominates the distribution of all goods and services, including land, living locations, skills and so on. But this involves bringing the substance of society under the dictates of the market as commodities. The result is a profound transformation of human society as traditionally conceived. e.g. the sedentary extended family collapses to the mobile nuclear family, the village beomes the dormitory suburb, education is transformed from personal maturation to saleable skill development, and so on. (But, on the other side, authority and information are somewhat less dominated by hereditary control, there is more choice of employment (subject to market constraints), more tolerance of cultural expressions of individuality, and so on). Importantly for policy, there are (strictly) no collective decisions imposed, collective policy results from aggregating individual choice and is coherent only to the extent that market-priceable consequences of individual actions are coherently transferable throughout the market. Good or bad, however one evaluates it, there is no doubt that choosing to conceive and organise society in these terms involves making the deepest possible value judgements. While the market functions independently of individual value judgements made in the market, choice of the market as the fundamental economic institution is clearly a fundamental value judgement. Similar kinds of remarks apply to the choice of the Classical or the Marxist social forms". [107]

The issue of importance is the rationality and objectivity of values. If evaluative reasoning is objective, then the issue of whether or not economics should have values judgement in it or not does not matter. Even radicals could accept the recommendations of a conservative such as Hancock about the extremely limited competence of economists: indeed we could welcome it. Economics could then be seen, in its rightful place as a form of applied mathematics, and ethics and political philosophy would arise to take their rightful role in the political arena as the real cognitive disciplines for the investigation of social policies. The role of economics, instead of being decisive, as in the popular doctrine of economic rationalism, would be only of marginal assistance in tackling the big questions of any society. They would be decided by philosophical debate, rather than blind acceptance of the justice of certain economic models. Economics would determine the <u>limits</u> of social action, not its precise <u>nature</u>.

According to Lionel Robbins, "Economics is the science which studies human behaviour as a relationship between ends and scarce means that have alternative uses". [108] For the moral and political philosopher reviewing this definition it is impossible to see how evaluative considerations could not be relevant to the study of the use of scarce means or resources, which have alternative uses, some of them moral and some of them not, because, "ends" presuppose social values. If human beings act on the basis of reason, knowledge and belief, rather than mechanical non-intentional stimulus-response behaviour, then an adequate causal account of their behaviour must include not only reference to the agent's values, but an understanding of the soundness of the agent's reasoning. [109]

Economics under Robbins' definition could very well be viewed as an evaluative enterprise, if it was not for an unscientific, irrational bias for methodological positivism.

Allowing ethics and political philosophy to penetrate into the domain of influence in public policy now occupied by economics would allow for questions such as: "how well does capitalism itself deal with the central economic problem of scarcity?" "Is the capitalist system good, just and rational, or should it be changed?" "Is there another economic system which is better?" These questions are <u>never</u> addressed by neo-classical economists for the very good reason, that if they do answer "yes" to them, they are suddenly in the dilemma of belonging to a paradigm in crisis. As well political philosophy would never accept a statement such as "Human wants always exceed existing goods and services" without investigating the very rationality, morality and sanity of the "wants" itself. Once again this task is outside the professional competence of neo-classical economics. Since so many important questions are outside the competence of economists, I suggest that their influence in society be replaced by the more comprehensive discipline of ethics and political philosophy. Plato was not wrong about everything.

M. Bookchin has given some useful insights into the nature of <u>moral economy</u>. In reflecting upon the significance of market forces upon our lives he gives the following passionate moral critique of the "expanding domain of economics": [110]

> "... economics, with its panoply of scientific pretensions, has muddled the entire issue of economics and morality. It is also hard to see because we tend to assume that the economic status quo is a given, a "natural state of affairs", that is assumed to be part of a fictitious "human nature". So deeply rooted is the market economy in our minds that its grubby language has replaced our most hallowed moral and spiritual expressions. We ... "invest" in our children, marriages, and personal relationships, a term that is equated with words like "love" and "care". We live in a world of "trade-offs" and we ask for the "bottom line" of any emotional "transaction". We use the terminology of contracts rather than that of loyalties and spiritual affinities". [111]

The alternatives to the market economy emerged in America after the Stock Market crash of 1929 - barter, sharing, communitarian values, mutual aid, self-reliance, and regionalism. Before the development of modern market economies a product's worthiness was morally integrated with the worthiness of the producer, crafter and seller; goodwill in the domain of business in past human ages encompassed the values of integrity, reliability, and public duty. The very idea of "planned obsolescence" would be an alien concept to pre-capitalist crafts-persons. Price was a moral bond reached between buyer and seller that reflected "justice" - hence the notion of a "just price". Again the idea of buyer and seller reaching an equilibrium price through the Newtonian forces of supply and demand, would be alien to the pre-capitalist world. Such is the nature of the moral economy:

> "A moral economy - a participatory system of distribution based on ethical concerns - is meant to dissolve the immorality that the modern mind identifies with economics as such. Its goal is to dissolve the antagonism between "buyer" and "seller", to show that in practice both "buyer" and "seller" form a community based on a rich sense of mutuality, not on the opposition of "scarce resources" to "unlimited needs". The object exchanged is secondary to the ethical values that are explicitly shared by the participants of a moral economy. For "buyer" and "seller" to care for each other's well-being, for them to feel deeply responsible to each other, and for them to be cemented by a deep sense of obligation for their mutual welfare, is to replace a strictly economic nexus with an ethical one - that is to <u>turn economics into culture</u> rather than to visualize it as the "circulation" of things. Where distribution becomes a form of complementarity, it ceases in fact to be economic in the usual meaning of the

word and the terms "buyer" and "seller" became meaningless". [112]

Bookchin's vision then is of a productive community of mutually interlocked social responsibility, where people exchange services at a price, which is not the unconscious outcome of the blind Newtonian crash of market forces, but a price which considers the welfare of agents as part of an integrated community, a kind of moral ecosystem. Bookchin openly admits that this sketch is utopian, for a true moral economy has never existed. Nevertheless, inspirations can be drawn from guilds and communes through the centuries, and today, as limited as these examples may be. [113]

4. Towards a Sustainable Future

It will no doubt be felt by many readers that the entire argument of this book - that the socia problems of AIDS and the wider health, poverty and socio-environmental can only be dealt with by radical national and global social change - is an utterly absurd dream. However, as that very famous modern song goes "I'm not the only one". In this concluding section a brief review of some international organisations and government leaders who have reached similar conclusions will be given.

Harold Coolidge, in the introduction to <u>Sustaining Tomorrow: A Strategy for World Conservation and Development</u> (1984) [114] points out the feeling of the World Conservation Strategy (backed by the International Union for Conservation of Nature and Natural Resources, UN Environment Programme and the World Wildlife Fund) of the value of "the unity of resource conservation and human development as mutually reinforcing tools for building a sustainable future". [115] The global environmental problems that threaten the biosphere, threaten life itself:

> "When the last of a wild species is destroyed, we should not only feel the loss of an irreplaceable aspect of the natural world, we should also feel the loss of the potential it may have had to provide new medicines, new crops, new products for a better human existence. Similarly, when the tropical forests are wantonly destroyed, we not only lose a great treasure of biological diversity, we also lose the stabilizing effect those forests have on our climate. Conservation and development are not only compatible, they are two expressions of the same need - to keep the earth as a sustaining home". [116]

In the executive summary of the World Conservation Strategy three main aims of the movement are listed:

(1) to maintain essential ecological processes and life-support systems

(2) to preserve genetic diversity

(3) to ensure sustainable utilization of species and ecosystems.

These objectives are believed to be urgent because

a) The carrying capacity of the planet is being reduced in both developing and developed countries because of soil destruction, deforestation, agricultural mismanagement and increasing urbanization (which buries 3,000 square kilometres of prime farmland under tar and concrete annually in just the developed countries).

b) Hundreds of millions of rural poor in the developing countries, of which there are at least 800 million destitute, are destroying forests to obtain firewood to keep themselves alive, or clearing forests to grow food to keep their families alive. 400 million tonnes of dung are burnt each year by the rural poor for fuel, not only contributing towards atmospheric pollution, but to increased soil erosion and the vicious cycle of decreased yields and the increased need to clear more forests. Human population will be over 6 billion by the year 2000. To feed these people at present levels will require a 50% increase in current production from agriculture and fisheries. However, due to soil destruction there is a substantial problem of increasing hunger.

c) The energy and financial costs of providing goods and services are growing especially in developing countries due to increased siltation and the devastation of crops from floods.

d) The resource bases of major industries are shrinking due to the contraction of tropical forests and the destruction and pollution of coastal support systems, threatening fishing industries.

Along with this, by the year 2000, unless present policies and activities are globally changed, tropical lowland forests will be largely gone and high-altitude, open forests and woodlands will be greatly reduced; one-third of the world's present cropland will be gone; the water regimes will be interrupted due to massive forest and vegetation loss, bringing floods in the wet season (increasing the vicious cycle of soil destruction), and drought in the dry (with loss of soil from wind). This will in turn reduce agricultural productivity further; the extinction of between 15% and 20% of all living species of plants and animals; the combination of ocean pollution and overfishing may lead to the collapse of today's major fisheries.

These problems were produced by a number of factors including: the failure to integrate conservation and development; an inability of decision makers to recognise the global significance of environmental problems; lack of environmental planning and appropriate laws; a lack of support for conservation.

The three organisations IUCN, UNEP and WWF have seven themes in their conservation plan:

1. Mobilizing an international network for conservation action.

2. Developing better means to monitor and analyse data.

3. Promoting conservation as part of economic development.

4. Conserving biological diversity.

5. Protecting habitats and ecosystems.

6. Presenting a world view of conservation concerns.

7. Identifying key conservation issues of the future.

Dasmann in the same report, lists three further essential concepts for World Conservation:

1. <u>Ecodevelopment</u> - development must be directed towards meeting the basic food, clothing and shelter needs of the poorest people in the world, before attending to the wants of the affluent. This means working at the grass roots level for rural and local development.

2. <u>Self-reliance</u> - development must not encourage reliance upon some metropolitan country. "It must increase local self-reliance, including relative self-sufficiency in some essentials such as food, but not total self-sufficiency in a sense that rules out the benefits of trade. Such self-reliance should be built from local knowledge, tradition, and skills, rather than the transfer of unsuited technology. It is self-reliance based upon appropriate technology - appropriate to the environment and appropriate to the background and knowledge of the people". [117]

3. <u>Sustainability</u> - an indefinite survival of the human species compatible with ecodevelopment and self-reliance (to this I would add: compatible also with the socio-moral ramifications of deep ecology/green philosophy).

Development on this position, is a socio-ethical concept, as it is put in the International Foundations for Development Alternatives, <u>Third System Report</u>:

"Some still consider that development refers to things and can be reduced to capital accumulation, economic growth and economic restructuring. But development fundamentally refers to human beings, the whole man, the whole woman. It is a human experience synonymous with the fulfilment of individual mental, emotional and physical potentiality. The society, its economy and polity ought to be organised in such a manner as to maximise for the individual the opportunities for self-fulfilment. There is development when people and their communities act as subjects and are not acted upon as objects, assert their autonomy, self-reliance and self-confidence, when they set out and carry out projects. To develop is to be or to become, not to have". [118]

Or more concisely, the words of K.K. S. Dadzie:

"Development is the unfolding of people's individual and social imaginations in defining goals and inventing ways to approach them. Development is the continuing process of the liberation of peoples in society. There is development when they are able to assert their autonomy, and in self-reliance carry out activities of interest to them". [119]

The idea of development as a moral concept was essential to the conceptual framework on The World Commission on Environment and Development <u>Our Common Future</u> (1987) [120] through the concept of <u>sustainability</u>. Two key concepts are featured in this:

"* the concept of 'needs' in particular the essential needs of the world's poor, to which overriding priority should be given; and

* the idea of limitations imposed by the state of technology and social organisation on the environment's ability to meet present and future needs". [121]

More recently in an interview published in 1989 in <u>New Perspectives Quarterly</u>, Ms. Gro Harlem Brundtland, Prime Minister of Norway and chair of the UN World Commission on Environment and Development, outlines the moral nature of sustainability in more detail:

"Fundamentally, 'sustainable development' is a notion of discipline. It means humanity must ensure that meeting present needs does not compromise the ability of future generations to meet their own needs. And that means disciplining our current consumption ... The industrial world has already used so much of the planet's ecological capacity that the sustainability of future life is in doubt. That can't continue ... Particularly since the emergence of the money economy, we have adopted a way of thinking which places only a present value on resources. The value of a natural resource is priced by market forces of supply and demand only in a very short term time frame. That kind of thinking is no longer possible when the depletion of finite resources - including our precious atmosphere - threatens to ruin our own long-term life basis". [122]

In reply to Brundtland, our blind opportunistic growth supporters would no doubt maintain that we can never be absolutely certain about any of this, so let's carry on as we are. Now there is, I think, a decisive philosophical argument that can be worked against those who demand absolute certainty. It was noted by Pascal, and is known as Pascal's Wager. He thought that in terms of practical rationality, belief in the Christian God was infinitely preferable to atheism because one choice led to heaven and the other to hell. As a pragmatic argument for Christian theism it is lacking because it fails to establish the uniqueness of Christianity: the Wager would work for any other religion. As well it is logically possible that God may choose to punish theists for being so self-interested! Nevertheless, this argument works well with less lofty topics, especially since the choice between sustainability and increasing economic growth is exhaustive. Consider then which of the alternatives we would most regret having taken, if in some time in the future we become absolutely certain about the environmental issue. The worse case scenario from the pro-growth position is environmental collapse, depleted resources and a polluted and dying planet. The worse-case scenario from the steady-state perspective (noting that nuclear war is theoretically possible under both, but more probable with massive global inequalities and politico-economic imperialism that is a natural outcome of our opponent's model) is that consumption and utility has been foregone for a number of generations. However, the global utility intergenerationally of humanity would be greater in our model than in the worse-case pro-growth scenario, because there would still be healthy people alive. So under uncertainty, sustainability wins by a TKO (technical knock-out)!.

Much ecocentric literature has been exclusively concerned with either general philosophical concepts (e.g. deep ecology, sustainability) or with global environmental problems, without much consideration of the sorts of political, social, legal and economic changes that will be needed to bring about sustainability within given nations, such as Australia. These sorts of problems can't be solved by general eco-philosophical ratiocination - they require the development of social and political movements. Such movements are <u>emergent</u> phenomena, they arise seemingly spontaneously. But, intellectual work can shape such movements to a certain extent. In the Australian context such intellectual work is badly needed by progressive and radical thinkers on the shape and structure of a good society - economically just, highly democratic - where the opinion of the ordinary working person counts, egalitarian, pluralistic at the individual level in life-style but united by common community values of justice and care, ecologically balanced and socially sane. [123] At a time when one needs an electron microscope to see the essential difference between the ALP and the Liberal Party [124], there is a need for a <u>Social and Green Alliance</u> (SAGA) that would unite the lost Democrats, the Greens, "Grey Power" the Labour movement, the Green Left of the ALP and the Rainbow Alliance. [125] Intellectuals can no more physically unite all of these groups, than they can part the sewerage from the sea at Bondi Beach with words from their lips. However, it is theoretically possible to work out how such an alliance could form, how to interest the public in the alternative, and more broadly what a sustainable Australia would be like. It may well be that all is hopeless and forlorn, that the sheer size of modern techno-industrial society has resulted in the emergence of a juggernaut with unstoppable inertia. If this is so, then clearly the human story will be full of sound and fury, but only for a very short time on the evolutionary scale of things. Humanity will be like a falling star, rather than like a comet. But remembering Smith's Wager, we can only know whether this is so by attempting to put on the brakes. If they do not work after frantic pumping, then the choice has been taken out of our hands.

This is a book about AIDS, society and philosophy, and therefore must conclude, as is the tradition, with a neat and philosophically profound message about that topic. My message is simply this: AIDS is but an interconnected part of an enormously complex socio-politico-environmental mess; if it, and any number of new "pandemics" that may face us in the twenty first century, are to be satisfactorily dealt with, then **NOW** is the time for bold thinking <u>both</u> globally <u>and</u> locally, and action with dignity, courage and ultimate concern for both human and Gaia's welfare, globally and locally as well.

NOTES AND REFERENCES

1. T. Roszak, *The Making of a Counter Culture*, (Faber and Faber, London, 1971), p. xiv.

2. A. Bloom, *The Closing of the American Mind*, (Penguin Books, London, 1987, p. 382).

3. P.M. Bhargava and C. Chakrabarti, "The Crisis of Civilization", *New Humanist*, Vol. 103, No. 1, 1988, pp. 7-10.

4. S. Kingman, "AIDS Conference Hears Demands for 'Bill of Rights'", *New Scientist*, Vol. 122, 10 June 1989, p. 9.

   Some facts about the World's Weapon industry:

   - 1/4 of the world's scientific research and development budget is spent on defense.

   - over 1/2 million scientists are engaged in the development of new military weapons.

   - SDI, strategic defense initiative costs $3,900 million a year.

   - US spends 73.09% of its scientific research and development budget each year on new military weapons, 2.0% on medical research; the U.K. 57.0% on military weapons research and also 2.0% on medicine; Canada surprisingly 7.8% on military weapons and 8.1% on health. (*New Internationalist*, No. 1982, April 1988) p. 16.

5. R. Ornstein and P. Ehrlich, *New World New Mind: Moving Toward Conscious Evolution*, (Doubleday, New York, 1989).

6. ibid p. 127.

7. ibid p. 130.

8. AAP, "Depletion of Ozone Linked to AIDS", *The Australian*, Tuesday May 16, 1989, p. 3.

9. D. O'Reilly, B. Stannard and B. Cohen, "The Greening of Australia", *The Bulletin with Newsweek*, June 6, 1989, pp. 48-56; S. Alterman (Brussels) "Green Tide on Rise in Europe", *The Advertiser*, Tuesday, June 20, 1989, p. 7.

10. R. MacDonald, "Survival", *Business Review Weekly*, March 31, 1989, pp. 46-49.

11. Editorial, "Charting a Future for the Planet", *The Advertiser*, Monday, June 5, 1989, p. 20. (World

Environment Day) cf. also Editorial, "Recognition of a World in Crisis", <u>The Advertiser</u>, Monday October 10, 1988, p. 20; J. Cribb, "World at Risk", <u>The Weekend Australian</u>, April 1-2, 1989, weekend 3; "Personal Action Guide for the Earth", <u>The Weekend Australian</u>, July 8-9, 1989.

12. L. Timberlake, "Sustained Hope for Development", <u>New Scientist</u>, Vol. 119, 7 July, 1988, pp. 60-63.

13. Comprehensive discussions of the vital signs of the earth include: The World Commission of Environment and Development, <u>Our Common Future</u>, (Oxford University Press, Oxford, 1987) and L. Brown (director), Worldwatch Institute, <u>State of the World 1988</u>, (W.W. Norton, New York, 1988).

14. D. Ellsberg (interview in <u>Not Man Apart</u>), Friends of the Earth, San Francisco, February 1980, quoted from F. Capra, <u>The Turning Point</u>, (Bantam Books, New York, 1983).

15. cf. W.U. Chandler, "Assessing SDI", in Brown, <u>State of the World 1988</u>, op.cit note 13, pp. 137-150; R. Sagdeev and A. Kokoshin, "Space - Strike Arms and International Security", in J. Holdren and J. Rotblout (eds.) <u>Strategic Defenses and the Futute of the Arms Race</u>, (Macmillan Press, London, 1987), pp. 37-79.

16. Capra op.cit note 14, p. 242.

17. A.B. Pitlock, <u>Beyond Darkness: Nuclear Winter in Australia and New Zeealand</u>, (Sun Books, Melbourne, 1987); G.F. Carrier, "Nuclear Winter: The State of the Science", <u>Issues in Science and Technology</u>, Vol. 1, 1985, pp. 114-117; M.M. May, "Nuclear Winter: Strategic Significance", ibid pp. 118-120; A. Gore, ibid pp. 120-123; G.W. Rathjens and R.H. Siegel, ibid pp. 123-127; T.A. Postol, ibid pp. 128-131; R.L. Wagner, ibid pp. 131-133; S.H. Schneider and S.L. Thompson, "Simulating the Climatic Effects of Nuclear War:, <u>Nature</u>, Vol. 333, 1988, pp. 221-227.

18. C. Flavin, "Reassessing Nuclear Power", in L. Brown (director), Worldwatch Institute, <u>State of the World 1987</u>, (W.W. Norton, New York, 1987), pp. 57-80.

19. R. and V. Routley, "Nuclear Energy and Obligations to the Future", <u>Inquiry</u>, Vol. 21, 1978, pp. 133-179; B.E. Wynne, "Nuclear Power - Is the Health Risk Too Great?" <u>Journal of Medical Ethics</u>, Vol. 8, 1982, pp. 78-85; C. Sweet, "The Hidden Costs of Nuclear Energy", <u>New Ecologist</u>, No. 1, Jan/Feb, 1978, pp. 17-19; C. Conroy, "Energy: We Can Do Better than Nuclear Power", in D.

Wilson (ed.) <u>The Environmental Crisis</u>, (Heinemann, London, 1984), pp. 93-112).

20. E.S. Deevey (et al) "Mayan Urbanism: Impact on a Tropical Karst Environment", <u>Science</u>, Vol. 206, 1979, pp. 298-306; J.D. Hughes and J.V. Thirgood, "Deforestation in Ancient Greece and Rome: A Cause of Collapse", <u>The Ecologist</u>, Vol. 12, 1982, pp. 196-208.

21. L. Brown, <u>Building a Sustainable Society</u>, (W.W. Norton, New York, 1981), p. 5.

22. J. Leggett, "The Biggest Mass - Extinction of Them All", <u>New Scientist</u>, Vol. 122, 10 June 1989, p. 44.

23. N.R. Sampson, <u>Farmland or Wasteland: A Time to Choose</u>, (Rodale Press, Emmaus, 1981); E. Eckholm, Planning for the Future: <u>Forestry and Human Needs</u>, (Worldwatch Paper 26, Worldwatch Institute, Washington D.C., 1979); M. Glantz (ed.) <u>Desertification: Environmental Degradation in and Around Arid Lands</u>, (Westview Press, Boulder, 1977); J. Cribb, "White Death", <u>The Weekend Australian Magazine</u>, April 29-30, 1989, pp. 8-16; J. Thornes, "Solutions to Soil Erosion", <u>New Scientist</u>, Vol. 122, 3 June, 1989, pp. 27-31.

24. Council on Environmental Quality and Department of State, <u>The Global 2000 Report to the President</u>, (GPO, Washington D.C. 1980) and <u>Global Future: Time to Act</u>(GPO, Washington D.C., 1981).

25. K. Forestier, "The Degreening of China", <u>New Scientist</u>, Vol. 123, 1 July 1989, pp. 24-27; J. Silvertown, "A Silent Spring in China", <u>New Scientist</u>, Vol. 123, 1 July 1989, pp. 27-30.

26. P.R. Ehrlich and A.H. Ehrlich, <u>Extinction</u> (Random House, New York, 1981) and F.W. King, "Preservation of Genetic Diversity", in F.R. Thibodeau and H.H. Field (eds.) <u>Sustaining Tomorrow: A Strategy for World Conservation and Development</u>, (University Press of New England, Hanover and London, 1984), pp. 41-55.

27. M. Cross, "Spare the Tree and Spoil the Forest", <u>New Scientist</u>, Vol. 120, 26 November 1988, pp. 24-25. An insight into Japan's anti-green super-growth mentality is seen in the comments of Sabura Okita, chairman of the WWF in Japan believes that tropical forests can only survive if they have an economic value which comes from commercial exploitation. For Okita, Japan should not stop the cutting. The rain forest, as conservationists such as Davie Suzuki has argued, is a mega-complex ecosystem that can't simply be replaced as one replaces one's Toyota, or a patch of tomatoes.

28. E.C. Wolf, *On the Brink of Extinction: Conserving the Diversity of Life*, Worldwatch Paper 78, June 1987, p. 9. cf. also S. Pastel and L. Heise, "Reforesting the Earth", in *State of the World 1988*, op.cit. note 13, pp. 83-100; D. MacKenzie and F. Pearce, "A Sudden Thaw in the Arctic", *New Scientist*, Vol. 122, 15 April 1989, pp. 25-26; J. Drewett, "Never Mind the Whale, Save the Insects", *New Scientist*, Vol. 120, 17 December 1988, pp. 32-35; J. Cribb and L. Taylor, "Graveyard Australia", *The Weekend Australian*, July 8-9, 1989, Weekend 3 and 6; M. Ahmad, "Bangladesh: How Forest Exploitation is Leading to Disaster", *The Ecologist*, Vol. 17, 1987, pp. 168-169; P. Hurst, "Forest Destruction in South East Asia", *The Ecologist*, Vol. 17, 1987, pp. 170-174; V. Plumwood and R. Routley, "World Rainforest Destruction - The Social Factors", *The Ecologist*, Vol. 12, 1982, pp. 40-22.

29. J.D. Nations and D.I. Komer, "Rainforests and the Hamburger Society", *The Ecologist*, Vol. 17, 1987, pp. 161-167; J.K. Skinner, "Bic Mac and the Tropical Forests", *Monthly Review*, Vol. 37, December 1985, pp. 25-32. Not only are such high tech hamburgers a poor source of nutrition, being high in fats, but in the light of these papers, they are unhealthy for the planet as a whole and provide few jobs for the majority of people in the tropics.

30. J. Petras and M. Morley, *The United States and Chile - Imperialism and the Overthrow of the Allende Government* (Monthly Review Press, London, 1975).

31. X. Smiley (Moscow) "Polluted Inland Soviet Sea 'Threatens the World'", *The Advertiser*, Friday June 23, 1989, p. 1. Heavy metal pollution extends global and is a problem in most cities of the world. For example at Port Pirie, South Australia, heavy metals have contaminated at least 400 square metres of coast and heavy metals from BHP steelworks at Whyalla have already altered the marine environment, according to the *Report of the Pollution Sub-Committee of the SA Fishing Industry Council* cited by C. Painter, "The Poisoning of our Gulf", *Sunday Mail*, June 11, 1989, pp. 4-5.

32. S. Hazarika, *Bhopal: The Lessons of a Tragedy*, (Penguin Books, Harmondsworth, 1986).

33. J. Bellini, *High Tech Holocaust*, (Greenhouse Publications, Victoria, 1987).

34. (Agence France-Presse) "Polluted Air in the U.S 'exceeds worst fears'," *The Advertiser*, March 25, 1989, p. 7.

35. S.J. Reaven, "The Methodology of Probabilistic Risk Assessment: Completeness, Subjective Probability, and

"The Lewis Report", Explorations in Knowledge, Vol. 5, No. 1, 1988, pp. 11-32.

36. cf. J.E. Cummins, "Extinction: The PCB Threat to Marine Mammals", The Ecologist, Vol. 18, 1988, pp. 193-195; M. MacQuitty, "Pollution Beneath the Goldern Gate", New Scientist, Vol. 118, 30 June 1988, pp. 62-66; T. Ruff, "Ne Mange Pas Les Poissons," Australian Society, July 1989, p. 32; "The Global Poison Trade: How Toxic Waste is Dumped on the Third World", Newsweek, November 7, 1988, pp. 8-11; J. Cribb, "Who is Poisoning Our Water?", The Weekend Australian, July 1-2, 1989, Weekend 17; S. Pastel, "Controlling Toxic Chemicals", in State of the World 1988, op.cit note 13, pp. 118-136.

37. J. Bone (New York), "Big Apple's Rotten Core is Becoming the Eighth Wonder", The Australian, Tuesday May 9, 1989, p. 11; K. Murphy (et al), "How Long Before We're All Up to Our Necks in Garbage?", The Bulletin with Newsweek, March 14, 1989, pp. 46-54.

38. F. Pearce, "Acid Rain", New Scientist, Vol. 116, 5 November 1987, pp. 1-4 and Acid Rain, (Penguin Books, Harmondsworth, 1987); N. Dudley, "Acid Rain and Pollution Control Policy in the U.K." The Ecologist, Vol. 16, 1986, pp. 18-23; S. Pastel, "Protecting Forests from Air Pollution and Acid Rain", in L. Brown (et al) State of the World 1985, (W.W. Norton, New York, 1985), pp. 97-123; S. Elsworth, Acid Rain, (Pluto Press, London, 1985).

39. J.G. Irwin and M.L. Williams, "Acid Rain: Chemistry and Transport", Environmental Pollution, Vol. 50, 1988, pp. 29-59; V.A. Mohnen, "The Challenge of Acid Rain", Scientific American, Vol. 259, August 1988, pp. 14-22; J.R. Kennedy, Acid Soil and Acid Rain, (John Wiley, New York, 1986).

40. Pearce, Acid Rain, op.cit note 38, p.9.

41. L.B. Love, "Controlling Acid Rain", Issues in Science and Technology, Vol. 5, 1989, pp. 109-111; J.L. Regens and R.W. Rycroft, The Acid Rain Controversy, (University of Pittsburgh Press, Pittsburgh, 1988); J.C. White (ed.), Acid Rain: The Relationship Between Sources and Receptors, (Elsevier, New York, 1988); R.K. Raufer and S.L. Feldman, Acid Raid and Emissions Trading, (Rowman and Littlefield, New Jersey, 1988).

42. J.L. Kulp, "Information Needs - Terrestrial", in White, ibid, pp. 95-100. For a balanced discussion of all aspects of the controversies cf. C.C. Park, Acid Rain: Rhetoric and Reality, (Methuen, London, 1987). Ozone is a strong oxidizing agent and is used in bleaching and sterilizing water. In the lower atmosphere it can

damage plants at a mere 50 pbb and make a working environment unsafe for humans at 80 ppb. In south-east England during the hot summer of 1976, ozone concentration peaked at 260 pbb. Ironically if <u>ground level</u> ozone levels double, there may be a greenhouse effect produced and levels of ozone throughout Europe dangerous for both humans and nature. This is compatible with a decrease in <u>stratospheric</u> ozone.

43. J.T. Mathews, "Global Climate Change: Toward a Greenhouse Policy", <u>Issues in Science and Technology</u>, Vol. 3, 1987, pp. 57-68; I.M. Mintzer, <u>A Matter of Degrees</u>, (World Resources Institute, 1987); B. Bolin (et al, eds.) <u>The Greenhouse Effect, Climatic Change and Ecosystems</u>, (John Wiley and Sons, New York, 1986); G.I. Pearman (ed.), <u>Greenhouse: Planning for Climate Change</u>, (CSIRO, Melbourne, 1988); T. Dendy (ed.) <u>Greenhouse '88: Planning for Climate Change</u>, (Department of Environment and Planning, Adelaide, 1989); A. Henderson-Sellers and R. Blong, <u>The Greenhouse Effect: Living in a Warmer Australia</u>, (New South Wales University Press, Kensington, N.S.W., 1989).

44. J. Gribbin, <u>The Hole in the Sky: Man's Threat to the Ozone Layer</u>, (Corgi Books, London, 1988); R.A. Kerr, "Stratospheric Ozone is Decreasing", <u>Science</u>, Vol. 239, 25 March 1988, pp. 1489-1491; R.S. Stolarski, "The Antarctic Ozone Hole", <u>Scientific American</u>, Vol. 258, 1988, pp. 20-26; J. Titus, <u>Effects of Changes in Stratospheric Ozone and Global Climate</u>, (EPA, Washington, 1986); R.R. Jones, "Ozone, Depletion and Cancer Risk", <u>The Lancet</u>, August 22, 1987, pp. 443-446; M. Jones, "In Search of the Safe CFCs", <u>New Scientist</u>, 26 May 1988, pp. 56-60; F.S. Rowland and D.G. Aldrich, "Chlorofluorocarbons, Stratospheric Ozone, and the Antarctic 'Ozone Hole'," <u>Environmental Conservation</u>, Vol. 15, 1988, pp. 101-115; D.D. Doniger, "Politics of the Ozone Layer", <u>Issues in Science and Technology</u>, Vol. 4, 1988, pp. 86-92; H.U. Dutsch, "The Antarctic 'Ozone Hole' and Its Possible Global Consequences", <u>Environmental Conservation</u>, Vol. 14, 1987, pp. 95-97; F. Pearce and I. Anderson, "Is There an Ozone Hole Over the North Pole?", <u>New Scientist</u>, Vol. 121, 25 February 1989, pp. 32-33; C. Woods, "Life Without a Sunscreen", Vol. 120, 10 December 1988, pp. 46-49.

45. S. Boyle, "Global Warming - A Paradigm Shift for Energy Policy?", <u>Energy Policy</u>, Vol. 17, 1989, pp. 2-5.

46. cf. H. Stretton, "Tasks for Social Democratic Intellectuals", in his <u>Political Essays</u>, (Georgian House, Melbourne, 1987), pp. 195-214; B. Head, "The Australian Intelligentsia: Beyond Dependency?", <u>Social Alternatives</u>, Vol. 6, 1987, pp. 61-65; A. Bloom, <u>The Closing of the American Mind</u>, op.cit. Note 2; G. Duncan,

"The Modern University", <u>Social Alternatives</u>, Vol. 7, 1989, pp. 7-8; J. McLaren, "Consuming Passions: Education - Liberal, Vocational and Technical", ibid pp. 13-15; S. Marginson, "Is There Life After Dawkins?, ibid pp. 30-36; N. Preston, "What Education is 'In the National Interest'? A Discussion of the Dawkins' Intiatives", ibid pp. 37-40; M. Macklin, "Opposing the Tertiary Tax", ibid pp. 43-45.

47. Editorial, "Dawkins Talks Through his Mortarboard", <u>The Australian</u>, Friday June 16, 1989, p.12; T. Abbott, "Vice-Chancellors Forsake Ideals for the Greater Glory of Bureaucracy", <u>The Australian</u>, Wednesday June 21, 1989, p. 18.

48. T. O'Riordan, <u>Environmentalism</u>, 2nd edition, (Pion Press, London, 1981); A. Jones, "The Violence of Materialism in Advanced Industrial Society: An Eco-Sociological Approach", <u>Sociological Review</u>, Vol. 35, 1987, pp. 19-47, citation p. 44; K. Sale, <u>Human Scale</u>, (Coward, McCann and Geoghegan, New York, 1980) and <u>Dwellers in the Land: The Bio-regional Vision,</u> (Sierra Club Books, San Francisco, 1985).

49. H. Stretton, <u>Capitalism, Socialism and the Environment</u>, (Cambridge University Press, Cambridge, 1976), p. 19.

50. J. Porritt, <u>Seeing Greening: The Politics of Ecology Explained</u>, (Basil Blackwell, Oxford, 1987), pp. 10-11; S. Irvine and A. Ponton, <u>A Green Manifesto: Policies for a Green Future</u>, (Macdonald Optima, London, 1988: "... the Green goal is to allow everyone the opportunity to live a fulfilling life, caring for and sharing with each other, future generations and other species, whilst living sustainably within the capacities of a limited world". (p.16)

51. An unsystematic sample includes: R. Dubos, <u>So Human an Animal</u>, (Sphere Books, London, 1973), <u>A God Within</u>, (Sphere Books, London, 1976) and with B. Ward, <u>Only One Earth</u>, (Penguin, Harmondsworth, 1982); M. Bookchin, <u>Towards an Ecological Society</u>, (Black Rose Books, Montreal, 1980); E. Eckholm, <u>Down to Earth</u>, (Pluto Press, London, 1982); D. Elgin, <u>Voluntary Simplicity</u>, (William Morrow, New York, 1981); H. Henderson, <u>The Politics of the Solar Age</u>, (Doubleday, New York, 1981); J. Schell, <u>The Fate of the Earth</u>, (Alfred A. Knopf, New York, 1982); N. Singh, <u>Economics and the Crisis of Ecology</u>, (Oxford University Press, Delhi, 1976); H. Skolimcwski, <u>Eco-Philosophy</u>, (Marion Boyars, London, 1981); D. Wilson (ed.), <u>The Environmental Crisis</u>, (Heinemann, London, 1984); F. Barnaby, (ed.) <u>The Gaia Peace Atlas Survival into the Third Millennium</u>, (Pan Books, London, 1988); E. Goldsmith and N. Hildyard (eds.) <u>Battle for the Earth: Today's Key Environmental</u>

Issues, (Child and Associates, Brookvale, NSW, 1988); V. Serventy, *Saving Australia: A Blueprint for Our Survival*, (Child and Associates, Brookvale, N.S.W., 1988); J. Seymour and H. Girardet, *Blueprint for a Green Planet*, (Angus and Robertson, North Ryde, N.S.W. 1987); P. Ehrlich and A. Ehrlich, *Earth*, (Thames and Methuen, London, 1987); P. Bunyard and F. Morgan-Grenville, *The Green Alternative*, (Methuen, London, 1987); E. Goldsmith (et al), *Blueprint for Survival*, (Penguin, Harmondsworth, 1972); J. Parritt and D. Winner, *The Coming of the Greens*, (Fontana, London, 1988); D. Hutton (ed.), *Green Politics in Australia*, (Angust and Robertson, North Ryde, 1987); T. Bendixson, *Instead of Cars*, (Temple Smith, London, 1974); D. Pirages, *Global Ecopolitics: The New Context for International Relations*, (Duxbury Press, North Scituate, 1978), and (ed.) *The Sustaintable Society: Implications for Limited Growth*, (Praeger, New York, 1977); A. Rotstein (ed.) *Beyond Industrial Growth*, (University of Toronto Press, Toronto, 1976); D. Worster, *Nature's Economy: The Roots of Ecology*, (Sierra Book Club, San Francisco, 1977); W.R. Catton and R.E. Dunlop, "Environmental Sociology: A New Paradigm", *American Sociologist*, 13, 1978, pp. 41-49; W. Ophuls, *Ecology and the Politics of Scarcity*, (Freeman, San Francisco, 1977); A. Schnaiberg, *The Environment: From Surplus to Scarcity*, (Oxford University Press, New York, 1980); K.E.F. Watt (et al), *The Unsteady State: Environmental Problems, Growth and Culture*, (University Press of Hawaii for the East-West Center, Honolulu, 1977); R. Barnet and R. Muller, *Global Reach: The Power of the Multinational Corporations*, (Simon and Schuster, New York, 1974); A. Roberts, *The Self Managing Envrionment*, (Allison and Busby, London, 1979); M Allaby and P. Bunyard, *The Politics of Self-Sufficiency*, (Oxford University Press, Oxford, 1980); E. Goldsmith, *The Stable Society*, (Wadebridge Press, Wadebridge, 1978); E. Morgan, *Falling Apart: The Rise and Decline of Urban Civilization*, (Souvenir Press, London, 1976); E. Goldsmith, "Gaia: Some Implications for Theoretical Ecology", *The Ecologist*, Vol. 18, 1988, pp. 64-74; J.D. Hughes, "Gaia: An Ancient View of Our Planet", *The Ecologist*, Vol. 13, 1983, pp. 54-60; A. Ette and J. Bower, "Reverence and Responsibility: The Need for Good Husbandry", *New Ecologist*, No. 3, 1978, pp. 82-83; G. Lawrence, "A Rural Renaissance? Towards Socialist Agriculture for Australia", *Social Alternatives*, Vol. 5, 1986, pp. 36-45; A. Jones, "From Fragmentation to Wholeness: A Green View of Science and Society (Part II)", *The Ecologist*, Vol. 18, 1988, pp. 30-34, and "Beyond Industrial Society", *The Ecologist*, Vol. 13, 1983, pp. 141-147; E. Goldsmith, "Deindustrialising Society", *The Ecologist*, Vol. 7, 1977, pp. 128-143; E. Waddell, "The Return to Traditional Agriculture", *The Ecologist*, Vol. 7, 1977, pp. 144-147; E. Goldsmith, "The Need for a New

Economics", *The Ecologist*, Vol. 9, 1979, pp. 196-199; K. Penny, "Economics for a Post-Industrial Society", *The Ecologist*, Vol. 9, 1979, pp. 200-208; P. Bunyard, "Gaia: The Implications for Industrialised Societies", *The Ecologist*, Vol. 18, 1988, pp. 196-206; J. Papworth, "Non-Local Government and Local Power", *The Ecologist*, Vol. 18, 1988, pp. 213-222; E. Goldsmith, "Can We Control Pollution?", *The Ecologist*, Vol. 9, 1979, pp. 273-290 and pp. 316-328; C.J. Hughes, "Gaia: A Natural Scientist's Ethic for the Future", *The Ecologist*, Vol. 15, 1985, pp. 92-95; cf. M. Satin (ed.) *New Age Politics*, (Dell Publishing, New York, 1978) for an extensive bibliography of the '70s antigrowth - anticonsumerism - antihierarhcy literature.

52. Sale op.cit., note 48.

53. V. Routley and R. Routley, "Social Theories, Self Management and Environmental Problems", in D. Mannison (et al., eds.) *Environmental Philosophy*, (Australian National University, Canberra, 1980), pp. 217332.

54. R. Bahro, *Socialism and Survival*, (Heretic, London, 1982) and *From Red to Green*, (Verson Books, London, 1984).

55. T. Roszak, *Person/Planet: The Creative Disintegration of Industrial Society*, (Doubleday, New York, 1979).

56. I. Pausacker and J. Andrews, *Living Better with Less*, (Penguine, Victoria, 1981).

57. A. Gorz, *Ecology as Politics*, (Pluto Press, London, 1987).

58. F. Capra, *The Turning Point*, (Bantam Books, New York, 1983).

59. E.L. Wheelwright, "The Socio-Economic Roots of the Environmental Problem", in *Radical Political Economy: Collected Essays*, (ANZ Books, Sydney, 1974), pp. 134-144. Citation p. 142.

60. R.E. Dunlap, "Paradigmatic Change in Social Science", *American Behavioral Scientist*, Vol. 24, 1980, pp. 5-14; W.R. Catton and R.E. Dunlap, "A New Ecological Paradigm for Post- Exurberant Sociology", *American Behavioral Scientist*, Vol. 24, 1980, pp. 15-47; W.R. Catton, *Overshoot: The Ecological Basis of Revolutionary Change*, (University of Illinois Press, Urbana, 1982).

61. D.H. Wrong, "The Oversocialized Concept of Man in Modern Sociology", *American Sociological Review*, Vol. 26, 1961, pp. 183-193.

62. Other works advancing the Dunlap-Catton thesis include J. Rodman, "Paradigm Change in Political Science: An Ecological Perspective", <u>American Behavioral Scientist</u>, Vol. 24, 1980, pp. 49-78; D.L. Hardesty, "The Ecological Perspective in Anthropology", <u>American Behavioral Scientist</u>, Vol. 24, 1980, pp. 107-124; D.B. Luten, "Ecological Optimism in the Social Sciences: The Question of Limits to Growth", <u>American Behavioral Scientist</u>, Vol. 24, 1980, pp. 125-151; T.R. Vale (ed.) <u>Progress Against Growth: Daniel B. Luten on the American Landscape</u>, (Guilford Press, New York, 1986); R. Hueting, <u>New Scarcity and Economic Growth</u>, (North-Holland, Amsterdam, 1980).

63. J.W. Smith, <u>Reductionism and Cultural Being</u>, (Martinus Nijhoff, The Hague, 1984).

64. Capra, <u>The Turning Point</u>, op.cit. Note 58.

65. cf. D. Bohm, <u>Wholeness and the Implicate Order</u>, (Routledge and Kegan Paul, London 1982) and with R. Weber, "Nature as Creativity", <u>Revision</u>, Vol. 5, 1982, pp. 35-40; J.S. Bell, <u>Speakable and Unspeakable in Quantum Mechanics</u>, (Cambridge University Press, Cambridge, 1987).

66. For a review cf. J.W. Smith, B.C. Goodwin and G. Webster, "Neo-Darwinism and Constructional Biology", <u>Explorations in Knowledge</u>, Vol. 4, 1987, pp. 29-40; M.W. Ho and P.T. Saunders (eds.) <u>Beyond Neo-Darwinism</u>, (Academic Press, London, 1984); R. Sheldrake, <u>The Presence of the Past: Morphic Resonance and the Habits of Nature</u>, (Collins, London, 1988).

67. cf. J.W. Smith, <u>Reason, Science and Paradox</u>, (Croom Helm, London, 1986), <u>Essays on Ultimate Questions</u>, (Gower, Aldershot, 1988) and <u>The Worms at the Heart of Things</u> (Forthcoming).

68. B. Jones, <u>Sleepers, Wake! Technology and the Future of Work</u>, (Oxford University Press, Melbourne, 1983).

69. Gorz, <u>Ecology as Politics</u>, op.cit. Note 57.

70. D. Ehrenfeld, <u>The Arrogance of Humanism</u>, (Oxford University Press, Oxford, 1978).

71. For some examples of cultural disasters of technocentrism cf. L.H. Instone, <u>Science, Technology and Western Domination</u>, (Monash University, Graduate School of Environmental Science, Environmental Paper No. 4, Victoria, 1985).

72. I. Illich, <u>Energy and Equity</u>, (Harper and Row, New York, 1974).

73. G. Lawrence, "A Rural Renaissance? Towards a Socialist Agriculture for Australia", Social Alternatives, Vol. 5, 1986, pp. 36-45.

74. F. Hirsch, Social Limits to Growth, (Routledge and Kegan Paul, London, 1977).

75. Two conditions are often cited as constituting Pareto optimality:

    (P1) A social optimum exists whenever it is not possible to make someone better off without making somebody worse off.

    (P2) Maximum social welfare occurs whenever it is possible to make somebody better off without making anybody worse off.

    Some economists believe that (P2) follows from (P1) - which is an invalid inference as (P1) is a negation of a possibility, whilst (P2) is a possibility statement with no negation. (P1) is consistent with egalitarianism, (P2) conflicts with it. For a counter-model consider:

    (Q1) It is not possible to make body x hotter without making any other body colder (thermodynamic equilibrium) in systerm S.

    (Q2) It is possible to make a body hotter without making any other body colder (in system S).

    (Q2) contradicts (Q1), thus it does not follow from it. Therefore (P2) does not follow from (P1).

76. Quoted from E.L. Wheelwright, "Introduction to Marxian Economics", in E.L. Wheelwright and F.J.B. Stilwell (eds.) Readings in Political Economy, Volume 1, (ANZ Books, Sydney, 1976), pp. 231-235. Citation p. 234.

77. D.H. Meadows (et al.) The Limits to Growth, (Earth Island Ltd., London, 1972).

78. F.E. Trainer, Abandon Affluence!, (Zed Boooks, London, 1985).

79. D. Pepper, "Determinism, Idealism and the Politics of Environmentalism - A Viewpoint," International Journal of Environmental Studies, Vol. 26, 1985, pp. 11-19. It is a frequent allegation in Australian exurberant social science, that ecological critiques are racist. For example if it is argued that Australia has the highest rate of population increase in the world (Appendix 2, Australian Immigration Department, Australia's Population Trends and Prospects) most of which is from immigration - and that there is massive damage occurring

to the environment from population consumption pressure including the destruction of agricultural land so that a drop in immigration is requir3d, then such socio-ecologists are "racist", "evil", "dangerous". These claims are made even if the restrictions are right across the board, not employing (physical) racial or (cultural) ethnic categories <u>at all</u>! The immigration lobby obviously believe that its intake of immigrants are obviously all poverty stricken which it is not with the present immigration emphasis being upon wealth for investment. But even if this was so, it is not an adequate response to Third World poverty because only a selected few get a lucky ticket to affluent Australia. Socio-ecologists at this point can play the same game played by exurberant social science - what could be more racist than we in Australia (this writer included) living as we do when many Aboriginal settlements lack adequate clean water and millions around the world die of starvation? Surely no humane philosopher can ignore this truly cruel racist paradox and the socio-ecology movement does not. cf. J.W. Smith, "Review of S. Castles (et al), <u>Mistaken Identity: Multiculturalism and the Demise of Nationalism in Australila</u> (Pluto Press, Sydney, 1988)", <u>Politics</u>, Vol. 24 (1), May 1989, pp. 126-127.

The random use of the term 'racist' is also made of any Australian who dares to criticise the economic activities of Asian super powers such as Japan. Even though there is a massive library of criticism of U.S. and U.S.S.R. economic and environmentally destrutive activities, Japan must remain criticism free, presumably because it might damage our trade relations. Now the racist allegation is wrong because the socio-ecology criticism is not made on the basis of race or ethnicity, but on the grounds of economic exploitation and environmental destruction (David <u>Suzuki</u>, perhaps the best known ecological critic of Japn could hardly be a racist about Japan10. Second the random use of the term 'racist' to any critic of capitalism will lead to the situation where real racism will grow in society because the charge will become drained of meaning. Finally there is an emerging anti-democratic "fascist" trend in exurberant sociology, which puts some topics "off limits". No topic is perhaps more "off limits" than the "dangerous" thought that business men/women, politicians and academics, executives and the stars of <u>Business Review Weekly</u>, have too much wealth. It is the role of intellectuals to question everything, including themselves.

80. P.E. O'Sullivan, "Shallow and Deep Envrionmental Science", <u>International Journal of Environmental Studies</u>, Vol. 30, 1987, pp. 91-98.

81. cf. Science Council of Canada, <u>Canada as a Conserver Society</u>, Report No. 27, Ottowa September 1977, pp. 13-14 and Science Council of Canada, <u>Natural Resource Policy Issues in Canada</u>, Report No. 19, 1973; D. Brooks, "Economics, Resources, and the Conserver Society", in R. Birrell (et al), <u>Quarry Australia? Social and Environmental Perspectives on Managing the Nation's Resources</u>, (Oxford University Press, Oxford, 1982), pp. 29-43.

82. H. Daly, "The Steady - State Economy: What, Why and How?", in <u>Quarry Australia</u>, ibid pp. 251-260, citation p. 252; H. Daly (ed.) <u>Economics, Ecology, Ethics: Essays Toward a Steady - State Economy</u>, (W.H. Freeman, San Francisco, 1980).

83. H. Daly, "Growth Economics and the Fallacy of Misplaced Concreteness", <u>American Behavioral Scientist</u>, Vol. 24, 1980, pp. 79-105. Citation p. 88.

84. P.A. Samuelson (et al) <u>Economics</u>, 2nd Australian edition, (McGraw-Hill, Sydney, 1975), p. 883.

85. N. Gworgescu-Roegen, "The Entropy Law and the Economic Problem", in <u>Energy and Economic Myths</u>, (Pergamon Press, New York, 1976), pp. 53-60. Citation p. 59; N. Georgescu-Roegen, "The Steady State and Ecological Salvation: A Thermodynamic Analysis", <u>BioScience</u>, Vol. 27, 1977, pp. 266-270.

86. J. Rifkin with T. Howard, <u>Entropy: A New World View</u>, (Bantam Books, New York, 1981).

87. ibid p. 170.

88. ibid p. 199.

89. I. Prigogine and I. Strengers, <u>Order Out of Chaos: Man's New Dialogue with Nature</u>, (Heinemann, London, 1984); W. Lepkowski, "The Social Thermodynamics of Ilya Prigogine", <u>Chemical and Engineeering News</u>, Vol. 57, 1979, pp. 30-33. For criticism cf. E. Goldsmith, "Superscience - Its Mythology and Legitimisation", <u>The Ecologist</u>, Vol. 11, 1981, pp. 228-241.

90. L. Brown, <u>Building a Sustainable Society</u>, (W.W. Norton, New York, 1981), p. 121.

91. R.G. Lipsey (et al) <u>Positive Economics for Australian Students</u>, (Weidenfeld and Nicolson, London, 1981).

92. D. Bell, "Are There 'Social Limits' to Growth", in K.D. Wilson (ed.), <u>Prospects for Growth</u>, (Praeger, New York, 1977), pp. 13-26.

93. C. Kaysen, "The Computer that Printed Out W*O*L*F", Foreign Affairs, Vol. 50, 1972, pp. 660-68.

94. P.P. McGuinness, The Australian, Thursday June 15, 1989, p. 2.

95. N. Georgescu-Roegen, "Energy and Economic Myths", in Energy and Economic Myths, op.cit. Note 85, pp. 3-36, citation p. 30.

96. G. Hardin, "The Tragedy of the Commons", Science, Vol. 162, 1968, pp. 1243-1248, The Limits of Altruism, (Indiana University Press, Bloomington, 1977); and J. Baden (eds.) Managing the Commons, (W.H. Freeman, San Francisco, 1977); R. DeYoung and S. Kaplan, "On Averting the Tragedy of the Commons", Environmental Management, Vol. 12, 1988, pp. 273-283.

97. cf. also M. Sagoff, The Economy of the Earth, (Cambridge University Press, Cambridge, 1988).

98. An unsystematic sample of the critiques of mainstream economics includes: F. Green and P. Nore (eds.) Economics: An Anti-Text, (Macmillan, London, 1977); K. Boulding, Beyond Economics, (University of Michigan Press, Ann Arbor, 1968); H. Henderson, Creating Alternative Futures, (Putnam, New York, 1978); R. Kuttner, "The Poverty of Economics", The Atlantic Monthly, Vol. 255, February 1985, pp. 74-84; R.M. Cyert and G. Pottinger, "Toward a Better Microeconomic Theory", Philosophy of Science, Vol. 46, 1979, pp. 204-222; A Rosenberg, "A Skeptical History of Microeconomic Theory", Theory and Decision, Vol. 12, 1980, pp. 79-93 and "If Economics Isn't Science, What is it?", Philosophical Forum, Vol. 14, 1983, pp. 296-314; J. Robinson, On Re-Reading Marx, (Student's Bookshop, Cambridge, 1953); M. Hollis and E. Nell, Rational Economic Man: A Philosophical Critique of Neo-Classical Economics, (Cambridge University Press, New York, 1985); H. Stretton, "Paul Streeten: An Appreciation", in S. Hall and F. Steward (eds.) Theory and Development: Essays in Honour of Paul Streeten, (Macmillan, London, 1985), pp. 1-27; E.K. Hunt and H.J. Sherman, Economics: An Introduction to Traditional and Radical Views, (Harper and Row, New York, 1978); M. Linder, The Anti-Samuelson; Vol. 1 Macroeconomics: Basic Problems of the Capitalist Economy; Vol. 2 Microeconomics: Basic Problems of the Capitalist Economy, (Urizen Books, New York, 1977); T. Balogh, The Irrelevance of Conventional Economics, (Weidenfeld and Nicolson, London, 1982); W. Leontieff, "Theoretical Assumptions and Non-Observed Facts", American Economic Review, Vol. LXI, 1971, pp. 1-7; P. Streeten (ed.) Unfashionable Economics: Essays in Honour of Lord Balogh, (Weidenfeld and Nicolson, London,

1970); M.A. Lutz and K. Lux, *The Challenge of Humanistic Economics*, (Benjamin/Cummings, Menlo Park, 1979).

99. For discussions (both for and against Marxism) of some of the outstanding problems of Marxism cf. B. Smart, *Foucault, Marxism and Critique*, (Routledge and Kegan Paul, London, 1983); P. Anderson, *Considerations on Western Marxism*, (New Left Books, London, 1976) and *Arguments within English Marxism*, (New Left Books, London, 1980); A. Wellmer, *Critical Theory of Society*, (Seabury Press, New York, 1974); R. Bahro, *The Alternative in Eastern Europe*, (New Left Books, London, 1978); D. Kellner, *Herbert Marcuse and the Crisis of Marxism*, (University of California Press, Berkeley, 1984); A.W. Gouldner, *Against Fragmentation: The Origins of Marxism and the Sociology of Intellectuals*, (Oxford University Press, New York, 1985); V. Burris, "The Discovery of the New Middle Class", *Theory and Society*, Vol. 15, 1986, pp. 317-349; M. Albert and R. Habnel, *Unorthodox Marxism*, (South End Press, Boston, 1978); D. Ward, *Towards a Critical Political Economics: A Critique of Liberal and Radical Economic Thought*, (Goodyear Publishing, California, 1977); J. Schwartz (ed.) *The Subtle Anatomy of Capitalism*, (Goodyear Publishing, California, 1977); P.M. Sweezy, "After Capitalism - What?", *Monthly Review*, Vol. 37, 1985, pp. 98-111; E.O. Wright, "A General Framework for the Analysis of Class Structure", *Politics and Society*, Vol. 13, 1984, pp. 383-423.

100. cf. J. Weeks, *Capital and Exploitation*, (Princeton University Press, Princeton, 1981).

101. H.J. Sherman, *Foundations of Radical Political Economy*, (M.E. Sharpe Inc., New York, 1987).

102. ibid p. 104.

103. It is difficult for even hard-nosed Marxist materialists to avoid value commitments. For example Ian Hunt, "A Critique of Roemer, Hodgson and Cohen on Marxian Exploitation", *Social Theory and Practice*, Vol. 12, 1986, pp. 121-171 says about Marx's theory of exploitation:

"...capitalist exploitation involves the coercive appropriation of surplus - value, so that wage - labor is a species of forced labor, no matter what the free wage contract may insinuate to the contrary". (p.123)

The notion of coercion though involves moral-evaluation, it is not a value-neutral economic conception. This being so, Marxian economics requires for its epistemological foundation, a moral-evaluative theory.

104. A. Etzioni, *The Moral Dimension: Toward a New Economics*, (Free Press, New York, 1988).

105. ibid pp. 3-4.

106. K. Hancock, "The Social Sciences: Economics", *Flinders Journal of History and Politics*, Vol. 2, 1970, pp. 28-34. Citation p. 30.

107. C.A. Hooker, "Hollis and Nell's *Rational Economic Man: A Philosophical Critique of Neo-Classical Economics*", *Philosophy of Science*, Vol. 46, 1979, pp. 470-490. Citation p. 489. More generally J.C. Gaia, "Moral Autonomy and the Rationality of Science", *Philosophy of Science*, Vol. 44, 1977, pp. 513-541; D.N. McCloskey, *The Rhetoric of Economics*, (University of Wisconsin Press, Madison, 1985) is even more critical "during their conversion to a mathematical way of talking the economists adopted a crusading faith, a set of philosophical doctrines, that makes them prone now to fanaticism and intolerance. The faith consists of scientism, behaviorism, operationalism, positive economics, and other quantifying enthusiasms of the nineteen-thirties. In the way of crusading faiths, these doctrines have hardened into ceremony, and now support many nuns, bishops, and cathedrals" (p. 4). cf. also David Collard, *Altruism and Economy: A Study in Non-selfish Economics* (Martin Robertson, Oxford, 1978).

108. L. Robbins, *The Nature and Significance of Economic Science*, (Macmillan, London, 1962), p. 16.

109. C. Dyke, "The Question of Interpretation in Economics", *Ratio*, Vol. XXV, 1983, pp. 15-29.

110. J. Hirshleifer, "The Expanding Domain of Economics", *American Economic Review*, Vol. 75, 1985, pp. 53-68; G. Radnitzky and P. Bernholz (eds.) *Economic Imperialism: The Economic Approach Applied Outside the Traditional Areas of Economics*, (Paragon House, New York, 1985).

111. M. Bookchin, *The Modern Crisis*, (Black Rose Books, Montreal, 1987).

112. ibid p. 90.

113. The most famous discussion of an alternative moral economics is still to be found in the works of E.F. Schumacher, *Small is Beautiful: A Study of Economics as If People Mattered*, (Sphere Books, London, 1974); *Good Work*, (Harper and Row, New York, 1979); G. Kirk (ed.) *Schumacher on Energy*, (Sphere Books, London, 1983); D. Dickson, *Alternative Technology*, (Fontana, London, 1974); N. Jequier (ed.) *Appropriate Technology: Problems and Promises*, (OECD, Paris, 1976); D. Burch,

"Appropriate Technology for the Third World; Why the Will is Lacking", <u>The Ecologist</u>, Vol. 12, 1982, pp. 52-66; R.S. Eckaus, "Appropriate Technology: The Movement has Only a Few Clothes On", <u>Issues in Science and Technology</u>, Vol. 3, 1987, pp. 62-71; F. Stewart, "The Case for Appropriate Technology: A Reply to R.S. Eckaus," <u>Issues in Science and Technology</u>, Vol. 3, 1987, pp. 101-109; W. Ophuls, "Buddhist Politics", <u>The Ecologist</u>, Vol. 7, 1977, pp. 82-86.

114. F.R. Thibadeau and H.H. Field (eds.) <u>Sustaining Tomorrow: A Strategy for World Conservation and Development</u>, (University Press of New England, Hanover and London, 1984).

115. ibid p. vii.

116. ibid pp. vii-viii.

117. R.F. Dasmann, "An Introduction to World Conservation", ibid, pp. 16-24. Citation p. 20.

118. International Foundations for Development Alternatives, <u>Third System Report</u>, (I.F.D.A. Dossier, Nyon, Switzerland, 1979), quoted from Dasmann, ibid, p. 21.

119. K.K.S. Dadzie, "Economic Development", <u>Scientific American</u>, Vol. 243, 1980, pp. 59-65, quoted from Dasmann p. 21.

120. The World Commission on Environment and Development, <u>Our Common Future</u>, (Oxford University Press, Oxford, 1987).

121. ibid p. 42.

122. G.H. Brundtland (et al.) "From the Cold War to a Warm Atmosphere", <u>New Perspectives Quarterly</u>, Vol. 6, 1989, pp. 4-8. Citation p. 5.

123. R. Aronson, "Social Madness", <u>Radical Philosophy</u>, No. 40, Summer, 1985, pp. 13-19.

124. P. Kelly, "Tweedle-Bob and Tweedle-Andy: The Absence of Choice in Australian Politics", <u>The Independent Monthly</u>, Vol. 1, No. 1, July 1989, pp. 8-10, for a view from the respectable right.

125. cf. Rainbow Alliance, <u>New Economic Directions for Australia: A Discussion Paper</u>, April 1988. Thinking on environmental issues in universities in Australia, outside of philosophy, is strongly influenced by technology worship and economic rationalism. It is becoming so that the highest human qualities, values and visions are things to be ashamed of, like a sexually transmitted disease. Can human beings survive with

psychological sanity in an antiseptic world of technical fixes and endless cost-benefit analyses? What is the worth of such a life, what is the point of such a world? These sorts of Socratic questions, which should be at the core of any society are lacking from Australian life, and certainly from Australian intellectual life. The time has come for Australian intellectuals to ask them once more.

Index

"Accommodators", 295
Abortion, 62-63, 93-95
AIDS, Africa, 4,6,124
  anal sex, 126-133
  biomedical aspect, 22-25
  capitalist exploitation, 3
  discrimination, 2,3,99
  homosexuality, 119-126
  medical confidentiality,
    198,221-229
  politics, 3,99
  prisons, 112-115
  schools and workplaces, 115-119
  social meaning, 2,3,18-22,99
  stigma and prejudice,2,3,99
  testing, 109-112
Allen, R., 5
Allocation of scarce medical
  resources,254-257
AZT, 17

Bayles, M., 278
Biotic impoverishment, 284
Blainey, G., 281
Bookchin, M., 314,315

Cloning, 92
Cognitive relativism, 82
Conway,D., 102,103
"Cornucopians", 294
"Crisis of Civilisation", 5, 283
Critical legal studies,39,79-80

Daly, H., 300
Davies, P., 55,87
Deconstructionism, 35-39,69-77
Deep ecocentrism, 295,297
Deep ecology, 294
Dialectics, 61
Drug abuse, philosophical
  aspects, 180-187
Duesberg, P., 12-16,26,27

Economic rationalism, 241
Egalitarianism, 216,238-268
Ehrlich, P., 283, 284
Ehrenfield, D., 299
Epidemics, 5,22,99
Etzioni, A., 311

Falsificationism, 50
Feyerabend, P., 40-47, 80-81, 298
Foucault, M., 33
Freedom and self-determination, 257-258

Georgescu-Roegen, N., 302
Greenhouse effect, 87, 88

Harris, J., 279
Henley, K., 280
Heroin, 165-167
  legalization, 167-172
  and case against, 173-180
Heterosexual transmission, 8-9
"High Tech Holocaust", 290-293
Hirsch, F., 299, 300, 332
Holistic health, 10-12
Homosexuality and
  Christianity, 133-144
Hospital funding crisis, 240

Iatrogenic disease, 2, 32
Induction, 48, 51, 85-86
IV drug use, social problems, 161-165
IVF, 63, 90-93, 95-97

Justice, 242
  and health care, 238

Kaplan, M., 278

Law of diminishing returns, 305
Legal paternalism, 100
Limits of medicine, 2

MacIntyre, A., 56-57
Mann, J.M., 4
Marxist economics, 311
Maxwell, N., 54-56
McCloskey, H.J., 243
Medicine, philosophical aspects, 30-35
Meritocracy, 260-264
Mill, J.S., 100-101, 301
Moral economy, 309-316
Multinationals, 290-291

Natural diversity, destruction of, 289-290

Natural law, 59
Needle exchange programmes, 162, 164
New ecological sociology, 298
Nielsen, K., 276
Nozick, R., 266-268
Nuclear energy, 286-287
Nuclear warfare, 286-287

Objectivity, 2
Ornstein, R., 283, 284

Philosophy, its appalling state, 53-54
Popper, K., 50, 86
Population pressure, 287-289
Postmodernity, 35-36, 69-77
Post-structuralism, 35-36, 69-77
Poverty, 239
Privacy, ideology, 196, 199
  critique, 206-211
Prostitution, 106-109
Putnam, H., 83-84

Quarantines, 103

Ramsey, P., 238
Rawls, J., 264-266
Relativism, 40-47
Rifkin, J., 302-303
Rorty, R., 37-38, 78
Russell, B., 47, 84

Singer, P., 63-64
Social opportunity cost, 304
Sociology of medicine, 34, 35
Soil destruction, 287-289
Steady-state economy, 300, 301
Strong programme of the sociology of knowledge, 35, 68
Sustainability, 316-321

Theories of truth, 47-48, 61
Trainer, T., 273, 300
Turner, B.S. 33-34, 35, 275

Utilitarianism, 213-214, 258-260

Walzer, M., 275
Williams, B., 56-57
Wisdom, 53-54